WITHDRAWN

American Public Health Association

VITAL AND HEALTH STATISTICS MONOGRAPHS

MORTALITY AND MORBIDITY IN THE UNITED STATES

MORTALITY AND MORBIDITY IN THE UNITED STATES

CARL L. ERHARDT
and
JOYCE E. BERLIN,
editors

1974 / HARVARD UNIVERSITY PRESS
Cambridge, Massachusetts

Library of Congress Catalog Card Number: 74–83140
ISBN 0-674-58740-5
Printed in the United States of America

CONTRIBUTORS

ODIN W. ANDERSON, Ph.D.
Professor and Director
Center for Health Administration Studies
University of Chicago
Chicago, Illinois

JOYCE E. BERLIN
Project Coordinator, Health Effects Study
Department of Epidemiology
School of Public Health
Harvard University
Boston, Massachusetts

JAMES O. CARPENTER, Ph.D.
Assistant Professor of Public Health Administration, and
Associate Director, Program in Health Gerontology
School of Public Health
University of Michigan
Ann Arbor, Michigan

PHILIP COLE, M.D.
Associate Professor
Department of Epidemiology
School of Public Health
Harvard University
Boston, Massachusetts

CARL L. ERHARDT, Sc.D.
Chief Research Scientist
New York City Health Research Council, and
Adjunct Associate Professor of Biostatistics
Columbia University
New York, New York
Chairman (1969-74), Committee on Vital and Health Statistics Monographs,
    Statistics Section, American Public Health Association, Washington, D.C.

IAN T. HIGGINS, M.D., F.R.C.P.
Professor of Epidemiology and Environmental and Industrial Health
School of Public Health
University of Michigan
Ann Arbor, Michigan

v

81-2252

BRIAN MACMAHON, M.D., Ph.D., D.P.H.
Professor and Chairman
Department of Epidemiology
School of Public Health
Harvard University
Boston, Massachusetts

RAY F. MCARTHUR, M.S.W., M.P.H.
Deputy Director of Medical Surveillance
Bureau of Health Care Administration
State Department of Health
Lansing, Michigan

JOHN F. NEWMAN, Ph.D.
Senior Analyst
Medicus Systems Corporation, and
Assistant Professor (Sociology)
College of Nursing and Allied Health Sciences
Rush University
Chicago, Illinois

CARL E. ORTMEYER, Ph.D.
Demographer
Appalachian Laboratory for Occupational Respiratory Diseases
National Institute for Occupational Safety and Health
Department of Health, Education, and Welfare
Morgantown, West Virgina

HERBERT I. SAUER, M.S.P.H.
Assistant Professor
Department of Community Health and Medical Practice
University of Missouri
Columbia, Missouri

MORTIMER SPIEGELMAN, M.E., M.B.A.*
Statistician, Metropolitan Life Insurance Company (Retired)
New York, New York
Chairman (1959-69), Committee on Vital and Health Statistics Monographs,
   Statistics Section, American Public Health Association, Washington, D.C.

*Deceased March 25, 1969.

PREFACE

This final volume of the Vital and Health Statistics Monographs presents a summary picture of mortality and morbidity in the United States, with brief international comparisons and particular emphasis on the decade of the 1960's. Of special concern are the health problems of the aged, infant mortality, mortality and morbidity within the United States by geographic variation and by marital status, and future needs for health resources. This general overview is an attempt to synthesize material presented in great detail in the preceding volumes of this monograph series:

Accidents and Homicide by Albert P. Iskrant and Paul V. Joliet
Infectious Diseases by Carl C. Dauer, Robert F. Korns, and Leonard M. Schuman
Trends and Variations in Fertility in the United States by Clyde V. Kiser, Wilson H. Grabill, and Arthur A. Campbell
Infant, Perinatal, Maternal, and Childhood Mortality in the United States by Sam Shapiro, Edward R. Schlesinger, and Robert E. L. Nesbitt, Jr.
Tuberculosis by Anthony M. Lowell, Lydia B. Edwards, and Carroll E. Palmer
The Epidemiology of Oral Health by Walter J. Pelton, John B. Dunbar, Russell S. McMillan, Palmi Moller, and Albert E. Wolff
Syphilis and Other Venereal Diseases by William J. Brown, James F. Donohue, Norman W. Axnick, Joseph H. Blount, Neal W. Ewen, and Oscar G. Jones
Marriage and Divorce: A Social and Economic Study by Hugh Carter and Paul C. Glick
Digestive Diseases by Albert I. Mendeloff and James P. Dunn
The Frequency of the Rheumatic Diseases by Sidney Cobb
Cardiovascular Diseases in the United States by Iwao M. Moriyama, Dean E. Krueger, and Jeremiah Stamler
Cancer in the United States by Abraham M. Lilienfeld, Morton L. Levin, and Irving I. Kessler
Mental Disorders/Suicide by Morton Kramer, Earl S. Pollack, Richard W. Redick, and Ben Z. Locke
Epidemiology of Neurologic and Sense Organ Disorders by Leonard T. Kurland, John F. Kurtzke, and Irving D. Goldberg
Differential Mortality in the United States: A Study in Socioeconomic Epidemiology by Evelyn M. Kitagawa and Philip M. Hauser

The authors of each of these volumes have our profound gratitude.

The editors of the present volume are greatly indebted to the contributing authors, who generously gave their time and energies to preparation of the various chapters. Included among these is Mortimer Spiegelman who, before his untimely death, had designed the general format and substance of the first three chapters, which were then updated and completed by Carl Erhardt.

vii

It is also fitting, in this final volume, to acknowledge the extensive and devoted assistance of Miss Teresa Hilb, who served as secretary and assistant to both Mr. Spiegelman and Dr. Erhardt. Her careful construction of the typed tables, her meticulous attention to details of the texts and figures, and her able maintenance of minutes and of files, preparation of drafts for reports, verification of data, and keeping of precise records of budget items, was inspiring. Without her contribution, completion of the series would have been infinitely more difficult.

Finally, the monograph series would not exist at all had it not been for Mortimer Spiegelman's initiation of the project and his devotion to it.

To all those involved go our thanks.

Carl L. Erhardt
Joyce E. Berlin

CONTENTS

TABLES

FIGURES

APPENDIX TABLES AND FIGURES

FOREWORD

Rapid advances in medical and allied sciences, changing patterns in medical care and public health programs, an increasingly health-conscious public, and the rising concern of voluntary agencies and government at all levels in meeting the health needs of the people necessitate constant evaluation of the country's health status. Such an evaluation, which is required not only for an appraisal of the current situation, but also to refine present goals and to gauge our progress toward them, depends largely upon a study of vital and health statistics records.

Opportunity to study mortality in depth emerges when a national census furnishes the requisite population data for the computation of death rates in demographic and geographic detail. Prior to the 1960 census of population there had been no comprehensive analysis of this kind. It therefore seemed appropriate to build up for intensive study a substantial body of death statistics for a three-year period centered around that census year.

A detailed examination of the country's health status must go beyond an examination of mortality statistics. Many conditions such as arthritis, rheumatism, and mental diseases are much more important as causes of morbidity than of mortality. Also, an examination of health status should not be based solely upon current findings, but should take into account trends and whatever pertinent evidence has been assembled through local surveys and from clinical experience.

The proposal for such an evaluation, to consist of a series of monographs, was made to the Statistics Section of the American Public Health Association in October 1958 by Mortimer Spiegelman, and a Committee on Vital and Health Statistics Monographs was authorized with Mr. Spiegelman as Chairman, a position he held until his death on March 25, 1969. The members of this committee and of the Editorial Advisory Subcommittee created later are:

Committee on Vital and Health Statistics Monographs

Carl L. Erhardt, Sc.D., Chairman
Paul M. Densen, D.Sc.
Robert D. Grove, Ph.D.
Clyde V. Kiser, Ph.D.
Felix Moore

George Rosen, M.D., Ph.D.
William H. Stewart, M.D.
 (withdrew June 1964)
Conrad Taeuber, Ph.D.
Paul Webbink
Donald Young, Ph.D.

Editorial Advisory Subcommittee

The early history of this undertaking is described in a paper presented at the 1962 Annual Conference of the Milbank Memorial Fund.[1] The Committee on Vital and Health Statistics Monographs selected the topics to be included in the series and also suggested candidates for authorship. The frame of reference was extended by the committee to include other topics in vital and health statistics than mortality and morbidity, namely fertility, marriage, and divorce. Conferences were held with authors to establish general guidelines for the preparation of the manuscripts.

Support for this undertaking in its preliminary stages was received from the Rockefeller Foundation, the Milbank Memorial Fund, and the Health Information Foundation. Major support for the required tabulations, for writing and editorial work, and for the related research of the monograph authors was provided by the United States Public Health Service (Research Grant HS 00572, formerly CH 00075 and originally GM 08262). Acknowledgment should also be made to the Metropolitan Life Insurance Company for the facilities and time that were made available to Mr. Spiegelman before his retirement in December 1966, after which he devoted his major time to administer the undertaking and to serve as general editor. Without his abiding concern over each monograph in the series and his close work with the authors, the completion of the series might have been in grave doubt. These sixteen volumes are a fitting memorial to Mr. Spiegelman's resolute efforts.

The New York City Department of Health allowed Dr. Carl L. Erhardt to allocate part of his time to administrative details for the series from April to December 1969, when he retired to assume a more active role. The National Center for Health Statistics, under the supervision of Dr. Grove and Miss Alice M. Hetzel, undertook the

---

[1] Mortimer Spiegelman, "The Organization of the Vital and Health Statistics Monograph Program," *Emerging Techniques in Population Research (Proceedings of the 1962 Annual Conference of the Milbank Memorial Fund*; New York: Milbank Memorial Fund, 1963), p. 230. See also Mortimer Spiegelman, "The Demographic Viewpoint in the Vital and Health Statistics Monographs Project of the American Public Health Association," *Demography*, 3:574 (1966).

sizable tasks of planning and carrying out the extensive mortality tabulations for the 1959-61 period. Dr. Taeuber arranged for the cooperation of the Bureau of the Census at all stages of the project in many ways, principally by furnishing the required population data used in computing death rates and by undertaking a large number of varied special tabulations. As the sponsor of the project, the American Public Health Association furnished assistance through Dr. Thomas R. Hood, its Deputy Executive Director.

Because of the great variety of topics selected for monograph treatment, authors were given an essentially free hand to develop their manuscripts as they desired. Accordingly, the authors of the individual monographs bear the full responsibility for their manuscripts, and their opinions and statements do not necessarily represent the viewpoints of the American Public Health Association or of the agencies with which they may be affiliated.

William H. McBeath, M.D., M.P.H.
Executive Director
American Public Health Association

NOTES ON TABLES AND FIGURES

1. Regarding 1959-61 mortality data:
   a. Deaths relate to those occurring in the United States, including Alaska and Hawaii;
   b. Deaths are classified by place of residence at death, unless otherwise stated;
   c. Fetal deaths are excluded;
   d. Deaths of unknown age, marital status, nativity, or other characteristics have not been distributed into the known categories, but are included in their totals;
   e. Deaths were classified by cause according to the *Seventh Revision of the International Statistical Classification of Diseases, Injuries, and Causes of Death* (Geneva: World Health Organization, 1957);
   f. Unless otherwise specified, all death rates are average annual rates per 100,000 population in the category specified, as recorded in the United States census of April 1, 1960;
   g. Age-adjusted rates were computed by the direct method using the age distribution of the total United States population in the census of April 1, 1940, as a standard.[1] The mortality tabulations prepared especially for this series included age-adjusted death rates for all ages, under 15 years, and 65 years and over. In tabulations by marital status, the age-adjusted groupings were 15 years and over, 15-64 years, and 65 years and over.
2. Regarding "crude" and "adjusted" rates:
   Unless otherwise specified, all rates are "crude" (unadjusted). However, in some instances crude rates have been so labeled intentionally for clarity, emphasis, or to avoid confusion with other similar tables or figures in which age-adjusted data are used.
3. Symbols used in tables of data:
   - - - Data not available;
   . . . Category not applicable;
   — Quantity zero;
   0.0 Quantity more than zero but less than 0.05.
   * Figure does not meet the standard of reliability or precision:
      a) Rate or ratio based on less than 20 deaths;
      b) Percentage or median based on less than 100 deaths;
      c) Age-adjusted rate computed from age-specific rates where more than half of the rates were based on frequencies of less than 20 deaths. For disorders sharply delimited by age, this criterion may give a spurious impression of imprecision; where feasible in such instances, numbers of deaths are also entabled.
4. Geographic classification:[2]
   a. Standard Metropolitan Statistical Area (SMSA): except in the New

[1] Mortimer Spiegelman and H.H. Marks, "Empirical Testing of Standards for the Age Adjustment of Death Rates by the Direct Method," *Human Biology*, 38:280 (September 1966).
[2] National Center for Health Statistics, *Vital Statistics of the United States, 1960* (Washington, D.C.: Public Health Service, 1963), vol. 2, *Mortality*, pt. A, sec. 7, p. 8.

England states, "an SMSA is a county or a group of contiguous counties which contains at least one city of 50,000 inhabitants or more or 'twin cities' with a combined population of at least 50,000 in the 1960 census. In addition, contiguous counties are included in an SMSA if, according to specified criteria, they are (a) essentially metropolitan in character and (b) socially and economically integrated with the central city or cities." In New England, the Division of Vital Statistics of the National Center for Health Statistics uses, instead of the definition just cited, Metropolitan State Economic Areas (MSEA's) established by the Bureau of the Census, which are made up of county units.

b. Metropolitan and nonmetropolitan: "Counties which are included in SMSA's, or, in New England, MSEA's are called metropolitan counties; all other counties are classified as nonmetropolitan."

c. Metropolitan counties may be separated into those containing at least one central city of 50,000 inhabitants or more or "twin cities" as specified previously, and into metropolitan counties without a central city.

d. Census regions: Nine geographic divisions of the United States as utilized by the Bureau of the Census, each region comprising a group of states (without reference to SMSA's), including as appropriate the District of Columbia, Alaska, or Hawaii.

5. The following sources in the Public Health Service, U.S. Department of Health, Education, and Welfare, were used in preparing the figures, text tables, and appendix tables referable to mortality data for the United States. Any additional sources are specified in the text tables and figures.

a. National Center for Health Statistics, special tabulations of deaths and death rates for the period 1959-61 for the American Public Health Association.

b. National Center for Health Statistics, *Vital Statistics of the United States*, Washington, D.C., issued annually.

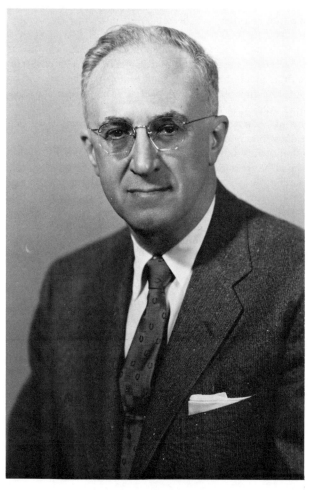

MORTIMER SPIEGELMAN
(1901–1969)

DEDICATION

This volume concludes the group of sixteen Vital and Health Statistics Mongraphs published under the sponsorship of the Statistics Section of the American Public Health Association. The early plan for the monographs was developed by Mortimer Spiegelman in the late 1950's. Its specific purpose was to develop a coordinated body of health information using population data which would derive from the 1960 census. Once the project became viable through financial support, Mr. Spiegelman began the onerous task of recruiting authors for specific volumes, coordinating their requests for special tabulations, and negotiating with the National Center for Health Statistics for the production of the necessary mortality data. Formidable as these tasks were, there followed the longer and more difficult ones of prodding completed manuscripts from authors who were already fully committed elsewhere, and of editing the manuscripts for publication. The series was not completed at the time of Mortimer Spiegelman's death in 1969, but his planning, groundwork, and perseverance made its ultimate achievement possible.

This volume is dedicated to Mortimer Spiegelman, initiator of the Vital and Health Statistics Monographs and chairman of the Monographs Committee until his death. He was a colleague of intellect, and a gentleman of great heart with compassion for his fellowmen.

Helen C. Chase, Dr.P.H.
Chairman, Statistics Section (1970–1972)
American Public Health Association

1 / MORTALITY AND LONGEVITY IN THE UNITED STATES

Mortimer Spiegelman
Carl L. Erhardt

The marked changes in the social, economic, and cultural patterns of American life today from those of the country's early history are well documented and tell a fascinating story. Lacking in this documentation, though, is the evidence needed for an adequate portrayal of the nation's health status in its formative years. Perhaps the most useful insight into the situation then as compared with the situation today is provided by the course of the death rate for New York City, which is plotted in Fig. 1.1. The trends may present, in a very general sense, a picture typical for the country over its history.

For most of the nineteenth century, the death rate in New York City ranged above a level of 25 per 1,000 population, with rather frequent outbreaks of yellow fever, smallpox, and cholera. However, this is only part of the infectious disease picture for that century: early in the second half (1861-65), Massachusetts, for example, had a death rate of 365 per 100,000 population for tuberculosis, 105 for typhoid and paratyphoid fever, 123 for diphtheria, 19 for measles, and 9 for smallpox.[1] In sharp contrast, in the United States one hundred years later, the death rate for tuberculosis is barely 4 per 100,000 population; deaths from typhoid fever, diphtheria, and measles have been reduced to almost negligible numbers; and to find a single case of smallpox is cause for alarm. The intervening period for these diseases was one of rapid decline. The most significant interruption in the decline during the current century was the 1918 epidemic of influenza. It is worth pointing out that death rates for Massachusetts from 1865 to 1900 suggest declines during that interval at ages 5-39 years, but the quality of these data is uncertain.[2]

The course of mortality in the United States for the present century is shown in Fig. 1.2. These rates relate to an expanding area that started with ten states and the District of Columbia in 1900 and extended to the whole country by 1933. Barring the extraordinary peak of 1918, the general course has been downward to a low point in 1954, with a practically level rate since then. Whereas the average

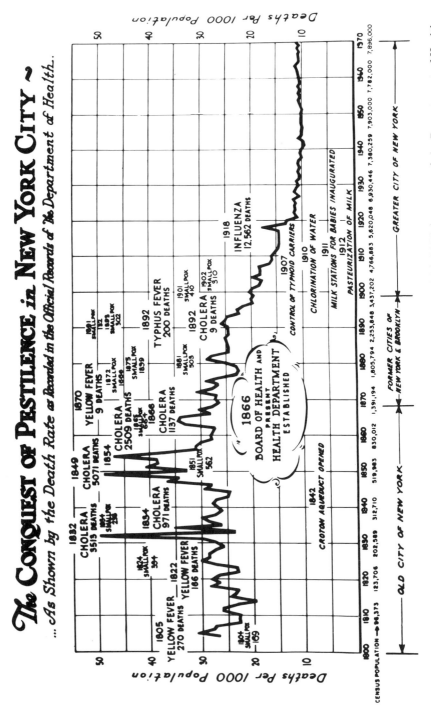

Figure 1.1 Crude death rate per 1,000 population: New York City, 1804–1970 (courtesy of the Department of Health, City of New York)

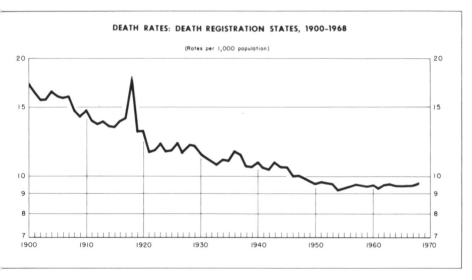

DEATH RATES: DEATH REGISTRATION STATES, 1900-1968

(Rates per 1,000 population)

Figure 1.2 Crude death rate per 1,000 population: United States, 1900–68 (courtesy of the National Office of Vital Statistics, U. S. Department of Health, Education and Welfare)

of the annual crude death rates for the five-year period 1900-04 was 16.2 per 1,000 population, that for 1963-67 was 9.5.

This chapter deals with mortality generally. Geographic variations are covered in Chapter 5, special problems of the aged in Chapter 6, the influence of marital status in Chapter 7, and particular problems among infants in Chapter 8.

Mortality by Age, Sex, and Color

Mortality varies strikingly with age. Quite generally, the death rate is relatively high in the first year of life and decreases rapidly to a minimum around age 10 or 11 years; it then proceeds to mount— slowly with added years until about age 45 or 50, and then at an accelerating pace for all but the last few years. Only a rare life extends beyond age 110. Over the span of human life, the benefit of mortality reduction in the course of time has been very uneven.[3],[4]

A convenient summary of the course of mortality in the United States during this century according to age, sex, and color is contained in Tables 1.1 and 1.2, in which averages have been formed of annual death rates for the expanding death registration states during successive five-year periods from 1900 to 1964. Comment will

Table 1.1   Average of annual death rates for successive five-year periods from 1900 to 1964 for white persons by age and sex: United States*

Sex; period	Death rate per 100,000 at ages—											
	All ages	Under 1	1-4	5-14	15-24	25-34	35-44	45-54	55-64	65-74	75-84	85 and over
Male												
1960-64	1,086.5	2,553.9	96.5	50.0	142.0	163.7	331.9	912.7	2,200.7	4,860.3	10,055.7	22,070.4
1955-59	1,082.2	2,808.3	105.6	54.9	152.2	165.0	335.7	913.4	2,207.1	4,761.7	10,197.2	20,833.3
1950-54	1,087.7	3,215.1	128.6	64.1	158.5	181.4	366.3	963.3	2,267.3	4,772.1	10,336.3	20,523.0
1945-49	1,143.9	4,063.8	171.2	85.6	186.6	224.9	429.5	1,035.5	2,319.2	4,833.8	10,700.9	22,793.4
1940-44	1,177.9	5,034.0	252.9	106.7	219.1	275.9	490.2	1,113.0	2,468.5	5,183.3	11,636.8	23,771.6
1935-39	1,171.8	6,162.4	393.1	142.8	237.4	330.6	577.7	1,211.4	2,541.9	5,358.2	12,470.9	24,143.6
1930-34	1,149.5	6,704.8	499.6	167.8	270.2	374.8	621.4	1,215.3	2,532.5	5,407.3	12,023.0	23,959.6
1925-29	1,204.0	7,631.9	628.8	201.9	315.9	420.6	692.6	1,252.4	2,506.7	5,651.0	12,839.3	26,693.0
1920-24	1,121.5	8,627.2	798.0	239.2	349.3	467.8	692.4	1,181.5	2,416.4	5,407.8	12,208.0	25,823.1
1915-19**	1,392.6	10,909.7	1,005.9	254.3	432.6	637.8	894.8	1,393.6	2,730.9	5,776.5	12,224.4	24,284.9
1910-14	1,449.5	12,575.7	1,195.8	269.6	441.9	634.9	952.3	1,455.3	2,765.3	5,774.0	12,436.0	24,800.8
1905-09	1,598.2	14,813.9	1,476.9	315.5	509.8	722.5	1,023.7	1,546.1	2,902.8	5,845.7	12,795.6	26,338.2
1900-04	1,686.3	15,467.4	1,719.9	357.1	539.2	783.1	1,056.8	1,555.5	2,900.4	5,885.4	12,752.2	26,639.7
Female												
1960-64	797.9	1,917.6	79.8	33.0	54.9	85.8	190.9	457.4	1,044.8	2,717.4	7,383.6	19,862.1
1955-59	788.9	2,116.1	88.9	35.3	57.2	88.1	192.2	461.3	1,105.0	2,867.2	7,802.9	19,397.9
1950-54	792.8	2,424.8	107.7	42.6	66.2	103.1	221.3	521.1	1,226.9	3,097.1	8,181.0	19,157.5
1945-49	838.8	3,112.2	142.1	56.3	92.1	142.3	275.2	605.8	1,408.7	3,434.1	8,852.9	20,908.4
1940-44	894.0	3,912.2	215.1	73.4	125.2	195.3	339.1	708.5	1,598.5	3,911.5	9,873.5	22,040.3
1935-39	948.4	4,755.4	341.5	108.0	179.1	277.6	430.4	833.5	1,816.9	4,280.0	10,862.7	22,606.0
1930-34	958.7	5,235.5	437.0	131.9	225.3	335.2	489.5	895.5	1,938.2	4,477.3	10,715.3	22,481.3
1925-29	1,043.0	5,925.9	561.0	160.2	290.9	400.3	573.3	987.0	2,041.9	4,813.5	11,631.2	26,710.5
1920-24	1,096.6	6,713.9	714.9	199.0	343.3	475.9	620.7	1,022.1	2,073.3	4,823.7	11,472.8	25,945.8
1915-19**	1,215.1	8,523.7	905.5	244.1	393.0	564.2	719.1	1,111.1	2,258.5	5,125.1	11,383.9	23,327.6
1910-14	1,266.7	10,064.2	1,089.9	244.1	384.1	555.9	738.3	1,136.7	2,274.0	5,101.7	11,491.6	23,908.0
1905-09	1,410.1	11,924.2	1,350.0	292.3	447.6	648.3	817.8	1,235.8	2,437.3	5,224.5	11,677.3	25,316.4
1900-04	1,521.8	12,479.4	1,591.1	340.9	518.9	747.8	914.1	1,330.5	2,519.4	5,248.5	11,674.5	25,012.2

*Death registration states.

**Excluding 1918 for all ages.

Table 1.2 Average of annual death rates for successive five-year periods from 1900 to 1964 for nonwhite persons by age and sex: United States*

Sex; period	Death rate per 100,000 at ages—											
	All ages	Under 1	1-4	5-14	15-24	25-34	35-44	45-54	55-64	65-74	75-84	85 and over
Male												
1960-64	1,126.2	4,674.9	185.0	70.6	211.9	397.5	750.7	1,539.6	3,105.8	5,963.2	8,190.8	15,304.5
1955-59	1,151.1	5,373.2	208.3	76.7	228.9	412.1	713.9	1,569.9	3,227.6	5,391.0	8,202.1	14,754.9
1950-54	1,224.7	5,859.1	253.9	92.1	278.9	469.6	813.2	1,792.2	3,477.7	5,319.6	8,606.0	15,612.6
1945-49	1,266.9	6,681.2	293.8	114.8	357.7	569.0	968.4	2,013.0	3,292.0	5,211.6	8,305.7	16,122.2
1940-44	1,434.4	8,813.9	470.7	154.2	468.5	768.9	1,217.9	2,294.1	3,471.1	5,784.0	9,559.5	18,971.5
1935-39	1,575.6	10,544.9	673.9	201.8	591.9	1,004.2	1,550.6	2,513.2	3,881.5	5,795.3	10,556.7	18,727.5
1930-34	1,609.4	11,226.9	851.0	237.9	694.3	1,109.2	1,601.5	2,445.9	3,842.6	6,034.3	10,994.7	20,545.4
1925-29	1,799.8	13,957.4	1,137.8	292.9	838.1	1,227.6	1,738.4	2,635.2	3,685.8	6,583.5	12,473.3	28,060.9
1920-24	1,682.2	14,627.3	1,313.3	305.2	867.4	1,114.1	1,460.8	2,116.0	3,100.6	5,826.9	11,599.6	26,784.7
1915-19**	2,005.4	16,893.6	1,826.6	402.1	1,045.5	1,348.1	1,725.0	2,239.5	3,821.2	6,706.2	12,275.7	23,225.6
1910-14	2,149.3	20,963.6	2,389.5	487.1	1,027.7	1,288.2	1,750.4	2,451.0	3,996.5	6,863.7	11,755.1	20,052.9
1905-09	2,431.0	28,725.5	3,519.3	664.1	1,157.3	1,374.8	1,722.6	2,522.5	4,099.4	6,942.8	12,087.8	20,959.4
1900-04	2,582.7	34,248.0	4,034.0	715.7	1,183.7	1,370.3	1,625.0	2,518.4	4,516.4	7,272.9	13,075.5	23,456.1
Female												
1960-64	853.2	3,725.0	159.8	49.9	104.3	251.5	537.9	1,096.1	2,367.8	4,090.4	6,423.9	13,118.0
1955-59	886.9	4,272.2	181.6	54.8	120.4	273.8	569.9	1,244.3	2,467.3	3,902.5	6,497.3	11,794.8
1950-54	948.8	4,537.0	215.5	66.4	178.5	341.2	683.9	1,480.7	2,683.3	4,024.7	6,715.2	12,449.6
1945-49	1,018.9	5,327.0	225.0	94.0	298.2	477.1	843.4	1,668.3	2,752.6	4,296.6	6,712.6	12,353.6
1940-44	1,176.3	7,080.2	413.5	130.1	442.0	654.5	1,080.0	1,933.6	3,098.7	4,802.0	7,519.9	14,508.4
1935-39	1,312.4	8,162.4	584.9	179.3	588.4	865.5	1,286.3	2,174.6	3,705.5	4,885.5	8,240.9	15,258.3
1930-34	1,396.9	8,927.7	744.9	223.4	702.0	1,005.6	1,384.9	2,312.0	3,863.7	5,457.9	8,641.4	16,417.1
1925-29	1,619.5	10,822.7	1,026.5	276.8	919.9	1,160.4	1,656.0	2,564.7	3,840.8	6,181.3	10,210.3	22,113.9
1920-24	1,599.6	11,658.6	1,208.1	312.3	954.0	1,131.9	1,498.4	2,323.0	3,544.3	5,895.0	9,999.4	22,489.5
1915-19**	1,879.1	13,355.2	1,685.4	439.9	1,107.2	1,320.3	1,649.4	2,407.6	4,063.8	6,408.6	10,802.5	21,222.5
1910-14	2,007.5	17,664.7	2,200.0	535.8	1,087.6	1,180.8	1,610.5	2,447.8	3,926.0	6,133.4	9,937.0	19,303.1
1905-09	2,291.4	24,568.2	3,206.2	768.8	1,206.6	1,279.6	1,604.6	2,424.7	4,008.7	6,414.8	9,979.1	19,219.9
1900-04	2,360.3	28,568.5	3,767.0	831.2	1,148.6	1,221.2	1,580.8	2,368.3	4,064.6	6,519.6	10,420.6	21,448.0

*Death registration states.
**Excluding 1918 for all ages and for ages up through 45-54.

be confined principally to the data for white persons, since the early data for nonwhites in the limited registration area may hardly be typical of their situation in the country as a whole.

Relative to the level of the death rates in 1900-04, childhood mortality decreased rapidly up to 1960-64, but the rate of decrease declined with advance in age. There was little difference between the sexes in rate of improvement at ages under 15; at the higher ages females made the better showing, often by a wide margin. For example, at ages 1-4, where the relative reduction in mortality was most rapid, the death rate for white males and females in 1960-64 was only one-twentieth of that for 1900-04. On the other hand, at ages 65-74, the death rate for white males in 1960-64 was about five-sixths of that for 1900-04, but for white females the ratio was not quite one-half. Year-by-year death rates according to age, sex, and color from 1930 through 1968 are shown in Figs. 1.3 and 1.4. A tendency toward leveling of the trend in death rates since about 1954 is evident for practically all age groups over 5 years, white and nonwhite.

Death rates for nonwhites are appreciably higher than those for the white population at all but the highest ages. Thus in 1960-64 the death rates for nonwhites at ages under 5 years were about twice those for white children. (See also the discussion of differential infant mortality in Chapter 8.) This ratio fell to about 1.5 at ages 5-14 and then rose to a peak at ages 25-34, where the death rate for nonwhite females was practically three times that for white females; among males, the corresponding ratio was nearly 2.5 to one. Although these ratios fell off with advance in age, they were consistently higher for females than for males up to age 85.[5]

Data are not available for an additional five-year interval, but the average of annual death rates per 100,000 by age, color, and sex for the four years ending in 1968 are provided in the table on page 7. These figures do not substantially affect the previous observations. However, it is notable that reversals of the earlier declines in mortality occur among several age groups beyond 14 years. This reversal holds for white males (15-44 and 55-74), white females (15-24, 35-44, and 85 and over), and nonwhite males (15-84). Only among nonwhite females have declines continued, except at ages 65-74.

To enhance comparability between the sexes and the two color categories, the sex-color-specific death rates for each year from 1900 through 1964 have been age adjusted and averaged for five-year

Age	White		Nonwhite	
	Male	Female	Male	Female
All ages	1,090	808	1,123	818
Under 1	2,295	1,718	4,070	3,328
1–4	85	70	155	130
5–14	50	30	70	45
15–24	160	60	248	103
25–34	170	85	475	250
35–44	342	193	858	533
45–54	905	463	1,633	1,030
55–64	2,240	1,023	3,195	2,143
65–74	4,958	2,630	6,638	4,495
75–84	9,930	6,933	8,205	6,035
85+	21,793	20,048	12,190	11,163

periods, with the results shown in Table 1.3. In the overall picture, the reduction in mortality from 1900-04 to 1960-64 was more rapid for females than for males among both color groups, while among males the rate dropped at a faster pace for nonwhite than for white persons. However, during the first half of this period there was relatively little variation in the rate of decline between the four color-sex categories. Most of the difference in mortality reduction among the categories occurred during the second half of the period under review and, except for white males, declines were sharper than for the first half. From 1930-34 to 1960-64, the declines in age-adjusted death rates amounted to 27.0 percent for white males, 46.8 percent for white females, 37.6 percent for nonwhite males, and 49.9 percent for nonwhite females.

The differences in trends of mortality just noted are reflected in the ratios of male to female age-adjusted death rates and of nonwhite to white rates. Prior to 1930, for both color categories, the excess of male mortality over that of females remained practically constant at an average level of 15 percent for whites and 7 percent for nonwhites. Because of greater mortality reductions among females since 1930, white male mortality by 1960-64 was 1.67 times that for white females; for nonwhites, the ratio rose to 1.38.

During all of the current century up through 1964, the ratio of nonwhite to white death rates for females has moved about a high, but fairly constant, level averaging 1.66. On the other hand, there has

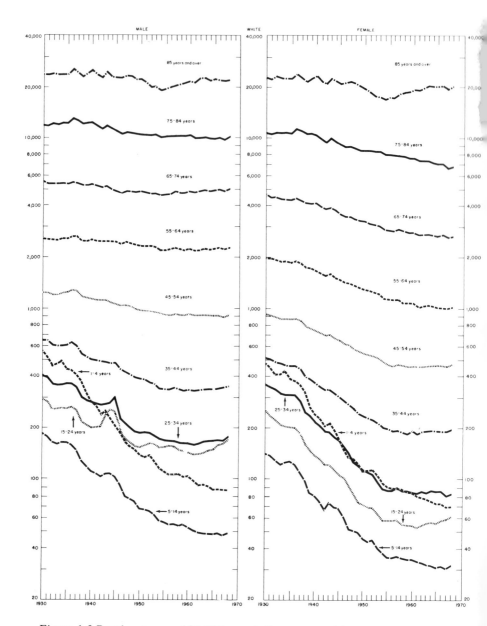

Figure 1.3 Death rates per 100,000 population among white persons, by sex and age: United States, 1930–68 (courtesy of the National Office of Vital Statistics, U. S. Department of Health, Education and Welfare)

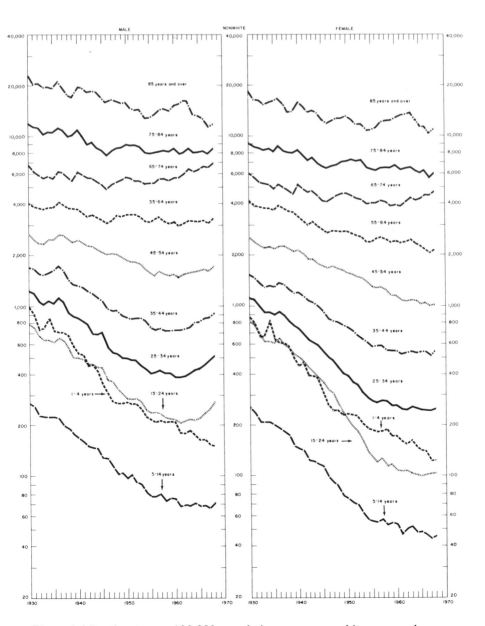

Figure 1.4 Death rates per 100,000 population among nonwhite persons, by sex and age: United States, 1930–68 (courtesy of the National Office of Vital Statistics, U. S. Department of Health, Education and Welfare)

Table 1.3   Average of annual age-adjusted death rates for all ages for successive five-year periods from 1900 to 1964 by color and sex, and ratios of male to female and of nonwhite to white death rates: United States

Period	Age-adjusted death rate, all ages			
	White		Nonwhite	
	Male	Female	Male	Female
1960-64	907.2	542.8	1,206.8	875.4
1955-59	910.0	566.3	1,204.7	911.0
1950-54	940.1	615.5	1,302.2	1,014.8
1945-49	1,014.5	706.6	1,375.4	1,139.2
1940-44	1,112.1	821.2	1,618.3	1,373.8
1935-39	1,210.5	952.8	1,848.9	1,595.1
1930-34	1,242.9	1,020.1	1,932.8	1,748.5
1925-29	1,332.8	1,140.7	2,149.7	2,013.2
1920-24	1,338.3	1,200.0	1,958.3	1,954.7
1915-19[a]	1,525.3	1,314.4	2,264.5	2,197.1
1910-14	1,586.2	1,357.8	2,399.4	2,243.9
1905-09	1,721.5	1,486.9	2,684.3	2,509.5
1900-04	1,777.1	1,579.8	2,874.6	2,611.2

From	Percent decrease in death rate			
1900-04 to 1960-64	49.0	65.6	58.0	66.5
1900-04 to 1930-34	30.1	35.4	32.8	33.0
1930-34 to 1960-64	27.0	46.8	37.6	49.9

	Ratio of rates			
	Male to female		Nonwhite to white	
	White	Nonwhite	Male	Female
1960-64	1.67	1.38	1.33	1.61
1955-59	1.61	1.32	1.32	1.61
1950-54	1.53	1.28	1.39	1.65
1945-49	1.44	1.21	1.36	1.61
1940-44	1.35	1.18	1.46	1.67
1935-39	1.27	1.16	1.53	1.67
1930-34	1.22	1.11	1.56	1.71
1925-29	1.17	1.07	1.61	1.76
1920-24	1.12	1.00	1.46	1.63
1915-19[a]	1.16	1.03	1.48	1.67
1910-14	1.17	1.07	1.51	1.65
1905-09	1.16	1.07	1.56	1.69
1900-04	1.12	1.10	1.62	1.65

Source: Data for 1900 through 1949 from Vital Statistics-Special Reports, vol. 43, no. 1, January 9, 1956; data from 1950 through 1964 from National Center for Health Statistics (unpublished).
[a]Average for four years excluding 1918.

been a marked tendency for nonwhite male mortality to converge with that of white males since 1930-34, when the ratio of the former to the latter was 1.56, compared with 1.62 for 1900-04 and 1.33 in 1960-64.

The reasons for the differentials in mortality reductions since 1930 are unclear. Within each color category males and females generally live in the same social environment and should share equally in improvements benefiting health. This assumption appears to be borne out by the similarity in mortality reduction noted previously for males and females under age 15. For the higher ages, however, the influences producing the divergence in trends are not apparent and leave room for conjecture. There is the possibility, for example, that the increasing availability and widening use of labor-saving appliances have eased the household work of women. Although men have undoubtedly gained by their improved work environment, it is possible that the stresses produced by economic pressures leave their mark. Growing differences in habits of personal health care may also enter the picture; for example, the weight-conscious attitude of women may contribute to their increasing mortality advantage. For the age group 15-24 years, it is possible to speak in more substantial terms. Table 1.1 shows that the two sexes had about the same death rates in 1900-04, but by 1960-64 the rate for males was more than 2.5 times that for females. At that stage of life maternal mortality has been brought to an extremely low level, but males have been disadvantaged by the rising death toll from motor vehicle accidents. Further general comment on sex differentials according to cause of death will be made in Chapter 2.

Longevity

The average length of life in the United States at the time of its founding was about 35 years, a level not far different from that for Sweden near the same time.[6,7] The quality of the United States figure, however, is uncertain since it is derived solely from death records at some time before 1789 in Massachusetts and New Hampshire. The next indication, on firmer ground, is provided by life tables for Massachusetts in 1850, with an average of 38.3 years for males and 40.5 years for females, as shown in Table 1.4. Compared with the apparently slow improvement in longevity during the early years of the country, the half-century from 1850 to 1900-02 was one of rapid gain, the rise amounting to about ten years. The next

Table 1.4   Expectation of life at birth and at ages 20, 40, and 60, by sex and color: United States, 1850 to 1968

Period; color	Male				Female			
	0	20	40	60	0	20	40	60
White								
1968[a]	67.5	49.9	31.6	15.8	74.9	56.7	37.6	20.2
1965[a]	67.6	50.2	31.7	16.0	74.7	56.6	37.5	20.1
1959-61[a]	67.6	50.3	31.7	16.0	74.2	56.3	37.1	19.7
1949-51[b]	66.3	49.5	31.2	15.8	72.0	54.6	35.6	18.6
1939-41[b]	62.8	47.8	30.0	15.1	67.3	51.4	33.3	17.0
1929-31[b]	59.1	46.0	29.2	14.7	62.7	48.5	31.5	16.1
1919-21[c]	56.3	45.6	29.9	15.3	58.5	46.5	30.9	15.9
1909-11[d]	50.2	42.7	27.4	14.0	53.6	44.9	29.3	14.9
1900-02[d]	48.2	42.2	27.7	14.4	51.1	43.8	29.2	15.2
1890[e]	42.5	40.7	27.4	14.7	44.5	42.0	28.8	15.7
1850[e]	38.3	40.1	27.9	15.6	40.5	40.2	29.8	17.0
Nonwhite[f]								
1968[a]	60.1	43.6	27.4	14.5	67.5	50.5	32.7	17.9
1965[a]	61.1	45.1	28.3	15.1	67.4	50.8	32.8	18.2
1959-61[a]	61.5	45.8	28.7	15.3	66.5	50.1	32.2	17.8
1949-51[b]	58.9	43.7	27.3	14.9	62.7	46.8	29.8	17.0
1939-41[b]	52.3	39.7	25.2	14.4	55.5	42.1	27.3	16.1
1929-31[b]	47.6	36.0	23.4	13.2	49.5	37.2	24.3	14.2
1919-21[c]	47.1	38.4	26.5	14.7	46.9	37.2	25.6	14.7
1909-11[d]	34.1	33.5	21.6	11.7	37.7	36.1	23.3	12.8
1900-02[d]	32.5	35.1	23.1	12.6	35.0	36.9	24.4	13.6

Sources: 1850 - J. C. G. Kennedy, The Seventh Census - Report of the Superintendent of the Census for December 1, 1852, Washington, 1853, pp. 11-13.

1890   G. W. Glover, United States Life Tables, 1890, 1901, 1910, and 1901-1910, Bureau of the Census, Washington, 1921.

1900-02 and later - National Center for Health Statistics, Vital Statistics of the United States, 1968, vol. 2, section 5, Washington, 1971.

[a]Total of 50 States and the District of Columbia.
[b]Conterminous United States.
[c]Death Registration States of 1920.
[d]Original Death Registration States.
[e]Total population in Massachusetts, of whom about one percent are nonwhite.
[f]For 1900-02 to 1929-31, figures for nonwhites relate only to Negroes.

half-century, to 1949-51, was one of extraordinary longevity improvement that can hardly be duplicated in the future. During this interval the average life-span rose by 18.1 years for white males and by 20.9 years for white females. Although the figures shown for nonwhites in the early years of this century may not be typical of their situation in the country as a whole, they point to a rise of 26.4 years for males and 27.7 years for females up to 1949-51.

A slower pace of improvement in longevity for the second half of the present century is evident in the data up to 1968, with signs of retrogression appearing for most groups except white females. Since 1949-51, the rise in average length of life has been only 1.2 years for white males, 2.9 years for white females, 1.2 years for nonwhite males, and 4.8 years for nonwhite females. For both the longer period since the beginning of the century and the shorter period since its midpoint, the data for average length of life show a greater gain for females than for males and also for nonwhites than for whites. These characteristics persist, generally, in the figures for expectation of life at the higher ages and reflect the course of mortality according to color and sex discussed previously, with more recent mortality rises likely to affect longevity figures adversely. Yet the low mortality rates observed in some areas of the country (Chapter 5) indicate that the potential exists for further inroads on overall mortality as well as for extension of life expectancy.

Cohort Mortality

The death rates in Tables 1.1 and 1.2 at ages 5 and over make it possible to observe the mortality of a generation as it progresses into higher ages. Consider, for example, the generation of white males at ages 15-24 in 1900-04; its average annual death rate then was 539.2 per 100,000. One decade later, the generation was 25-34 years old and its death rate was 634.9. If we proceed by decades diagonally toward the upper right of the table, we find that when the generation attained ages 65-74 in 1950-54 its death rate was 4,772.1 per 100,000. Finally, at ages 75-84 in 1960-64, its death rate reached 10,055.7.

The acceleration, or rate of rise, in mortality of a generation as it ages may be studied from the ratios of death rates for successive age groups. Thus for the generation just cited the ratio of the death rate at ages 75-84 to that at ages 65-74 is 2.11. Ratios derived in this way from the death rates in Table 1.1 for white males and females are shown in Table 1.5, which has a number of noteworthy features.

(*a*) Whereas the death rates for each period in Table 1.1 show a minimum at ages 5-14 years and a continued rise thereafter, the ratios in Table 1.5 give clear indication of another low in mortality for many generations at ages 25-34. This will be noted for generations of females reaching that age range during 1930 to 1959 and of males in 1925-29 and from 1945 to 1959. In fact, for white females

Table 1.5   Ratio of death rates by sex for white persons at stated ages in specified periods to the rates at ages ten years younger in a period ten years earlier: United States

Sex; period	15-24	25-34	35-44	45-54	55-64	65-74	75-84	85 and over
Male								
1960-64	2.22	1.03	1.83	2.49	2.28	2.14	2.11	2.14
1955-59	1.78	0.88	1.49	2.13	2.13	1.99	2.11	1.95
1950-54	1.49	0.83	1.33	1.97	2.04	1.93	1.99	1.76
1945-49	1.31	0.95	1.30	1.79	1.97	1.90	2.00	1.83
1940-44	1.31	1.02	1.31	1.79	2.03	2.05	2.15	1.98
1935-39	1.18	1.05	1.37	1.75	2.03	2.14	2.21	1.88
1930-34	1.13	1.07	1.33	1.76	2.14	2.24	2.22	1.96
1925-29	1.24	0.97	1.09	1.40	1.80	2.07	2.22	2.18
1920-24	1.30	1.06	1.09	1.27	1.66	1.96	2.11	2.08
1915-19	1.37	1.25	1.24	1.36	1.77	1.99	2.09	1.90
1910-14	1.24	1.18	1.19	1.38	1.78	1.99	2.11	1.94
Female								
1960-64	1.29	1.30	1.85	2.07	2.00	2.21	2.38	2.43
1955-59	1.02	0.96	1.35	1.68	1.82	2.04	2.27	2.19
1950-54	0.90	0.82	1.13	1.54	1.73	1.94	2.09	1.94
1945-49	0.85	0.79	0.99	1.41	1.69	1.89	2.07	1.92
1940-44	0.95	0.87	1.01	1.45	1.79	2.02	2.21	2.06
1935-39	1.12	0.95	1.08	1.45	1.84	2.10	2.26	1.94
1930-34	1.13	0.98	1.03	1.44	1.90	2.16	2.22	1.96
1925-29	1.33	1.02	1.02	1.37	1.84	2.13	2.27	2.35
1920-24	1.41	1.24	1.12	1.38	1.82	2.12	2.25	2.26
1915-19	1.34	1.26	1.11	1.36	1.83	2.10	2.18	2.00
1910-14	1.13	1.07	0.99	1.24	1.71	2.02	2.19	2.05

Note: The average of death rates for 1915-19 excludes the rates for 1918, the year of the influenza pandemic, for ages up through 45-54 years. Underlining indicates those ratios at midlife since 1945 that are higher than that for either the preceding or following age group.

who reached that age period during 1940 to 1954, the death rates for the generations were even lower than at ages 5-14 years. In most instances the generation death rates at ages 15-24 and 25-34 were not far different. In other words, there is a tendency for the generation curve of mortality to show a small peak at ages 15-24. These observations are illustrated in Fig. 1.5, where the death rates over their lifetime thus far are presented for females who were 5-14 years old in 1910-14. In contrast, the age-specific death rates for 1960-64 indicate the improvement in mortality at specific ages since the time when the cohort of 1910-14 reached those ages. The two curves converge and meet at 55-64, since the 1960-64 rate is established by

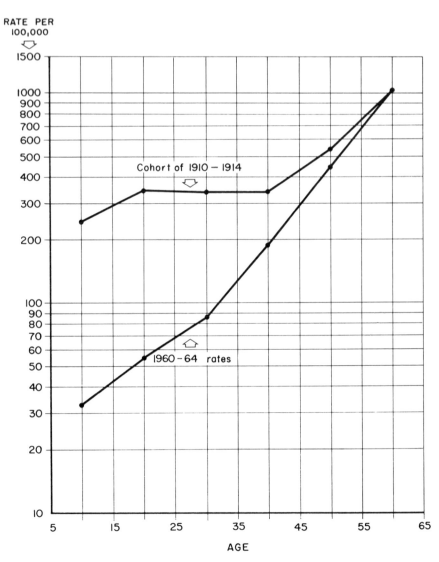

Figure 1.5 Death rates per 100,000 population among the cohort of white females 5–14 years old in 1910–14 at successive ten-year intervals and age-specific death rates of females, by age, in 1960–64: United States

the cohort of women who have now reached that age. In opposition to the idea of a constantly increasing death toll as one goes through life, it is clear now that specific generations in the past have experienced a fairly constant mortality over long periods.

(b) With advance in age, the generation mortality of males since

1930 tends to rise at a greater rate than that for females, but only up to entry into old age; at the very high ages female mortality increases at a greater rate.

(c) Before 1945 for males and 1960 for females, generation mortality between ages 25 and 85 rises with advance in age at a steadily increasing pace, as can be seen by reading across the rows in Table 1.5. Since those years, the rate of increase in generation mortality was greater upon entry into midlife (45-54) than upon entry into several higher age groups; that is, a greater relative increase in mortality rates has, in recent periods, been occurring at ages 45-54 or 55-64 in comparison with the rates for these persons ten years earlier than has been observed among others aging ten years during the same interval. In fact, for males the rate of rise in generation mortality upon entry into midlife increased rapidly with time; since 1955, it has been greater than at any other period of life. The midlife ratios since 1945 that are higher than those for immediately preceding or following ages have been underlined in Table 1.5.

(d) Despite the decline of usually calculated age-specific mortality rates in midlife (Tables 1.1 and 1.2), there has been a tendency for the generation curve of mortality to rise more steeply. Table 1.5 shows an upward trend in the ratios of death rates between ages 35 and 65 (reading up the columns).

(e) Statements of age at the upper extreme of life are generally unreliable and have sometimes been considered to understate mortality.[8] How this affects the death rates at ages 75-84 and ages 85 and over in Table 1.1 is not known. If we accept the rates as given, the ratios shown in Table 1.5 result. The interesting feature is that, in most instances, the ratio of the death rate at ages 85 and over—which may be taken to represent that at ages 85-94—to the death rate at 75-84 for the same generation is lower than the ratio preceding it. This would indicate that the rise in mortality at the extreme ages tends to taper off, a feature which, although suspect because of the uncertain quality of the data, finds confirmation in some annuity records and also in theoretical studies.[9-11] This feature may arise out of the heterogeneity of a population at any age with regard to its states of health, which may range from excellent by any standard to moribund. In passing from one age to the next, the relatively unhealthy lives will be lost by death at a greater rate than the relatively healthy lives; at the same time, many of the healthy will lose their state of well-being and enter the ranks of the unhealthy. At the extreme ages of life, it seems likely that the rate of loss of unhealthy lives is so much greater than the rate of accretion that the proportions of unhealthy persons among the very old tend then to decrease with advance in years. The net result would be a tapering off of the rise in death rates with advance in age at that stage of life.

Demographic, Social, and Economic Consequences of Mortality Trends

Without the long-term decline in mortality, the rate of natural increase—excess of birth rate over death rate—in the population of the United States would have been much smaller than actually experienced and its population growth not so great. Differentials in mortality trends according to age, sex, and color have an important role in the changing demographic structure of the country. Reductions in mortality and the accompanying improvements in longevity have raised appreciably the chances of survival from birth to the young adult ages, to midlife, and to the usual retirement ages. For example, according to the life table for all persons based upon mortality during 1900-02, the chances of surviving from birth to attain age 18 years were 78 per 100, compared with 97 per 100 on the basis of the life table for 1965. The corresponding chances of surviving to reach age 50 were 60 and 89 per 100, respectively; to reach age 65, the like figures were 40 and 71 per 100. These improved chances of survival have increased the numbers brought to the later ages of life, thereby enlarging the problems of the country relative to the social, economic, and medical care needs of the aged; the problems are being accentuated by the rise in the longevity of the aged. Although the chances of survival to the older ages are now greater, and the numbers of survivors have risen, their proportion in the total population depends also upon the course of the birth rate and of migration. Thus the fact that the proportion of total population at ages 65 and over rose from 4.1 in 1900 to 9.3 percent in 1965 cannot be ascribed to mortality reductions alone. These considerations and the unique problems of the aged are covered in Chapter 6.

Changes in the ratio of males to females in the population are influenced by sex differentials in mortality trends, by trends in immigration with its predominance of males, and by losses from war deaths. The net effect of the shifts in these influences over time has been to raise the sex ratio from 104.4 males per 100 females in 1900 to a high of 106.0 in 1910, after which it fell until the two were almost equal in number in 1940; by 1970, there were only 95 males per 100 females. Since the sex ratio at the younger ages is affected principally by the ratio at birth and by mortality differentials, at ages under 15 males outnumbered females in 1970, with a ratio of 104 to 100, but at ages 45-64 the ratio fell to 92 males to 100 females, and at ages 65 and over to 72.[12]

Although improved longevity has lengthened the period of married life, the greater gain for women than for men has added to the problems of widowhood by increasing both the chance that it will occur and the expected years spent in that state. For the average couple with a husband aged 30 and a wife aged 25, the joint expectation of life before the death of the first of the pair was 28.0 years according to life tables for 1900-02 and 37.0 years on the basis of those for 1959-61; this computation does not take divorce into account. Also, the expectation of life for women aged 25 increased from 40.1 years to 50.8 years over the same period. Accordingly, the expected years of widowhood rose from 12.1 years in 1900-02—40.1 minus 28.0—to 13.8 years in 1959-61—50.8 minus 37.0; this estimate includes the probability that the wife may die before the husband. On the basis of these life tables, the chance of widowhood rose from 60 to 70 in 100. Thus the likelihood of becoming a widow has increased, but the event itself has been postponed.[13,14]

The problems of orphanhood for both the individual and the community have been greatly reduced by lengthening the period of married life. It has been estimated that the number of orphaned children near the midcentury would have been doubled if mortality were then as it was at the start of the century.[13,14] The children spared parental loss have not only received the benefits of family life, but have also relieved the community of the burden of the many broken families that would have become indigent. Because of the slower gain in male longevity, among the children who have lost one or both parents the proportion without a father has increased.

Discussion

The course of the death rate in the United States has been generally downward since the beginning of the century. Declines have been registered for each age, sex, and color group, although to varying degrees. The rate of decline has considerably lessened in most recent years, and the trend has even been reversed for some age-sex-color groups. Data on longevity reflect these mortality changes.

It is no accident that reductions in mortality and improvement in longevity since the early years of the century have paralleled economic progress. Continuing development of agricultural and industrial efficiency creates wealth that may be turned to promote public and personal health and also release manpower needed for the tasks involved. It follows, from improvement in longevity, that the average years of working lifetime have increased, as have cumulative earnings during those years. At the same time, the family has benefited by a rise in the money value of the wage earner to his dependents, that is, the balance left from gross earnings after the needs of the breadwinner are provided.[15] Chapter 4 deals with the relation of illness and disability to income.

Advances in the medical and allied sciences have brought a stream of health goods and services of widening scope, improved quality, and enlarged quantity. Accompanying this flow is a steady improvement in the training of medical and allied personnel, not only during their formative years but also throughout their professional lifetimes. Less tangible as influences in the trend toward lower mortality are the benefits that accrue from the spread of medical care costs among the population. The growth of health insurance programs for the self-supporting and of welfare programs (including Medicare and Medicaid) for the fully and medically indigent has made it possible for many to seek medical care early and also has given them access to a better quality of care, although skyrocketing costs and unavailability of medical personnel and facilities in areas where they are desperately needed have lessened the potential impact of these programs. At the same time, as a result of medical advances made known by various mass media, the public has become more health conscious; self-appraisal of health status and attitudes toward health maintenance and the use of existing health services have been such as to favor mortality reductions. Less tangible still are the advantages to health that a higher standard of living may bring by way of improved body stamina.

Not of least influence, perhaps, are improvements that public health efforts have brought to bear. Development and application of vaccines, pasteurization of milk, chlorination and other protection of water supplies, improvement of waste disposal, protection against importation of nonendemic diseases, improvement of housing (including central heating), supervision, augmentation, and enrichment of food supplies, and more recently introduction of air conditioning have also played their parts.

Despite these advances in public health, which to a marked extent influenced the course of mortality early in the century, despite the development of sulfonamides and antibiotics during the thirties and forties, which greatly reduced mortality from infectious diseases not amenable to preventive measures, and despite other more recent dramatic medical and surgical procedures, it is somewhat paradoxical that the vast investments in insurance and medical care have not yielded commensurate improvement in mortality and longevity during the more recent years. Actual increases in age-specific rates among adults lend credence to the charge that there still are serious deficiencies in medical care delivery.

2 / MORTALITY IN THE UNITED STATES BY CAUSE

Mortimer Spiegelman
Carl L. Erhardt

In this chapter attention is given to only a few essential features in the trend of death rates by cause during this century, since such trends for specific conditions are discussed in various other volumes of this series. A ready picture is provided by the crude death rates in Table 2.1, which show data for selected causes for stated periods since 1900. Essentially the picture is one of rapid reduction in mortality from the infectious diseases, growing importance of the chronic diseases, a high death toll in recent decades from motor vehicle accidents, and a decrease in fatalities from other types of accidents.

Most significant in the general reduction in mortality during this century is the decline in the death rate for tuberculosis from a level of 184.8 per 100,000 in 1900-04 to only 4.1 in 1963-67. Over the same interval typhoid fever, diphtheria, and whooping cough have been virtually eliminated as causes of death, and measles has been brought almost to that point. The death rate for syphilis in 1963-67 was about one-tenth of that for 1940-44. For gastritis, duodenitis, enteritis, and colitis the death rate in 1963-67, at 4.1 per 100,000, had declined by 96 percent since the beginning of the century. At that time the level of the death rate for influenza and pneumonia was practically identical to that for tuberculosis. Although the improvement since then for tuberculosis has been much more spectacular, the rate for influenza and pneumonia in 1963-67 declined to less than one-fifth that of 1900-04.

A much different picture is presented by the chronic and degenerative diseases. The major cardiovascular-renal diseases, a broad category always outstanding among causes of death, recorded a rise from a death rate of 359.2 per 100,000 in 1900-04 to 518.2 in 1963-67. Over the same period the death rate from malignant neoplasms reached a level of 153.7 in 1963-67, more than two and one-quarter times the rate for 1900-04. The death rate for ulcer of the stomach and duodenum increased at almost the same pace, although its level is much lower. Cirrhosis of the liver recorded a

Table 2.1 Crude and age-adjusted death rates per 100,000 population for specified causes for total persons of all ages: United States death registration states, 1900-04 and 1920-24, and total country, 1940-44 and 1963-67

Cause of death	Crude death rate				Age-adjusted death rate*			
	1963-67	1940-44	1920-24	1900-04	1963-67	1940-44	1920-24	1900-04
All causes	945.2	1,062.0	1,198.0	1,622.3	743.1	1,017.1	1,327.8	1,698.1
Tuberculosis, all forms	4.1	43.4	97.1	184.8	3.6	43.0	102.4	188.5
Syphilis and sequelae	1.3	12.6	17.5	12.9	1.0	12.3	19.1	--
Typhoid fever	0.0	0.6	7.4	26.8	0.0	0.7	7.5	26.8
Diphtheria	0.0	1.0	13.8	32.8	0.0	0.9	13.2	27.3
Whooping cough	0.0	2.2	9.0	10.7	0.0	2.0	6.6	8.0
Measles	0.1	1.1	7.2	10.0	0.1	1.1	5.8	8.1
Malignant neoplasms	153.7	123.1	86.8	67.6	127.8	118.4	108.2	83.9
Diabetes mellitus	17.3	26.2	17.0	12.2	13.7	25.1	20.8	14.6
Cardiovascular-renal diseases	518.2	490.4	369.4	359.2	381.8	469.1	473.9	437.2
Diseases, cardiovascular system	512.7	418.3	288.0	275.0	377.2	399.9	370.0	335.5
Vascular lesions of c.n.s.	104.1	91.7	93.4	106.3	73.2	87.6	122.2	134.2
Diseases of heart	368.8	301.9	166.1	147.7	276.3	288.9	210.4	180.8
Chronic and unsp. nephritis	5.5	72.1	81.4	84.2	4.7	69.2	103.9	101.6
Influenza and pneumonia	32.3	63.7	141.0	184.4	23.7	60.3	147.3	190.9
Ulcer of stomach and duodenum	5.6	6.8	4.8	2.8	4.4	6.6	5.6	3.3
Gastritis, enteritis, etc.	4.1	9.8	43.2	115.6	3.2	8.9	34.0	91.6
Cirrhosis of liver	12.9	9.0	7.2	13.2	12.3	8.7	9.0	15.9
Congenital malformations	9.9	11.5	14.7	12.6	8.1	11.5	14.7	12.6
Motor vehicle accidents	25.4	22.7	12.8	--	26.6	22.6	13.3	--
All other accidents	30.4	50.3	57.9	79.1	26.8	49.0	61.9	83.1
Suicide	10.9	11.9	11.5	10.9	11.2	11.7	13.0	12.1
Homicide	5.7	5.7	7.8	1.2	6.4	5.7	7.9	1.2
Symptoms, senility, ill defined	12.3	22.7	29.9	94.3	10.1	22.7	29.9	94.3

Source: National Center for Health Statistics, Vital Statistics - Special Reports, vol. 43 (1956) and unpublished data; Vital Statistics of the United States, Vol. II, Part A, Table 6-4, 1963-1967 and Part B, Table 7-6, 1963 and Table 7-7, 1964-1967.

* Adjusted on the basis of the age distribution of the total population of the U.S. Census of April 1, 1940.

death rate of only 7.2 in 1920-24, but the rate rose to 12.9 by 1963-67.

The chronic diseases, in large measure affecting older persons in the population, have rates that are considerably influenced by the steady increase over the years in the proportion of aged. As will be discussed below, other population characteristics obviously have a bearing as well, but because of the marked influence of age Table 2.1 also presents age-adjusted rates. For the infectious diseases in general, it makes little difference whether crude or age-adjusted rates are considered. However, among the chronic diseases, the upward trend is not nearly so steep when age-adjusted rates are considered. For example, the crude rate for malignant neoplasms rose by 127 percent, whereas the age-adjusted rate shows an increment of only 52 percent. For vascular lesions of the central nervous system, an actual decline of 45 percent is seen for age-adjusted rates compared to very little change in the crude rates.

Problems of Interpretation

The interpretation of mortality trends for specific causes of death over long periods presents many difficulties. From the demographic viewpoint alone, the course of the crude death rate may be strongly influenced by the changing age, sex, and color composition of the population. For example, crude death rates for the chronic and degenerative diseases, as already seen, tend upward because of the rise in the proportion of aged persons in the population that has been experienced by the United States since 1900. The growth of the death registration states from a limited area in 1900 to the entire country in 1933 brought with it increased proportions of nonwhite population having a mortality above that of the white population. On the other hand, the slow but steady rise in the proportion of females in the population, with their lower mortality than that of males, tends to temper the course of the crude death rate. Obviously a better insight into the course of cause-specific mortality is obtained from age-adjusted death rates separately for whites and nonwhites of each sex. Other volumes of this series present such information.[1,2]

The comparability of death rates for specific causes over a long period may be markedly affected, moreover, by the decennial revisions of the International Classification of Diseases and by the form of the death certificate. Many considerations enter into these revisions of classification, with the result that the detailed disease entities included in a cause of death rubric may vary from one decade to another even though the title of the rubric may not be changed.[3] To enhance comparability, the National Center for Health Statistics has developed ratios on the basis of causes of death classified according to both the new and the previous revisions of the International Classification.[4] Such ratios, however, were not used to adjust the data in Table 2.1. Problems of comparability may also arise from changes in coding procedure in the vital statistics office as a result of rules introduced to amplify or modify the International Classification in current use. The quality of the result is also affected, of course, by the training received by the nosologists. Since the latter are necessarily guided by the information on the death certificate, any important change in its format may affect the interpretation of its content. Such was the case with the change from the Fifth to the Sixth Revision of the International List. This revision required a form of death certificate on which the physician was expected to enter the underlying cause as the final condition in a sequence of events leading to death. Previously in the United States, the nosologist selected the primary cause of death from among several conditions mentioned on the death certificate by referring to a "joint cause manual" wherein the precedence of one condition over another had been predetermined.

Particularly significant in the interpretation of mortality trends for specific causes of death are advances in medical science and practice. With new developments, there are changes in diagnostic concepts. New diagnostic tools aid in the more precise recognition of disease, and improvements in financing medical care have made its services accessible to larger proportions of the population, with benefit to the recognition of disease. Perhaps the best indicator of the total efforts to improve cause of death statistics is the course of the death rate for the residual category designated as "Symptoms, senility, and ill-defined conditions." This rate declined from 94.3 per 100,000 in 1900-04 to 12.3 in 1963-67. Whereas the category accounted for 5.8 percent of all deaths in the earlier period, that proportion was reduced to 1.3 percent in the latter period.

Rank of Causes of Death, 1967 and 1900

The trend data described previously gave some indication of the leading causes of death at the beginning of this century compared with those near the start of its last third. Notwithstanding the qualifications just cited regarding comparability of causes of death over the long period, the changes in rank from 1900 to 1967 shown in Table 2.2 are informative as a summary. In 1900, three infectious conditions—influenza and pneumonia, tuberculosis, and gastroenteritis—led the list of causes of death, accounting for 31.4 percent of all deaths. Following in order were three cardiovascular-renal conditions—diseases of the heart, cerebral hemorrhage, and chronic nephri-

Table 2.2   The ten leading causes of death: United States, 1967 and 1900

Rank	Cause of death	Rate per 100,000	Percent of all deaths
	1967		
	All causes	935.7	100.0
1	Diseases of heart	364.5	39.0
2	Malignant neoplasms	157.2	16.8
3	Cerebral hemorrhage[a]	102.2	10.9
4	Accidents, total	57.2	6.1
5	Influenza and pneumonia[b]	28.8	3.1
6	Certain diseases of early infancy[c]	24.4	2.6
7	General arteriosclerosis	19.0	2.0
8	Diabetes mellitus	17.7	1.9
9	Other diseases of circulatory system	15.1	1.6
10	Other bronchopulmonic diseases	14.8	1.6
	1900		
	All causes	1,719.1	100.0
1	Influenza and pneumonia[b]	202.2	11.8
2	Tuberculosis	194.4	11.3
3	Gastroenteritis	142.7	8.3
4	Diseases of heart	137.4	8.0
5	Cerebral hemorrhage[a]	106.9	6.2
6	Chronic nephritis	81.0	4.7
7	Accidents, total	72.3	4.2
8	Malignant neoplasms	64.0	3.7
9	Certain diseases of early infancy[c]	62.6	3.6
10	Diphtheria	40.3	2.3

Source: National Center for Health Statistics, Facts of Life and Death, Public Health Service Publication no. 600, Washington, 1970, Table 12.

[a]And other vascular lesions affecting central nervous system.
[b]Except pneumonia of newborn.
[c]Birth injuries, asphyxia, infections of newborn, ill-defined diseases, immaturity, etc.

tis—to which were ascribed only 18.9 percent of the total deaths. At that time the first ten causes included 64.1 percent of all deaths.

In marked contrast to 1900, the leading causes of death in 1967 were headed by three chronic conditions—diseases of the heart, malignant neoplasms, and cerebral hemorrhage—to which were attributed 66.7 percent of the deaths that year. Tuberculosis, gastroenteritis, and diphtheria disappeared from the list of the first ten causes of death; influenza and pneumonia was reduced from first rank in 1900 to fifth rank by 1967. Added to the list of the first ten causes in the later year were general arteriosclerosis, diabetes mellitus, a category called "other diseases of the circulatory system," and another category of "other bronchopulmonic diseases." With but minor exceptions among the last category, these conditions are chronic in nature. It is noteworthy that despite the decline in the death rate from accidents, they now represent the fourth leading cause of death. The first ten causes of death in 1967 accounted for 85.6 percent of all deaths.

Rank of Causes of Death by Color, Sex, and Age

Table 2.3, based on 1959-61 data, extends the ranking to the 15 causes of death for each color-sex category. In this way, it accounts for more than 90 percent of the white deaths and more than 85 percent of the nonwhite deaths. All but nonwhite females are alike with regard to the ranking of the first four causes of death; the exceptions for nonwhite females are not particularly marked. By extending the list, tuberculosis is brought back into the picture, ranking eighth for nonwhite males, fourteenth for nonwhite females, fifteenth for white males, and still lower for white females. Among white deaths, cirrhosis of the liver ranked tenth and eleventh for males and females respectively; for nonwhites, the respective ranks were fourteen and fifteen. Diabetes mellitus, which ranked seventh and eighth for nonwhite and white females respectively, was twelfth among white males and thirteenth for nonwhite males. Suicide is largely a problem of the white population, among whom it held eighth rank for males and thirteenth for females. On the other hand, the incidence of homicide among the nonwhite population is high; it ranked seventh for males and twelfth for females.

The variation in the five leading causes of death when age is taken into account, in addition to color and sex, is evident in Table 2.4. The numbers involved become too small for rankings of more than

Table 2.3 Rank of 15 leading causes of death and their death rates per 100,000 according to color and sex, all ages: United States, 1959-61

Cause of death	White Males Rank	White Males Rate	White Females Rank	White Females Rate	Nonwhite Males Rank	Nonwhite Males Rate	Nonwhite Females Rank	Nonwhite Females Rate
All causes		1,084.9		793.2		1,127.5		858.8
Diseases of heart (400-402, 410-443)	1	450.2	1	303.9	1	317.7	1	253.9
Malignant neoplasms (140-205)	2	165.9	2	139.7	2	134.5	3	108.9
Vascular lesions affecting c.n.s. (330-334)	3	102.1	3	110.0	3	115.5	2	120.9
Accidents (E800-E962)	4	69.7	4	31.1	4	92.5	6	37.4
Motor vehicle (E810-E835)		31.5		11.1		34.2		10.2
Other (E800-E802, E840-E962)		38.2		20.0		58.3		27.2
Certain diseases of early infancy[a] (760-776)	5	38.5	6	26.0	5	89.9	4	66.4
Influenza and pneumonia[b] (480-493)	6	34.7	5	26.0	6	63.8	5	43.6
General arteriosclerosis (450)	7	19.6	7	21.6	11	13.5	9	11.8
Suicide (E963, E970-E979)	8	17.5	13	5.2	--	--	--	--
Other bronchopulmonic diseases (525-527)	9	15.4	--	--	--	--	--	--
Cirrhosis of liver (581)	10	15.3	11	7.4	14	12.5	15	8.1
Other diseases of circulatory system (451-468)	11	13.8	10	8.2	15	11.6	13	9.3
Diabetes mellitus (260)	12	13.5	8	18.9	13	13.0	7	22.7
Ulcer of stomach and duodenum (540,541)	13	9.8	--	--	--	--	--	--
Congenital malformations (750-759)	14	9.0	9	10.8	9	15.4	8	12.1
Tuberculosis, all forms (001-019)	15	7.6	--	--	8	18.2	14	8.5
Other hypertensive disease (444-447)	--	--	12	6.3	12	13.5	10	11.7
Chronic and unspecified nephritis and other renal sclerosis (592-594)	--	--	14	5.2	10	13.8	11	11.6
Hernia and intestinal obstruction (560, 561, 570)	--	--	15	5.1	--	--	--	--
Homicide (E964, E980-E985)	--	--	--	--	7	34.3	12	9.4

[a]Birth injuries, asphyxia, infections of newborn, ill-defined diseases, immaturity, etc.
[b]Except of newborn.

Table 2.4 Rank of five leading causes of death and their death rates per 100,000 according to age, color, and sex: United States, 1959-61

Cause of death	Age	White				Nonwhite			
		Male		Female		Male		Female	
		Rank	Rate	Rank	Rate	Rank	Rate	Rank	Rate
All causes	1-4		101.6		83.7		197.8		167.4
Accidents		1	31.6	1	22.4	1	57.5	1	50.4
Motor vehicle			10.9		8.2		12.5		8.7
Other			20.7		14.2		45.0		41.7
Malignant neoplasms		2	12.4	4	10.1	5	7.3	4	6.6
Congenital malformations		3	11.9	2	12.1	3	14.5	3	14.0
Influenza and pneumonia		4	11.7	3	10.7	2	39.4	2	33.1
Gastritis, enteritis, colitis, etc.		5	2.9	5	2.3	4	8.8	5	5.9
All causes	5-14		52.9		34.3		73.5		51.6
Accidents		1	24.6	1	10.0	1	37.3	1	18.9
Motor vehicle			10.2		5.1		11.5		5.8
Other			14.4		4.9		25.8		13.1
Malignant neoplasms		2	8.4	2	6.3	2	5.0	2	4.8
Congenital malformations		3	3.9	3	3.4	4	3.8	4	3.2
Influenza and pneumonia		4	2.2	4	2.1	3	4.1	3	3.9
Diseases of heart		5	1.0	5	0.9	5	2.7	5	2.8
All causes	15-24		143.3		54.3		213.5		109.2
Accidents		1	92.4	1	19.3	1	95.8	1	19.9
Motor vehicle			62.8		15.2		49.2		11.8
Other			29.6		4.1		46.6		8.1
Malignant neoplasms		2	10.4	2	6.5	3	9.5	5	7.0
Suicide		3	8.2	5	2.3	5	6.5		...
Homicide		4	4.2		...	2	44.4	3	11.5
Diseases of heart		5	4.0	3	2.9	4	9.0	4	9.0
Congenital malformations			...	4	2.5		...		...
Complications of pregnancy, etc.			...		...		...	2	11.9

45–64

Cause								
Accidents	1	63.8	3	14.8	1	107.0	4	26.6
Motor vehicle		33.4		9.1		47.9		11.3
Other		30.4		5.7		59.1		15.2
Diseases of heart	2	63.5	2	18.6	2	99.7	1	72.6
Malignant neoplasms	3	32.8	1	43.7	4	43.7	2	62.9
Suicide	4	18.4	4	6.9	...	...	...	...
Homicide	...	...	...	...	3	77.4	5	20.6
Cirrhosis of liver	5	8.0	...	...	...	...	...	...
Vascular lesions affecting c.n.s.	...	...	5	6.9	5	29.4	3	33.8
All causes		1,467.9		722.8		2,153.6		1,627.5

65–74

Cause								
Diseases of heart	1	683.4	2	223.5	1	762.5	1	570.8
Malignant neoplasms	2	285.4	1	242.6	2	366.0	2	317.4
Vascular lesions affecting c.n.s.	3	82.5	3	63.5	3	254.0	3	266.5
Accidents	4	76.7	4	24.9	4	126.0	...	...
Motor vehicle		31.9		13.0		48.0		...
Other		44.9		11.9		78.1		...
Cirrhosis of liver	5	41.4	...	...	...	...	...	...
Diabetes mellitus	...	...	5	20.8	...	...	4	67.2
Influenza and pneumonia	...	...	...	...	5	82.8	5	42.2
All causes		4,764.7		2,755.4		5,537.2		3,907.1

75 and over

Cause								
Diseases of heart	1	2,265.7	1	1,220.1	1	2,195.5	1	1,620.9
Malignant neoplasms	2	886.5	2	563.9	2	920.8	3	540.9
Vascular lesions affecting c.n.s.	3	494.1	3	384.2	3	850.4	2	807.9
Influenza and pneumonia	4	123.0	5	59.5	4	219.8	5	115.8
Accidents	5	116.1	...	...	5	138.7	...	...
Motor vehicle		45.7		...		48.8		...
Other		70.4		...		89.9		...
Diabetes mellitus	...	...	4	104.0	...	...	4	140.9
All causes		11,896.6		9,687.4		9,510.3		7,817.9

Cause								
Diseases of heart	1	5,590.3	1	4,596.9	1	3,929.9	1	3,437.5
Vascular lesions affecting c.n.s.	2	1,886.7	2	1,861.3	2	1,609.7	2	1,624.0
Malignant neoplasms	3	1,477.1	3	996.3	3	1,135.8	3	692.0
General arteriosclerosis	4	511.5	4	489.2	5	368.3	4	330.4
Influenza and pneumonia	5	491.1	5	370.8	4	454.2	5	307.9

five. Data are not shown for the first year of life because the mortality picture changes rapidly during its course and the factors involved are considered in detail in Chapter 8 and elsewhere.[5] It is also of interest to compare these mortality findings with morbidity data in Chapter 4, particularly Table 4.5.

An outstanding feature of Table 2.4 is that accidents rank first as a cause of death for each age group under 25 years for both whites and nonwhites of each sex. Relative to other causes of death, accident fatalities were most prominent among white males at ages 15-24, where they accounted for almost two-thirds of all deaths. Among both white and nonwhite males accidents retained their first place among the causes of death at ages 25-44 years, fell to fourth place at ages 45-64, to fifth at ages 65-74, and were not among the first five at the higher ages. The role of motor vehicle accidents is especially noteworthy. If such accidents were considered a separate "cause" in ranking, they alone would constitute the leading cause of death for each sex-color group at ages 15-24, and the second leading cause for each group at ages 5-14 as well as among white males at ages 25-44. Except among nonwhite females aged 25-44, motor vehicle accidents by themselves would remain one of the five leading causes of death for every age-sex-color group below the age of 45. The same is usually true for accidents of other types.

Malignant neoplasms are prominent in the mortality picture at all stages of life. They rank first among the causes for white females at ages 25-44 and again at ages 45-64. At ages 1-4 they take second place among white males and assume this same rank within each color-sex category at ages 5-14. Beyond that age, they usually rank second or third.

From fifth in rank at ages 5-14, diseases of the heart rose, by ages 25-44, to first rank for nonwhite females and to second rank for the other color-sex categories. For the age groups at 45 and over, diseases of the heart uniformly led all other causes, except for white females at 45-64, among whom they were second to malignant neoplasms. Another cardiovascular condition—vascular lesions affecting the central nervous system—enters the leading causes of death at ages 25-44 excepting only white males. It reaches at least third rank for ages 45-64 and 65-74, and rises to second at ages 75 and over. In the oldest age group, another cardiovascular condition—general arteriosclerosis—assumes fourth place among the causes of death for three of the four color-sex categories; among nonwhite males it was preceded only by influenza and pneumonia, which combination was fifth in rank for the other color-sex groups. Diabetes mellitus entered the ranks of the first five causes of death among both white and nonwhite females at ages 45-64 and 65-74.

The category "influenza and pneumonia" was among the first five causes at ages 1-4 and 5-14 for each color-sex category and again at ages 65-74 and 75 and over. Congenital malformations occupied a similar position for the age groups under 15 years. Cirrhosis of the liver held fifth place among deaths of white males at ages 25-44 and 45-64.

Suicide and homicide assume an important role in the mortality of young adults, the former particularly among white males and the latter among nonwhite males. Homicide is second in rank, following accidents, as a cause of death for nonwhite males at ages 15-24; although it falls to third rank at ages 25-44 years, its death rate is appreciably higher. Among nonwhite females, this cause ranks third for the younger age group and fifth for the older group. Homicide occupies fourth place among the causes of death for white males at ages 15-24, with a rate only one-tenth that for nonwhite males. Suicide enters prominently in the mortality picture of both white males and females at ages 15-24 and 25-44 years; but among nonwhites only males at ages 15-24 show it as high as fifth in rank.

Mortality among males at the young adult ages in the United States is heavily weighted by violent death. Accidents, homicide, and suicide taken jointly account for almost three-fourths of the deaths of white males at ages 15-24 and for over two-thirds of nonwhite male deaths at these ages. The combined death rate, however, is appreciably greater for nonwhite males, namely 146.7 per 100,000 compared with 104.8 for white males.

Probability of Dying from Specified Causes

Another measure of mortality according to cause of death is provided by the probability of eventually dying from specific causes. This concept is based upon the assumption that the death rates and the life table for which the computation is made will continue into the future without change. Although this is a hypothetical picture, it is nevertheless an informative one. The results of a computation based upon data for 1959-61 are shown in Table 2.5.[6]

According to these results for 1959-61, about three-fifths of newly born babies will eventually die of a cardiovascular-renal condition. Most significant among these is arteriosclerotic heart disease, which

Table 2.5 Chances per 1,000 of eventually dying from specified causes, by color and sex, at birth and at age 40: United States, 1959-61

Cause of death	Birth				Age 40			
	White		Nonwhite		White		Nonwhite	
	Male	Female	Male	Female	Male	Female	Male	Female
Major cardiovascular-renal diseases	593.7	644.7	520.7	611.5	634.3	672.2	588.4	665.0
Vascular lesions affecting c.n.s.	106.8	158.9	126.1	175.5	114.4	165.7	143.7	191.6
Diseases of heart	438.1	423.7	337.2	370.8	468.3	442.2	381.8	404.4
Arteriosclerotic heart disease	351.6	297.1	202.2	195.9	376.8	311.0	230.9	216.0
General arteriosclerosis	23.0	36.7	18.9	25.0	24.9	38.5	22.0	27.8
Chronic and unspecified nephritis and other renal sclerosis	6.2	6.3	14.0	14.8	5.9	6.2	14.8	15.1
Malignant neoplasms	152.6	154.6	131.3	123.8	159.0	156.0	146.9	129.8
Digestive system	53.8	56.6	51.1	41.2	57.5	58.7	58.1	44.9
Respiratory system	35.1	7.1	27.2	5.6	37.4	7.3	30.9	6.0
Certain diseases of early infancy[a]	16.3	11.9	26.9	21.4	0.0	0.0	0.0	0.0
Influenza and pneumonia[b]	32.4	33.9	47.6	39.8	31.5	32.8	42.8	34.1
Tuberculosis	6.8	2.7	16.2	7.9	7.0	2.5	16.2	6.4
Diabetes mellitus	12.7	22.6	12.6	27.1	13.1	23.3	13.7	29.2
Cirrhosis of liver	12.8	7.0	10.3	7.0	13.2	6.9	9.8	5.8
Ulcer of stomach and duodenum	9.0	4.0	6.2	2.6	9.5	4.1	6.6	2.7
Congenital malformations	6.4	5.6	5.5	4.6	1.0	0.9	0.9	0.6
Motor vehicle accidents	23.7	9.2	25.0	7.5	12.0	5.8	14.0	4.4
Other accidents	30.5	24.9	40.2	23.4	22.3	23.2	26.2	18.2
Suicide	14.3	4.5	6.0	1.6	12.1	3.5	4.1	1.1
Homicide	2.7	1.1	25.2	6.7	1.4	0.6	11.5	2.7

Source: F. Bayo, "United States Life Tables by Causes of Death: 1959-61" Life Tables: 1959-61, vol. 1, no. 6, National Center for Health Statistics, Washington, May 1968.
aBirth injuries, asphyxia, infections of newborn, ill-defined diseases, immaturity, etc.
bExcept of newborn.

includes diseases of the coronary arteries. On the basis of these data, the chances per 1,000 for eventual death from arteriosclerotic heart disease are 351.6 for white males, 297.1 for white females, 202.2 for nonwhite males, and 195.9 for nonwhite females. The outlook at birth for eventual death from the malignant neoplasms is also high, averaging somewhat over 150 per 1,000 for white persons and in the neighborhood of 130 per 1,000 for nonwhites. In view of the association repeatedly reported between smoking and cancer of the lung, it is noteworthy that the chances of eventual death from cancer of the respiratory system are, for a newborn child, about 30 per 1,000 for males and 6 per 1,000 for females. The chances of an ultimate violent death for the newborn child are considerable, namely 96.4 per 1,000 for nonwhite males and 71.2 for white males; the chances for white and nonwhite females are about equal, somewhat under 40 per 1,000. Table 2.5 shows detail separately for motor vehicle accidents, all other accidents, suicide, and homicide. The chances of eventual death from specified causes after age 40 are set forth at the right of Table 2.5. For the most part these chances are higher than at birth for the chronic conditions, and lower for the acute conditions and the violent causes.

Gain in Longevity by Eliminating Specified Causes

The room for further improvement in longevity may be gauged by considering the increase in life expectancy that would result from the elimination of various causes of death. This concept also is hypo-thetical in nature, since it is based upon mortality data recorded for some period without considering the possibility of change. The results in Table 2.6 are derived from life tables and cause of death data for 1959-61. In the computation it is assumed that deaths from the cause in question are not present and that the lives so saved are subject to death from the remaining causes. It follows that the gains for specific causes are not additive.

For many causes of death, complete elimination would add only a fraction of a year to expectation of life at birth. For example, elimination of tuberculosis as a cause of death for white males would add only one-tenth of a year to their average length of life; for ulcer of the stomach and duodenum it is only 0.11 year and for diabetes mellitus, 0.15 year. Most significant for lengthening average lifetime span would be elimination of the cardiovascular-renal diseases, particularly arteriosclerotic heart disease, which would increase

Table 2.6 Increase in expectation of life in years resulting from elimination of specified causes of death by color and sex, at birth and at age 40: United States, 1959-61

Cause of death	Birth				Age 40			
	White		Nonwhite		White		Nonwhite	
	Male	Female	Male	Female	Male	Female	Male	Female
Major cardiovascular-renal diseases	10.85	10.47	10.44	12.53	11.33	10.74	11.30	13.08
Vascular lesions affecting c.n.s.	0.99	1.43	1.60	2.34	1.03	1.45	1.74	2.45
Diseases of heart	6.51	5.04	5.40	5.78	6.79	5.18	5.82	6.03
Arteriosclerotic heart disease	4.88	3.13	2.82	2.54	5.13	3.25	3.11	2.73
General arteriosclerosis	0.15	0.21	0.15	0.19	0.16	0.22	0.17	0.21
Chronic and unspecified nephritis and other renal sclerosis	0.09	0.08	0.20	0.22	0.07	0.07	0.18	0.19
Malignant neoplasms	2.12	2.43	1.98	2.18	2.00	2.24	2.05	2.08
Digestive system	0.63	0.68	0.70	0.59	0.65	0.69	0.76	0.62
Respiratory system	0.49	0.11	0.42	0.09	0.51	0.11	0.46	0.09
Certain diseases of early infancy[a]	1.12	0.90	1.70	1.45	0.00	0.00	0.00	0.00
Influenza and pneumonia[b]	0.46	0.42	1.05	0.90	0.28	0.25	0.51	0.38
Tuberculosis	0.10	0.05	0.29	0.19	0.09	0.04	0.24	0.11
Diabetes mellitus	0.15	0.27	0.18	0.42	0.14	0.26	0.18	0.42
Cirrhosis of liver	0.22	0.15	0.22	0.18	0.21	0.13	0.17	0.12
Ulcer of stomach and duodenum	0.11	0.05	0.10	0.04	0.11	0.05	0.09	0.04
Congenital malformations	0.37	0.36	0.30	0.27	0.02	0.02	0.02	0.01
Motor vehicle accidents	0.78	0.30	0.75	0.25	0.19	0.10	0.24	0.08
Other accidents	0.77	0.35	1.18	0.59	0.29	0.19	0.41	0.21
Suicide	0.31	0.12	0.15	0.05	0.20	0.07	0.07	0.02
Homicide	0.09	0.04	0.80	0.24	0.03	0.01	0.24	0.06

Source: F. Bayo, "United States Life Tables by Causes of Death: 1959-61" Life Tables: 1959-61, vol. 1, no. 6, National Center for Health Statistics, Washington, May 1968.
[a]Birth injuries, asphyxia, infections of newborn, ill-defined diseases, immaturity, etc.
[b]Except of newborn.

expectation of life at birth for white males by 4.88 years. The malignant neoplasms, accounting for a calculated gain of 2.12 years, and the category of "certain diseases of early infancy," with 1.12 years gained by their elimination, also offer considerable potential for improvement. For the other color-sex categories, gains of similar magnitude might be expected.

Cohort Mortality: Specified Causes

Because studies of mortality for specific causes of death over an extended period involve the problems of comparability cited previously, changes in generation experience are confined for present purposes to the period from 1950-54 to 1960-64.

Comparability ratios were used to adjust the recorded death rates for specific causes for 1950-54, which are based upon the Sixth Revision of the International List, to correspond to the Seventh Revision used for 1960-64. Otherwise the computation procedure followed that used for all causes in Chapter 1. The age-specific death rates in 1960-64 for the selected causes are shown in Table 2.7, and the ratio of these rates to those for persons ten years younger in 1950-54 appear in Table 2.8.[7] It must be kept in mind, in reviewing these data, that Table 2.8 demonstrates only what happened during a specific ten-year interval in the life of each generation. The figures are not intended to convey the relative risks at succeeding ages for any single cohort.

Whereas the death rates for tuberculosis in 1960-64 in Table 2.7 rose steadily with advance in age, a different picture is presented by the ratios of cohort mortality in Table 2.8. The latter indicate, for each age group and for each sex, a decrease in the death rate in proceeding from one age group to that succeeding, at least for the ten-year interval covered. For example, the ratio of the tuberculosis death rate for white males at ages 25-34 in 1960-64 to their rate at ages 15-24 in 1950-54 was 0.35. Although the ratios of generation death rates for both white males and white females from this cause showed a rise with advance in age for this ten-year period, they were consistently less than one.

The ratios of generation death rates for the major cardiovascular-renal diseases, and diseases of the heart in particular, are especially informative. For the latter, the ratios show that the current rate of increase for white males was most rapid in passing from the age group 25-34 years to ages 35-44, with a declining rate of increase

Table 2.7 Death rates for selected causes for white persons by age and sex: United States, 1960-64

Sex; cause of death	Death rate per 100,000 at ages —							
	15-24	25-34	35-44	45-54	55-64	65-74	75-84	85 and over
Male								
Tuberculosis	0.2	0.9	3.1	9.0	19.2	32.1	45.1	52.8
Major cardiovascular-renal	7.5	24.9	126.5	466.9	1,241.3	2,981.7	6,824.9	16,152.6
Vascular lesions of c.n.s.	1.6	3.8	11.1	39.3	133.8	478.8	1,491.1	3,756.3
Diseases of the heart	3.5	16.6	106.7	404.1	1,039.2	2,299.1	4,729.1	10,314.2
General arteriosclerosis	0.0	0.0	0.2	2.1	11.5	61.4	319.9	1,481.3
Chronic nephritis, etc.	1.8	2.9	3.8	6.5	11.3	22.0	54.1	139.4
Malignant neoplasms	10.2	18.3	47.1	164.2	453.2	914.5	1,400.0	1,862.0
Diabetes mellitus	0.6	2.8	5.0	10.7	30.3	75.5	144.9	194.2
Cirrhosis of the liver	0.2	2.5	13.6	37.2	51.7	58.2	45.2	37.5
Female								
Tuberculosis	0.2	0.8	2.0	3.1	3.6	6.7	13.9	21.9
Major cardiovascular-renal	6.0	14.8	44.6	148.5	492.5	1,678.2	5,319.9	15,376.8
Vascular lesions of c.n.s.	1.4	3.5	10.5	32.8	94.7	366.9	1,365.8	3,907.5
Diseases of the heart	2.5	7.6	27.7	102.6	364.5	1,197.5	3,488.1	9,513.9
General arteriosclerosis	0.0	0.0	0.1	0.9	5.9	41.9	271.3	1,470.5
Chronic nephritis, etc.	1.2	1.7	2.3	3.9	7.1	15.1	37.4	96.0
Malignant neoplasms	6.8	18.9	65.4	174.1	324.0	560.3	901.3	1,314.7
Diabetes mellitus	0.8	2.0	3.0	8.5	34.2	101.2	178.3	204.7
Cirrhosis of the liver	0.3	1.7	8.8	19.4	20.5	20.5	20.4	21.6

Table 2.8   Ratio of death rates from selected causes by sex for white persons at stated ages in 1960-64 to the rates at ages ten years younger in 1950-54[a]:   United States

Sex; cause of death	25-34	35-44	45-54	55-64	65-74	75-84	85 and over
Male							
All causes	1.03	1.83	2.49	2.28	2.14	2.11	2.14
Tuberculosis	0.35	0.43	0.54	0.58	0.62	0.64	0.68
Major cardiovascular-renal	2.08	4.09	3.41	2.49	2.27	2.24	2.25
Vascular lesions of c.n.s.	2.11	3.17	3.09	2.64	2.71	2.68	2.39
Diseases of the heart	2.41	5.03	3.58	2.49	2.15	2.07	2.14
General arteriosclerosis	-	b	b	b	4.87	3.93	3.49
Chronic nephritis, etc.	1.07	0.95	1.18	0.91	0.94	1.01	0.92
Malignant neoplasms	1.68	2.69	3.64	2.95	2.20	1.75	1.38
Diabetes mellitus	3.11	2.27	2.68	3.09	2.44	1.96	1.38
Cirrhosis of the liver	-	6.48	3.00	1.76	1.38	0.90	0.73
Female							
All causes	1.30	1.85	2.07	2.00	2.21	2.38	2.43
Tuberculosis	0.23	0.26	0.34	0.40	0.60	0.71	0.65
Major cardiovascular-renal	1.48	2.18	2.47	2.44	2.68	2.69	2.60
Vascular lesions of c.n.s.	2.33	3.18	2.73	1.82	2.53	2.88	2.64
Diseases of the heart	1.43	2.27	2.64	2.76	2.74	2.59	2.50
General arteriosclerosis	-	b	b	b	6.16	5.01	4.31
Chronic nephritis, etc.	0.89	0.96	0.87	0.76	0.81	0.84	0.82
Malignant neoplasms	2.55	3.19	2.40	1.77	1.59	1.51	1.31
Diabetes mellitus	1.67	1.58	3.15	3.14	2.03	1.46	1.07
Cirrhosis of the liver	-	4.63	2.52	1.49	1.22	0.98	0.76

[a]The recorded death rates for 1950-54, which were based upon the sixth revision of the International List, were adjusted to correspond to the seventh revision used for 1960-64 by means of comparability ratios.   See Vital Statistics - Special Reports, vol. 51, p. 245, March 1965.

[b]The death rates are too low for the ratio to be meaningful.

thereafter. However, for white females the rate of rise was relatively stable from entry into ages 45-54 and did not drop off substantially even at advanced ages. In the case of malignant neoplasms, the most rapid acceleration in death rates among white males occurred in passing from ages 35-44 to ages 45-54, but for white females it came ten years earlier.

Aside from the substantial jump at ages 25-34, when the rates were relatively low, death rates from diabetes mellitus for white males recorded their greatest rate of rise in midlife—in passing from ages 45-54 to ages 55-64. However, for white females this high rate of increase extended over the wider age range of 45-64 years in

1960-64. For cirrhosis of the liver, the rise in death rates decelerated rapidly with advance in age for both sexes.

Discussion

Since the turn of the century, mortality from infectious diseases has declined rapidly, while chronic diseases and motor vehicle accidents have assumed greater importance as causes of death. The changes in leading causes of death between 1900 and 1967 illustrate the point.

The significance of accidents is clear from their standing generally as the leading cause of death at each age under 25 years and for males to age 45. Malignant neoplasms are also of high rank at every age, but are consistently among the first three causes, regardless of color or sex, beginning at age 45. Suicide and homicide loom important among young adults, particularly males. Influenza and pneumonia appear among the five leading causes at each end of the age scale, while diseases of the heart assume prime importance after age 45.

Based on current mortality rates, the probability is highest that a newborn infant will eventually die of arteriosclerotic heart disease. The probability is greater than one-half that the infant will die of this condition, a malignant neoplasm, or an accident. The elimination of either of the first two could add materially to length of life, especially to expectation at age 40.

Viewing mortality as it affects a cohort provides a somewhat different picture than review of current age-specific mortality rates. Although the latter frequently indicate increasing mortality by age, cohort analysis suggests that, for some conditions, the risk declines as the cohort ages.

3 / INTERNATIONAL COMPARISONS OF MORTALITY AND LONGEVITY

Mortimer Spiegelman
Carl L. Erhardt

The United Nations has estimated that the total number of deaths in the world averaged 51 million annually during 1960-64, with a corresponding crude death rate of about 16 per 1,000 population.[1] These estimates are necessarily rough since the basic data—population and deaths—are not directly available for a large part of the world. In developing countries the rates must be estimated by sample surveys, other techniques, even conjecture. International comparisons must be viewed with caution, since the level of a crude death rate is affected by the age structure of the population to which it relates; a bias toward a low level occurs if a large proportion of a country's people is at the young ages where mortality typically is near its minimum. Comparisons of crude death rates are informative, nevertheless, because large differences are very likely indicative of wide divergences in health conditions.

A general view of mortality variations throughout the world, provided by Table 3.1, has several interesting features.[2] First, it shows a substantial and consistent variation in the levels of crude death rates among the regions of the world. The lowest rates were found in economically developed areas, which include Northern America, Australia and New Zealand in Oceania, most of Europe, the USSR, and Japan, with an average of about 9 per 1,000 population for 1960-68. The developing areas, on the other hand, had mortality rates about twice that level for the most part, as may be noted for much of Asia and Africa; for Latin America, the average was somewhat above that for the developed areas, but there was considerable variation for subareas. Second, all areas gave evidence of a mortality reduction from 1937 to 1955-59; this was rather substantial for the USSR and Japan, two economically developed countries, but the extent to which this decline may have resulted from a changed age composition was not measured. Third, the developing countries continued their move toward lower death rates from 1955-59 to 1960-66, but most of the developed countries did

Table 3.1   Estimated crude death rates for regions of the world, 1937, 1955-59, and 1960-68

Region	Crude death rates per 1,000 population		
	1960-68	1955-59	1937
World total	15	19	24-27
Northern America	9	9	11
Oceania	10	9	11
Australia and New Zealand	9	---	---
Melanesia	19	---	---
Polynesia and Micronesia	10	---	---
Europe (excluding USSR)	10	10	14
USSR	7	8	18
Latin America	11	19	20-25
Tropical South America	12	---	---
Middle America (Mainland)	11	---	---
Temperate South America	8	---	---
Caribbean	14	---	---
Asia (excluding USSR)	18	23	30-35
Japan	7	8	17
Africa	21	27	30-35
Western	26	---	---
Eastern	18	---	---
Northern	19	---	---
Middle	23	---	---
Southern	16	---	---

Sources: United Nations, Demographic Yearbook, 1968, New York, 1969, Table 1; Population Bulletin of the United Nations, no. 6, 1962, New York, 1963, p. 17.

not experience any improvement. This lack of improvement for the more recent period has already been noted for the United States in Chapter 1. Corresponding to these wide variations in crude death rates over time are the figures for expectation of life at birth. These range, according to data around 1960-65, from rough approximations of about 35 years for most of the new countries of Africa to levels of over 70 years for the Scandinavian countries and the Netherlands. The other economically developed countries generally show averages for expectation of life of more than 65 years for about the same period.[3]

Mortality in Developed Countries since 1920

As in the United States, for many countries of historically low mortality in Western Europe and for the major English-speaking countries elsewhere the downward trend of death rates came to a halt by about 1955. This may be noted in the crude death rates for quinquennial periods since 1920 in Table 3.2. Of the twenty countries listed, eight showed a record of continuing improvement into 1967. Three of them—France, Portugal, and Spain—started at a very high level in 1920-24. Four others—Canada, Australia, New Zealand, and Switzerland—may have benefited from a large recent influx of healthy migrants at the ages of low mortality.[4]

The tendency toward a halt in the decline of the crude rate in countries of traditionally low mortality apparently is not reflected in the downward trend of their infant mortality rates (Table 3.3). The latter are not strictly comparable because of differences among countries and changes over the years in their definitions of live births and infant deaths. For each period, however, with rare exception, the rates show an improvement over time.[5,6]

Specificity by Age and Sex

A better insight into the health standing of the United States relative to other economically developed countries, at least as indicated by mortality records, is provided by an examination of death rates specific for age and sex. Such a comparison is made in Table 3.4, which presents 1960 data for selected countries of low mortality.[7] To reduce the volume of detail, age-adjusted rates were computed by the direct method for four broad age groups and for all ages, using the total population of the United States in the 1950 census as the standard.

These mortality data generally show the most favorable situation for the Scandinavian countries and the Netherlands. For the 19 countries under review, the average of the adjusted rates for all ages was 10.3 per 1,000 for males and 7.0 for females. White males in the United States had a somewhat higher rate, 10.5 per 1,000, but white females had a considerably lower rate, 6.4 per 1,000. The 1960 averages according to age and sex for this group of countries are lower than those for 1950 for all but males at ages 65 and over.

The general decrease in mortality among these developed countries was accompanied by a lessening in their variation. The pertinent

Table 3.2 Average annual crude death rates per 1,000 for all causes: United States and selected countries of low mortality, 1920-1967

Country	1967	1960-64	1955-59	1950-54	1945-49	1935-39	1920-24
United States	9.4	9.5	9.4	9.5	10.0	11.0	12.0
Canada	7.4	7.7	8.1	8.7	9.4	9.9	11.9
England and Wales	11.3	11.8	11.6	11.6	11.5	12.0	12.3
Scotland	11.5	12.1	12.1	12.2	12.3	13.2	14.0
Australia	8.7	8.7	8.8	9.4	9.9	9.6	9.8
New Zealand	8.4	8.9	9.1	9.3	9.8	9.6	9.0
Union of So.Africa (white)	8.6[a]	8.9	8.6	8.6	8.9	9.8	10.1
Ireland	10.8	11.8	12.0	12.6	13.7	14.3	14.6
Netherlands	7.9	7.8	7.6	7.5	9.4	8.7	11.0
Belgium	12.1[a]	12.1	11.9	12.2	13.4	13.2	13.7
France	11.0	11.2	11.8	12.7	13.9	15.7	17.3
Switzerland	9.1	9.5	9.9	10.1	11.1	11.6	12.9
West Germany	11.2	11.1	11.0	10.7	11.3[b]	11.9[c]	13.9[c]
Denmark	10.3[a]	9.7	9.1	9.0	9.6	10.7	11.4[b]
Norway	9.6[a]	9.5	8.8	8.6	9.3	10.2	11.8
Sweden	10.1	10.0	9.6	9.7	10.4	11.7	12.4
Finland	9.4	9.2	9.1	9.7	11.8	13.3	15.6
Portugal	10.2	10.8	11.5	11.8	14.0	15.9	21.5
Italy	9.6[a]	9.8	9.6	9.9	11.2[b]	13.9	17.5[b]
Spain	8.7	8.8	9.4	10.2	12.0	17.9	21.0

Source: Demographic Yearbook, 1966, United Nations, New York, 1967, Table 17, and Demographic Yearbook, 1968, United Nations, New York, 1969, Table 18.

[a]1966.
[b]Four-year average.
[c]Germany before World War II.

Table 3.3 Deaths under one year of age per 1,000 live births: United States and selected countries of low mortality, 1920-1967

Country	1967	1960-64	1955-59	1950-54	1945-49	1935-39	1920-24
United States	22.4	25.3	26.4	28.1	33.3	53.2	76.7
Canada	22.0	26.6	30.5	37.0	46.6	68.5	93.9[a]
England and Wales	18.3	21.2	23.2	27.9	39.4	55.3	77.1
Scotland	21.0	25.7	28.7	34.6	50.5	75.5	92.0
Australia	18.3	19.7	21.4	23.8	28.0	39.1	61.0
New Zealand	18.0	20.9	23.8	26.6	30.7	42.7	---
Union of So.Africa (white)	23.2[b]	29.7	29.5	33.6	37.0	55.7	77.7
Ireland	24.4	28.4	34.6	42.1	61.5	69.6	71.5
Netherlands	13.4	16.5	19.3	24.7	40.4	37.4	74.4
Belgium	24.7[b]	27.8	35.4	46.3	71.2	83.4	108.2
France	20.7	25.5	33.9	46.2	72.0	71.1	97.1
Switzerland	17.5	20.5	23.9	29.5	37.9	45.3	70.3
West Germany	22.8	29.3	37.3	49.3	74.8[c]	66.3[d]	127.2[c,d]
Denmark	16.9[b]	20.2	23.7	28.5	41.2	64.2	82.4[c]
Norway	14.6[b]	17.5	20.2	24.2	32.6	40.4	53.3
Sweden	12.9	15.4	17.0	20.0	25.7	43.2	61.4
Finland	14.8	19.5	26.3	35.2	55.5	67.8	97.9
Portugal	59.2	77.4	87.7	91.8	111.2	139.4	152.8
Italy	34.7	40.4	48.7	61.0	79.4[c]	102.7	128.8[e]
Spain	33.2	42.2	51.6	62.5	80.5	124.5	---

Source: Demographic Yearbook, 1966, United Nations, New York, 1967, Table 14, and Demographic Yearbook, 1968, United Nations, New York, 1969, Table 17.
[a]One year only.
[b]1966.
[c]Four-year average.
[d]Germany before World War II.
[e]Three-year average.

standard deviations are shown at the bottom of Table 3.4. Although the mortality reductions from 1930 to 1960 have been substantial and their variation has been reduced, the ranking of these countries according to their mortality level has changed relatively little. For all ages combined, the coefficient of rank correlation between 1950 and 1960 was 0.92 for males and practically the same for females, while that between 1930 and 1950 was at a somewhat lower level (0.83 for each sex), as might be expected for the longer interval.

A noteworthy feature in the right-hand panel of Table 3.4 is the steady rise in the ratio of the average of male to female mortality from 1930 to 1960 for each broad age group. This rise indicates that the reduction in death rates during this period was generally more rapid for females than for males. For each of the three years of comparison, the advantage of females over males in mortality was relatively greatest at ages 45-64 in this group of countries, and least at ages 65 and over.

Table 3.4 Age-adjusted death rates[a] per 1,000 in broad age groups by sex: selected countries of low mortality, 1960

Country	Death rates per 1,000										Ratio of male to female death rates				
	Males					Females									
	All ages	Ages under 25	Ages 25-44	Ages 45-64	Ages 65 & over	All ages	Ages under 25	Ages 25-44	Ages 45-64	Ages 65 & over	All ages	Ages under 25	Ages 25-44	Ages 45-64	Ages 65 & over
U. S., white	10.5	2.3	2.4	15.0	70.9	6.4	1.5	1.3	7.3	48.4	1.6	1.5	1.8	2.1	1.5
England and Wales	10.5	2.0	1.7	13.4	78.6	6.6	1.4	1.2	7.0	51.9	1.6	1.4	1.4	1.9	1.5
Scotland	11.7	2.3	2.1	16.1	84.4	7.9	1.7	1.5	8.6	61.5	1.5	1.4	1.4	1.9	1.4
Australia[b]	10.6	2.1	2.2	13.5	77.7	6.7	1.5	1.4	7.3	51.3	1.6	1.3	1.6	1.8	1.5
New Zealand[c]	9.4	1.8	1.8	11.9	70.0	6.3	1.4	1.1	6.7	49.3	1.5	1.3	1.6	1.8	1.4
Canada	9.9	2.6	2.2	12.8	67.8	6.6	1.8	1.3	7.0	49.3	1.5	1.4	1.7	1.8	1.4
Union of South Africa[d]	12.3	3.2	3.5	16.8	80.2	7.8	2.2	1.8	9.2	55.1	1.6	1.5	1.9	1.8	1.5
Ireland	9.9	2.4	2.0	12.0	71.6	7.6	1.8	1.6	8.6	57.3	1.3	1.3	1.3	1.4	1.2
Netherlands	8.1	1.7	1.5	9.7	60.5	6.0	1.2	1.0	5.7	49.8	1.4	1.4	1.5	1.7	1.4
Belgium	11.2	2.7	2.2	14.4	79.9	7.3	1.9	1.3	7.1	57.7	1.5	1.4	1.7	2.0	1.5
France	10.6	2.4	2.5	14.0	73.5	6.4	1.7	1.3	6.7	47.9	1.7	1.4	1.8	2.1	1.5
Switzerland	9.7	2.3	2.0	11.4	72.0	6.7	1.4	1.1	6.5	54.6	1.4	1.6	1.8	1.8	1.3
Germany, Fed. Rep.	11.2	3.0	2.3	13.4	80.2	7.8	2.1	1.5	7.3	61.7	1.4	1.4	1.5	1.8	1.2
Denmark	8.6	1.9	1.6	10.1	65.3	6.7	1.3	1.3	6.8	54.5	1.3	1.5	1.8	1.8	1.2
Norway	8.0	1.9	1.8	9.2	59.0	5.8	1.2	0.9	5.2	48.3	1.4	1.6	2.0	1.5	1.2
Sweden	8.3	1.7	1.6	9.2	64.8	6.3	1.1	1.1	6.1	52.8	1.3	1.5	1.5	1.5	1.2
Finland	12.5	2.2	3.3	17.3	86.4	7.9	1.4	1.4	7.6	65.4	1.6	1.6	2.4	2.3	1.3
Portugal	12.8	6.5	3.0	13.1	79.9	9.5	5.5	1.8	7.0	64.5	1.3	1.2	1.7	1.9	1.2
Italy	10.5	3.5	2.1	12.3	72.6	7.5	2.8	1.4	6.7	55.8	1.4	1.3	1.5	1.8	1.3

Average – 1960	10.3	2.6	2.2	12.9	73.4	7.0	1.8	1.3	7.1	54.6	1.5	1.4	1.6	1.8	1.3
1950	11.1	3.8	2.8	13.6	73.2	8.5	3.0	2.1	8.7	59.6	1.3	1.3	1.3	1.6	1.2
About 1930	14.4	7.5	5.1	16.0	79.7	12.2	6.5	4.5	12.4	69.6	1.2	1.2	1.1	1.3	1.1
Stand. deviation 1960	1.4	1.0	0.5	2.3	7.5	0.9	1.0	0.2	0.9	5.4	0.12	0.11	0.27	0.21	0.12
1950	1.7	1.8	0.9	2.7	7.1	1.1	1.7	0.6	1.0	4.5	0.11	0.12	0.20	0.21	0.11
About 1930	2.4	2.5	1.5	3.1	8.7	1.7	2.5	1.0	1.7	5.7	0.07	0.06	0.14	0.19	0.08
Coefficient of variation – 1960	0.14	0.41	0.25	0.18	0.10	0.12	0.52	0.18	0.13	0.10	0.08	0.08	0.16	0.11	0.09
1950	0.15	0.48	0.31	0.20	0.10	0.13	0.58	0.28	0.11	0.08	0.08	0.09	0.15	0.13	0.09
About 1930	0.16	0.34	0.29	0.19	0.11	0.14	0.39	0.21	0.14	0.08	0.06	0.05	0.13	0.15	0.07
Coefficient of rank correlation[e] 1960 vs.1950	0.92	0.91	0.86	0.93	0.75	0.93	0.83	0.86	0.90	0.84					
1950 vs.1930	0.83	0.86	0.81	0.80	0.71	0.83	0.89	0.69	0.61	0.44					

[a] Adjusted on the basis of the age distribution of the total population of the U.S., Census of April 1, 1950.
[b] Excludes full-blooded aboriginals.
[c] Excludes Maoris.
[d] Europeans only.
[e] Spearman coefficient comparing ranks of countries.

Note: The statistical measures for 1950 and about 1930 were taken from M. Spiegelman, An International Comparison of Mortality Rates at the Older Ages, Proceedings of the World Population Conference, Rome, 1954, vol. 1, p. 289, United Nations Department of Economic and Social Affairs, New York (1955). Data for Spain were then omitted since a population base was not available for the computation of rates.

The general tendency among these countries was for the rate of mortality reduction to decline with advance in age; this was the pattern of change from 1930 to 1950 and again from 1950 to 1960, as is evident in Table 3.5. However, for 7 of these 19 countries, the age-adjusted rates for males at ages 65 and over were higher in 1960 than in 1950; for females, only Portugal showed such a change.

Rank of Death Rates for the United States

On the basis of adjusted death rates for all ages in 1960, shown in Table 3.4, among the 19 countries considered the United States white population ranked ninth for low mortality in the case of males and fifth for females. The relative position of white males in the United States in 1960 was about the same as in 1950, when they ranked eighth. However, for both of these years their standing was poorer than in 1930 when they ranked third. On the other hand, white females in the United States improved their relative position considerably: in 1960 they ranked fifth, rising from eleventh in rank in 1950, and ninth about 1930.

This ranking for all ages obscures a more interesting picture when detailed age groupings are examined, as is evident in Fig. 3.1. First, for each five-year age group under 70, white females in the United States had a better relative position than white males among the nations being compared in 1930, 1950, and again in 1960—the early childhood ages excepted for the last. Second, the general picture is one of steady regression in the relative position of the United States from the early ages up through midlife, with some improvement in the later years. The relatively poor position of the United States in 1960 at ages 15-24 for males may be attributed to a very high accident mortality. In large measure the favorable situation for the United States at the younger ages reflects its control over the infectious diseases, while the shift from that position in the later years emphasizes the growing importance to the country of the chronic degenerative conditions that take their greatest toll in late maturity, midlife, and old age.

A low mortality for a nation among its young persons does not necessarily mean that its population at the older ages will have the same advantage. The shift in rank among the countries under review is evident from the coefficient of rank correlation between the age-adjusted rates for ages under 25 and ages 65 and over. Whereas an unchanged array of ranks for the two age groups would yield a

Table 3.5 Ratio of death rates in 1960 to those in 1950 by age and sex: selected countries of low mortality

Country	Males					Females				
	All ages	Ages under 25	Ages 25-44	Ages 45-64	Ages 65 & over	All ages	Ages under 25	Ages 25-44	Ages 45-64	Ages 65 & over
United States, white	0.95	0.82	0.86	0.97	0.98	0.85	0.79	0.76	0.84	0.90
England and Wales	0.92	0.74	0.74	0.92	0.97	0.83	0.67	0.63	0.83	0.88
Scotland a	0.95	0.68	0.75	0.95	1.03	0.83	0.61	0.54	0.84	0.92
Australia a	0.95	0.78	0.92	0.94	0.98	0.86	0.79	0.78	0.84	0.90
New Zealand b	0.93	0.78	0.95	0.98	0.94	0.83	0.82	0.65	0.79	0.86
Canada	0.98	0.70	0.92	0.99	1.06	0.85	0.64	0.65	0.82	0.92
Union of South Africa c	1.04	0.91	1.06	1.01	1.09	0.91	0.85	0.78	0.93	0.94
Ireland	0.84	0.60	0.61	0.87	0.93	0.75	0.51	0.46	0.80	0.87
Netherlands	0.96	0.71	0.88	1.07	0.98	0.82	0.67	0.71	0.79	0.86
Belgium	0.93	0.60	0.71	0.96	1.04	0.82	0.58	0.59	0.78	0.94
France	0.88	0.59	0.76	0.94	0.95	0.78	0.53	0.61	0.79	0.88
Switzerland	0.89	0.70	0.80	0.86	0.96	0.82	0.61	0.61	0.76	0.90
Germany, Fed. Republic	0.99	0.64	0.79	1.06	1.11	0.86	0.58	0.71	0.85	0.96
Denmark	0.92	0.70	0.84	0.98	0.97	0.84	0.68	0.81	0.83	0.87
Norway	0.95	0.68	0.90	1.03	0.99	0.85	0.60	0.64	0.80	0.93
Sweden	0.92	0.77	0.84	0.92	0.96	0.83	0.73	0.69	0.78	0.87
Finland	0.89	0.54	0.73	0.89	0.99	0.83	0.47	0.56	0.82	0.95
Portugal	0.84	0.61	0.59	0.87	1.03	0.83	0.59	0.51	0.78	1.09
Italy	0.95	0.63	0.75	0.98	1.10	0.82	0.57	0.64	0.82	0.95
Average of ratios	0.93	0.69	0.81	0.96	1.00	0.83	0.65	0.65	0.82	0.92
Standard deviation	0.05	0.03	0.11	0.02	0.02	0.03	0.11	0.09	0.04	0.05
Coefficient of variation	0.05	0.04	0.14	0.02	0.02	0.04	0.16	0.14	0.05	0.06
Indices of Change: 1950 from about 1930 d										
Average of ratios	0.77	0.49	0.54	0.85	0.92	0.69	0.44	0.46	0.70	0.86
Standard deviation	0.07	0.09	0.08	0.09	0.08	0.06	0.08	0.08	0.07	0.08
Coefficient of variation	0.08	0.17	0.14	0.11	0.09	0.08	0.19	0.18	0.10	0.09

a Excludes full-blooded aboriginals.
b Excludes Maoris.
c Europeans only.
d Excludes Germany.

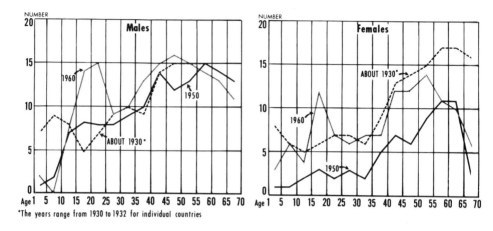

Figure 3.1 Number of Western European and English-speaking countries else-where (18 total) with age-specific death rates lower than those for white persons in the United States: 1960, 1950, and about 1930 (reproduced from *Proceedings of World Population Conference, 1965,* Vol. II, United Nations, New York, 1967, p. 375)

coefficient of óne, in this case the coefficient was 0.58 for males and 0.47 for females. An explanation for this shift is not apparent. However, it is worth considering the hypothesis that the country with the better control of its mortality in early life carries forward into the later years a large proportion of persons with physical impairments. The presence of relatively large contingents with higher mortality risk at the older ages in a country or community may tend to raise its total mortality at that stage of life above the mortality of other areas.[8]

Cohort Mortality

Thus far the comparison of mortality among nations has been concerned with the existing situation for specific years or periods. A further and perhaps more penetrating insight is obtained from study of the mortality experiences of generations of population as they age in the course of time.[9] For the present purpose, study is restricted to a comparison of the age- and sex-specific death rates for 1960 in the 19 economically developed countries under consideration with the record for the same cohorts when they were ten years younger in 1950. The data in Table 3.6 do not, therefore, reflect the experience of a single cohort over the age span given, but rather the experience

Table 3.6 Ratio of death rates by age and sex for white persons in 1960 to the rates at ages ten years younger in 1950: United States and 18 selected countries of low mortality

Age in 1960	Males					Females				
	United States ratio	Number of countries with lower ratios	Average of ratios			Number of countries with lower ratios	United States ratio	Average of ratios		
			All countries other than U.S.	Other English-speaking countries	Scand-inavian countries and the Netherlands			All countries other than U.S.	Other English-speaking countries	Scand-inavian countries and the Netherlands
15-19	1.86	18	1.19	1.33	1.15	18	1.00	0.68	0.75	0.66
20-24	2.43	16	1.98	2.29	1.88	16	1.50	1.16	1.25	1.17
25-29	1.15	10	1.14	1.09	1.21	15	1.17	0.90	0.91	1.16
30-34	1.00	13	0.94	0.99	0.99	17	1.25	0.87	0.92	1.05
35-39	1.47	16	1.18	1.43	1.17	16	1.50	1.08	1.20	1.30
40-44	2.10	18	1.60	1.86	1.68	17	1.85	1.31	1.49	1.47
45-49	2.45	18	1.98	2.27	2.07	17	1.95	1.56	1.69	1.72
50-54	2.51	13	2.33	2.59	2.46	14	1.93	1.78	1.88	1.88
55-59	2.31	7	2.37	2.53	2.56	13	1.89	1.82	1.83	1.88
60-64	2.27	5	2.41	2.47	2.64	9	2.06	2.03	2.07	2.08
65-69	2.15	4	2.39	2.36	2.66	3	2.13	2.26	2.22	2.38
70-74[a]	2.11	0	2.44	2.31	2.68	2	2.22	2.49	2.32	2.60
75-79[b]	2.15	1	2.49	2.37	2.73	2	2.43	2.62	2.46	2.76
80-84[c]	2.26	2	2.50	2.30	2.73	5	2.53	2.62	2.46	2.74

Source for basic data: United Nations, Demographic Yearbook, 1957, Table 11; World Health Organization, Annual Epidemiological Report, 1950 and 1960.

aUnion of South Africa (white) excluded at this and higher ages.
bPortugal and Italy excluded at this and higher ages.
cAustralia excluded.

over a ten-year period of a series of cohorts each of which attained a given age in 1960. Table 3.6 shows, for example, that the death rate for white males in the United States at ages 15-19 in 1960 was 1.86 times their death rate when they were 5-9 years old in 1950. Each of the other 18 countries had a lower ratio and their average was 1.19. The English-speaking countries other than the United States had an average ratio of 1.33, while the ratio for the Scandinavian countries and the Netherlands was only 1.15. In each instance, and for both sexes, these ratios of generation mortality reached a first peak at ages 20-24. As was seen in Chapter 1, the observation is not peculiar to this ten-year period, since several generations exhibit the same characteristic in their cohort mortality (Table 1.5 and Fig. 1.5).

At the higher ages the generation ratios of death rates for the United States during this ten-year interval continued to be above those for most countries up to age 55 in the case of males and to age 65 for females. In other words, to about these ages mortality of the generations in the United States was rising more rapidly, in proceeding up the age scale, than in most other economically developed countries. This feature conforms to the pattern described from cross-section mortality data in Fig. 3.1. Beyond these ages the ratios of mortality of these generations in the United States fell below the averages of those for the other countries. Among males, both the United States and the other English-speaking countries (as shown by their averages) had in common decreasing ratios among those who had passed age 54—a feature not shared by the Scandinavian countries or by the averages for all other countries.

Causes of Death in Developed Countries

In addition to limitations on interpretation of cause-of-death statistics within a country, as outlined in Chapter 2, international comparisons of the levels of death rates for specific causes present additional technical problems. There are differences to be considered not only in the vital statistics systems of the various countries, but also in the social and economic habits of their populations.[10,11]

Although death registration is virtually complete in the economically developed countries, there may be considerable variation in technique. Some may exclude from their count those infants who died within the first 24 hours or before their births were registered. At each step in the vital statistics system, procedures may differ not only among the various countries, but also from one time to another within a single country. What goes on the death certificate will be influenced by the health habits of the population, the stage of illness at which medical care is sought, the system of medical care and the training of its personnel, and even the legal structure. The picture of mortality by specific causes is also affected by the quality of the personnel responsible for classifying the information for statistical purposes and of those carrying out the tabulation procedures. Furthermore, at any one time the several countries may be using different versions of the International Classification of Diseases. Table 3.7 shows the revision of the ICD in use by each of the countries under consideration from 1950 through 1967, and Table 3.8 contains the code numbers used in these revisions for the several causes discussed subsequently.

The predominance of the chronic diseases in the current mortality picture in the economically developed countries is another source of difficulty in international comparisons. There may be differences of opinion among medical certifiers, both among countries and also within them, with regard to the train of morbid events culminating in death.

Table 3.7   International lists of causes of death used by selected countries of low mortality from 1950 to 1967

Country	5th Revision 1938	6th Revision 1948	7th Revision 1955
United States	-	1950-57	1958-67
England and Wales	-	1950-57	1958-67
Scotland	-	1950-57	1958-67
Australia	-	1950-57	1958-67
New Zealand	-	1950-57	1958-67
Canada	-	1950-57	1958-67
Union of South Africa (white)	-	1950-60	1961-67
Ireland	-	1950-58	1959-67
Netherlands	-	1950-57	1958-67
Belgium	1950-51	1952-60	1961-67
France	-	1950-57	1958-67
Switzerland	1950	1951-61	1962-67
West Germany	1950-51	1952-61	1962-67
Denmark	1950	1951-57	1958-67
Norway	1950	1951-61	1962-67
Sweden	1950	1951-57	1958-67
Finland	1950	1951-61	1962-67
Portugal	1950-51	1952-65	1966-67
Italy	1950	1951-61	1962-67
Spain	1950	1951-65	1966-67

Table 3.8   International codes used for causes of death

Cause of death	5th Revision	6th and 7th Revisions
Tuberculosis	A 6, 7	B 1, 2
Malignant neoplasms	A 15*	B 18
Diabetes	A 18**	B 20
Cardiovascular-renal diseases	A 22, 24, 25, 33*	B 22, 24 to 29, 38
Influenza and pneumonia	A 10, 27	B 30, 31
Cirrhosis of liver	--	B 37
Motor vehicle accidents	A 42	BE 47
All other accidents	A 43	BE 48
Suicide	A 40	BE 49

*Not strictly comparable with 6th and 7th Revisions.
**Not comparable with 6th and 7th Revisions.

Lastly, international comparability of death rates is problematical when crude death rates are used in place of age-adjusted rates. Table 3.9 indicates how the comparability of crude death rates for causes of death for a specified country may be affected, in the course of time, by the aging of its population, increased medical care, and improved certification of causes of death. It will be noted, for example, that in 1960 every country but New Zealand had a larger proportion of population at ages 65 and over and of deaths at ages 45 and over than in 1950. In Canada the proportion of the population in the oldest age group decreased slightly, but the percent of deaths at ages 45 and over nevertheless increased. Only two countries—Spain and Switzerland—had a larger number of persons per physician in 1960 than in 1950. Every country, except for the Union of South Africa, showed a smaller proportion of its deaths assigned to senility, ill-defined, and unknown causes in 1960 than in 1952. However, it is unlikely that an improved assignment of the extent indicated would have an appreciable effect upon the trends of the more specific causes among which they are distributed. These data also provide a clue to the possible variations in the quality of medical certification of causes of death among countries. Thus, in 1960 less than 2 percent of the total deaths were attributed to senility, ill-defined, and unknown causes in each English-speaking country—except the Union of South Africa and Ireland—and in Switzerland, Denmark, and Sweden. On the other hand, such deaths comprised more than 10 percent of the total in Belgium, France, Portugal, and Spain.

Table 3.9   Population at ages 65 and over, deaths at ages 45 and over, deaths due to senility, ill-defined, and unknown causes, and population per physician: selected countries of low mortality, about 1950 and about 1960

Country	Population at ages 65 and over, percent of total		Deaths at ages 45 and over, percent of total		Population per physician		Deaths due to senility, ill-defined, and unknown causes, percent of total	
	1950	1960	1950	1960	1950	1960	1952	1960
United States	8.1	9.3c	80.4	84.2c	790	780c	1.5	1.3
Canada	7.7	7.6c	74.8	80.5c	970	910	1.8	1.0
England and Wales	10.9	11.9c	87.8	91.7c	1,100b	960	1.6	1.4
Scotland	10.0	10.4c	84.3	90.1c	930d	760	3.1	1.2
Australia	8.1	8.5	82.7	85.2c	1,000d	860	2.1	1.0
New Zealand	9.4	8.7	84.6	84.5c	800	690c	1.0	0.8
Union of So.Africaa	6.4	6.6	72.9	78.0	2,100e	2,000	4.6	5.3
Ireland	10.7b	11.2c	80.5	88.9c	1,000b	950c	12.7	7.8
Netherlands	7.7	9.1c	81.5	88.1c	1,300	900	5.5	4.3
Belgium	11.1	12.0	83.5	90.2	1,000b	740c	15.3	11.9
France	11.8	12.1c	82.0	88.6c	1,100d	930	18.4	14.6
Switzerland	9.6	10.3c	84.1	88.2c	730b	750c	2.0	1.5
West Germany	9.3	10.6	80.0	87.5c	750d	690	9.4	6.7
Denmark	9.1	10.6	84.8	89.9	960	830g	2.1	1.5
Norway	9.6	10.9	84.4	89.6	950b	840	8.3	6.9
Sweden	10.2	11.9c	88.1	91.9	1,400	1,100	7.2	1.9
Finland	6.6	7.4	72.7	85.7c	2,000	1,600	6.8	2.3
Portugal	7.0	7.6	55.4	64.7c	1,500	1,200c	17.0	15.6
Italy	8.3b	9.2	72.1	82.8	820b	610	9.5	5.0
Spain	7.2	8.3	64.7	76.7c	990f	1,000c	13.3	12.7

Source: United Nations, Demographic Yearbook, annual volumes, and World Health Organization, World Health Statistics, annual (formerly Annual Epidemiological and Vital Statistics).

a White only.
b 1951.
c 1961.
d 1952.
e Total for Asiatic, white, and colored.
f 1953.
g 1959.

The many qualifications just cited bear upon the comparability of the levels of death rates among countries but fortunately do not wholly negate comparisons of their trends. For broad cause of death groupings, such as the cardiovascular-renal diseases and the neo-plasms, the nature of the qualifications for any one country is not likely to change substantially from one year to the next in most instances, nor is there apt to be a marked variation in the age and sex composition. The crude death rates for selected causes of death in the more economically developed countries of Western Europe, and in English-speaking countries elsewhere, are shown in Tables 3.10 to 3.14 for a succession of four-year periods from 1950 through 1965. It should be noted at this point that, for almost all years, the crude death rates are based upon estimates of population.

All Causes

The recent trend of mortality from all causes has already been considered. The interesting feature of Table 3.10, in connection with the halt in the decline in the death rate since about 1954 or 1955, is the change in signs from 1950 through 1965. Only two countries had a higher crude death rate in 1954-57 than in 1950-53. The number of such countries rose to seven in passing from 1954-57 to 1958-61. On the other hand, for all but three countries, the crude death rate for 1962-65 was higher than for 1958-61.

Cardiovascular-Renal Diseases

About one-half of the deaths from all causes were attributed to the cardiovascular-renal diseases in the English-speaking countries—the Union of South Africa excepted—the Scandinavian countries, and Finland. On the other hand, these diseases accounted for only about one-third of the total deaths in Belgium, France, Portugal, and Spain. It is significant that each of the latter had a relatively high proportion of its deaths classified among the ill-defined and un-known causes and senility; with a more adequate classification of causes of death many of these undoubtedly would be included among the cardiovascular-renal diseases, thereby reducing inter-national variability of rates in this category.

A record of continued rise in cardiovascular-renal mortality from one period to the next within the interval 1950 to 1965 was established by half of the countries considered here. Falling in this class is Scotland, but not England and Wales, where the rates were fairly stable. Only Canada and New Zealand were consistent in showing declines; it is noteworthy that these countries were the only ones to show decreases from 1950 to 1960 in the proportions of persons 65 or more years old in their populations. For the other countries it is difficult to discern any definite trend in mortality from cardiovascular diseases. The crude death rates for these condi-tions for the United States were practically stationary from one

Table 3.10   Crude death rates from all causes and the cardiovascular-renal diseases: selected countries of low mortality, 1950 to 1965

Country	Average annual death rate per 100,000				Percent change			
	1962 -65	1958 -61	1954 -57	1950 -53	1958-61 to 1962-65	1954-57 to 1958-61	1950-53 to 1954-57	1950-53 to 1962-65
All causes								
United States	947	941	936	962	+0.6	+0.5	-2.7	-1.6
Canada	767	788	820	884	-2.7	-3.9	-7.2	-13.2
England and Wales	1173	1169	1154	1172	+0.3	+1.3	-1.5	+0.1
Scotland	1214	1209	1197	1216	+0.4	+1.0	-1.6	-0.2
Australia	880	861	899	945	+2.2	-4.2	-4.9	-6.9
New Zealand	881	894	910	924	-1.5	-1.8	-1.5	-4.7
Union of So. Africa[a]	880[b]	874	852	857	+0.7	+2.6	-0.6	+2.7
Ireland	1171	1198	1207	1267	-2.3	-0.7	-4.7	-7.6
Netherlands	790	756	758	751	+4.5	-0.3	+0.9	+5.2
Belgium	1217	1181	1209	1221	+3.0	-2.3	-1.0	-0.3
France	1119	1113	1212	1227	+0.5	-8.2	-5.1	-8.8
Switzerland	952	951	1008	1017	+0.1	-5.7	-0.9	-6.4
West Germany	1121	1100	1101	1068	+1.9	-0.1	+3.1	+5.0
Denmark	988	935	899	902	+5.7	+4.0	-0.3	+9.5
Norway	962	905	862	863	+6.3	+5.0	-0.1	+11.5
Sweden	1008	973	964	979	+3.6	+0.9	-1.5	+3.0
Finland	942	892	920	988	+5.6	-3.0	-6.9	-4.7
Portugal	1066	1058	1145	1186	+0.8	-7.6	-3.5	-10.1
Italy	994	945	971	1003	+5.2	-2.7	-3.2	-0.9
Spain	884[c]	863	949	1037	+2.4	-9.1	-8.5	-14.8
Cardiovascular-renal diseases								
United States	488	488	483	488	0	+1.0	-1.0	0
Canada	367	377	384	403	-2.7	-1.8	-4.7	-8.9
England and Wales	566	571	568	560	-0.9	+0.5	+1.4	+1.1
Scotland	624	623	616	597	+0.2	+1.1	+3.2	+4.5
Australia	459	439	451	465	+4.6	-2.7	-3.0	-1.3
New Zealand	428	429	437	468	-0.2	-1.8	-6.6	-8.5
Union of So. Africa[a]	351[b]	339	330	320	+3.5	+2.7	+3.1	+9.7
Ireland	567	571	550	505	-0.7	+3.8	+8.9	-0.7
Netherlands	339	315	311	280	+7.6	+1.3	+11.1	+21.1
Belgium	403	345	357	465	+16.8	-3.4	-23.2	-13.3
France	361	359	380	384	+0.6	-5.5	-1.0	-6.0
Switzerland	413	416	439	437	-0.7	-5.2	+0.5	-5.5
West Germany	431	407	403	364	+5.9	+1.0	+10.7	+18.4
Denmark	454	423	406	389	+7.3	+4.2	+4.4	+16.7
Norway	465	421	374	331	+10.5	+12.6	+13.0	+40.5
Sweden	472	473	461	443	-0.2	+2.6	+4.1	+6.5
Finland	476	419	402	384	+13.6	+4.2	+4.7	+24.0
Portugal	332	307	316	299	+8.1	-2.8	+5.7	+11.0
Italy	434	396	394	364	+9.6	+0.5	+8.2	+19.2
Spain	282[c]	261	276	303	+8.0	-5.4	-8.9	-6.9

[a] White only.
[b] 1962 only.
[c] Average for 1962-63.

period to the next. This picture changes when the death rates for each year from 1950 through 1965 are age adjusted; both white and nonwhite females then show considerable improvement during the interval, but the rates for males were relatively stable from 1959.[12,13]

Malignant Neoplasms

As a cause of death, the malignant neoplasms rank second to the cardiovascular-renal diseases in importance in the countries under review. In only two countries of those in Table 3.11, the Netherlands and Denmark, does this category account for more than 20 percent of the deaths, and then only by a small margin. And in only two countries, Portugal and Spain, were these deaths fewer than 15 percent of the total. Each of these latter countries still has a relatively high death rate from the infectious diseases and also a large proportion of its deaths resulting from senility, ill-defined, and unknown causes, situations which would depress the relative importance of the malignant neoplasms.

Except for New Zealand and Switzerland, each country listed had a higher crude death rate for malignant neoplasms during 1962-65 than for 1950-53; for most, the interim rise was continuous. On the whole, the rise was more rapid in the earlier years of the period from 1950 to 1965 than in its later years. Although the aging of population undoubtedly has contributed to these rising rates, improved diagnosis also has had a role. Such data as are available indicate that most countries of the West have experienced a sharp rise in death rates from cancer of the respiratory system.[14,15] On the other hand, the death rate from cancer of the female genital organs appears to be stationary in some countries and declining in others. A reduction is also evident for cancer of the digestive system, but this may reflect more accurate determination and certification of the primary site of the malignancy.[16,17]

Diabetes Mellitus

At ages 65 and over, when diabetes mellitus takes its greatest death toll, it ranked among the first ten causes of death in 1963 for each country listed in Table 3.11, except the Union of South Africa and Spain for which ranked data are not available.[18] With the exception of New Zealand, the average annual crude death rate for 1962-65 was

Table 3.11 Crude death rates from malignant neoplasms and diabetes mellitus: selected countries of low mortality, 1950 to 1965

Country	Average annual death rate per 100,000				Percent change			
	1962 -65	1958 -61	1954 -57	1950 -53	1958-61 to 1962-65	1954-57 to 1958-61	1950-53 to 1954-57	1950-53 to 1962-65
Malignant neoplasms								
United States	152	148	147	142	+2.7	+0.7	+3.5	+7.0
Canada	133	129	129	128	+3.1	0	+0.8	+3.9
England and Wales	220	215	207	197	+2.3	+3.9	+5.1	+11.7
Scotland	225	213	207	195	+5.6	+2.9	+6.2	+15.4
Australia	134	130	130	128	+3.1	0	+1.6	+4.7
New Zealand	145	143	146	149	+1.4	-2.1	-2.0	-2.7
Union of So. Africa[a]	135[b]	137	132	123	-1.5	+3.8	+7.3	+9.8
Ireland	174	167	161	148	+4.2	+3.7	+8.8	+17.6
Netherlands	179	166	157	150	+7.8	+5.7	+4.7	+19.3
Belgium	234	220	208	159	+6.4	+5.8	+30.8	+47.2
France	203	195	185	176	+4.1	+5.4	+5.1	+15.3
Switzerland	186	191	190	187	-2.6	+0.5	+1.6	-0.5
West Germany	219	205	195	179	+6.8	+5.1	+8.9	+22.3
Denmark	221	209	194	174	+5.7	+7.7	+11.5	+27.0
Norway	169	163	160	156	+3.7	+1.9	+2.6	+8.3
Sweden	190	181	165	155	+5.0	+9.7	+6.5	+22.6
Finland	156	153	148	143	+2.0	+3.4	+3.5	+9.1
Portugal	107	93	82	65	+15.1	+13.4	+26.2	+64.6
Italy	159	146	131	115	+8.9	+11.5	+13.9	+38.3
Spain	126[c]	112	99	81	+12.5	+13.1	+22.2	+55.6
Diabetes mellitus								
United States	17.0	16.3	15.7	16.4[d]	+4.3	+3.8	-4.3	+3.7
Canada	12.4	11.5	11.0	10.9	+7.8	+4.5	+0.9	+13.8
England and Wales	8.4	7.6	7.1	7.4	+10.5	+7.0	-4.1	+13.5
Scotland	10.2	10.8	9.2	9.0	-5.6	+17.4	+2.2	+13.3
Australia	12.8	11.6	12.3	12.6	+10.3	-5.7	-2.4	+1.6
New Zealand	11.3	11.8	10.8	12.2	-4.2	+9.3	-11.5	-7.4
Union of So. Africa[a]	9.8[b]	10.0	9.0	8.5	-2.0	+11.1	+5.9	+15.3
Ireland	8.8	8.2	7.1	6.9	+7.3	+15.5	+2.9	+27.5
Netherlands	14.8	14.7	12.8	11.3	+0.1	+14.8	+13.3	+31.0
Belgium	26.0	23.7	24.0	18.6	+9.7	-1.3	+29.0	+39.8
France	15.6	12.1	12.0	11.2	+28.9	+0.8	+7.1	+39.3
Switzerland	18.8	13.9	13.5	14.4	+35.3	+3.0	-6.3	+30.6
West Germany	15.3	12.9	11.3	11.1	+18.6	+14.2	+1.8	+37.8
Denmark	7.2[e]	7.3	6.3	5.2	-8.9	+15.9	+21.2	+38.5
Norway	8.5	7.9	6.8	6.6	+7.6	+16.2	+3.0	+28.8
Sweden	15.7	12.9	10.4	11.5	+21.7	+24.0	-9.6	+36.5
Finland	11.0	9.9	6.5	6.1	+11.1	+52.3	+6.6	+80.3
Portugal	8.4	6.7	6.3	5.2	+25.4	+6.3	+21.2	+61.5
Italy	17.0	12.5	11.5	9.8	+36.0	+8.7	+17.3	+73.5
Spain	10.7[c]	8.4	7.5	6.3	+27.4	+12.0	+19.0	+69.8

[a] White only.
[b] 1962 only.
[c] Average for 1962-63.
[d] Average for 1952-53.
[e] Average for 1962-64.

greater than that for 1950-53. However, only half of these countries recorded a continued rise from one time interval to the next. Although diabetes mellitus ranks high among the causes of death, mortality data are hardly indicative of its importance as a morbid condition, since many with the disease have their deaths attributed to its complications, chiefly those of the circulatory system.

Tuberculosis

Without exception, the death rate for tuberculosis for each country listed in Table 3.12 recorded a reduction from one time interval to the next during 1950 to 1965, even though the 1950 rate was already markedly lower than in earlier years in many countries. For 11 countries the death rate in 1962-65 was about one-fourth or less than that in 1950-53, and for most of the others the later rate was only about one-third of the earlier level. Within the period from 1950 to 1965 the rate of reduction was relatively greatest in its early years, from 1950-53 to 1954-57, for each country but New Zealand. Notwithstanding these reductions, tuberculosis still ranks among the first ten causes in Belgium, Finland, France, West Germany, Ireland, Italy, and Portugal; the ranking for Spain is not known.[19]

Influenza and Pneumonia

Influenza and pneumonia, as a class, ranked either fourth or fifth among the causes of death in the countries in Table 3.12 during 1962-64, except for Scotland where it ranked sixth; its position is not known for the Union of South Africa and Spain. The pattern of trend of death rates from this class during 1950 to 1965 was mixed for the countries under review; there was, however, an outbreak of influenza in western Europe in 1951 and a more general epidemic in 1957. It is interesting to note, nevertheless, that a rather consistent downward trend in death rates was recorded for the block of countries consisting of the Netherlands, Belgium, West Germany, France, Switzerland, and Italy. Falling in this category also are Finland, Canada, and Australia. Only New Zealand and Sweden showed a pattern of consistent rise. A feature of importance regarding outbreaks of influenza is the elevation they may produce in the death rates from some other causes, particularly the cardio-vascular-renal diseases. This would be a consequence of the adverse effect of such outbreaks upon persons weakened by these diseases.[20]

Table 3.12   Crude death rates from tuberculosis and influenza and pneumonia:
.   selected countries of low mortality, 1950 to 1965

Country	Average annual death rate per 100,000				Percent change			
	1962 -65	1958 -61	1954 -57	1950 -53	1958-61 to 1962-65	1954-57 to 1958-61	1950-53 to 1954-57	1950-53 to 1962-65
Tuberculosis								
United States	4.6	6.2	8.9	17.7	-25.8	-30.3	-49.7	-74.0
Canada	3.8	5.1	8.6	20.2	-25.5	-40.7	-57.4	-81.2
England and Wales	5.7	8.3	13.8	28.0	-31.3	-39.9	-50.7	-79.6
Scotland	8.0	10.9	17.7	38.4	-26.6	-38.4	-53.9	-79.2
Australia	3.7	5.0	7.9	16.2	-26.0	-36.7	-51.2	-77.2
New Zealand	4.0	6.3	11.6	17.7	-36.5	-45.7	-34.5	-77.4
Union of So. Africa[a]	6.0[b]	7.2	8.3	17.1	-16.7	-13.3	-51.5	-64.9
Ireland	14.0	17.5	28.2	61.8	-20.0	-37.9	-54.4	-77.3
Netherlands	2.1	3.4	6.1	14.2	-38.2	-44.3	-57.0	-85.2
Belgium	12.3	16.9	23.8	34.2	-27.2	-29.0	-30.4	-64.0
France	16.9	22.5	30.1	49.6	-24.9	-25.2	-39.3	-65.9
Switzerland	9.6	13.7	20.2	30.0	-29.9	-32.2	-32.7	-68.0
West Germany	13.2	16.0	20.0	31.6	-17.5	-20.0	-36.7	-58.2
Denmark	2.9	4.2	5.9	11.7	-31.0	-28.8	-49.6	-75.2
Norway	4.6	6.5	11.8	22.3	-29.2	-44.9	-47.1	-79.4
Sweden	5.3	7.5	10.5	19.1	-29.3	-28.6	-45.0	-72.3
Finland	16.1	27.6	39.7	69.9	-41.7	-30.5	-43.2	-77.0
Portugal	33.6	47.2	61.6	108.2	-28.8	-23.4	-43.1	-68.9
Italy	14.2	17.9	22.2	34.1	-20.7	-19.4	-34.9	-58.4
Spain	22.6[c]	25.9	34.7	73.8	-12.7	-25.4	-53.0	-69.4
Influenza and pneumonia								
United States	33.2	32.8	29.2	31.3	+1.2	+12.3	-6.7	+6.1
Canada	31.0	34.6	36.8	42.2	-10.4	-6.0	-12.8	-26.5
England and Wales	72.0	67.1	55.2	61.1	+7.3	+21.6	-9.7	+17.8
Scotland	46.4	49.9	43.0	48.3	-7.0	+16.0	-11.0	-3.9
Australia	31.6	32.8	34.9	36.3	-3.7	-6.0	-3.9	-12.9
New Zealand	51.6	44.3	37.4	26.0	+16.5	+18.4	+43.8	+98.5
Union of So. Africa[a]	58.5[b]	56.0	53.0	57.3	+4.5	+5.7	-7.5	+2.1
Ireland	54.8	59.2	50.3	67.3	-7.4	+17.7	-25.3	-18.6
Netherlands	19.0	26.3	28.2	35.8	-27.8	-6.7	-21.2	-46.9
Belgium	32.1	35.7	37.4	50.8	-10.1	-4.5	-26.4	-36.8
France	41.6	46.9	61.7	82.0	-11.3	-24.0	-24.8	-49.3
Switzerland	31.8	33.1	41.0	41.5	-3.9	-19.3	-1.2	-23.4
West Germany	37.0	44.8	49.9	60.7	-17.4	-10.2	-17.8	-39.0
Denmark	29.1	29.6	24.9	42.4	-1.7	+18.9	-41.3	-31.4
Norway	55.8	50.7	45.6	51.9	+10.1	+11.2	-12.1	+7.5
Sweden	49.4	47.9	47.2	40.9	+3.1	+1.5	+15.4	+20.8
Finland	33.0	37.7	52.3	56.8	-12.5	-27.9	-7.9	-41.9
Portugal	94.8	85.8	87.3	83.6	+10.5	-1.7	+4.4	+13.4
Italy	44.6	47.5	57.9	71.9	-6.1	-18.0	-19.5	-38.0
Spain	59.4[c]	56.1	71.5	91.4	+5.9	-21.5	-21.8	-35.0

[a]White only.
[b]1962 only.
[c]Average for 1962-63.

Cirrhosis of the Liver

Except for New Zealand and the Union of South Africa, the death rates from cirrhosis of the liver for the countries listed in Table 3.13 were higher in 1962-65 than in 1950-53. The importance of this disease is made evident by the rank it holds at ages 45-64, where it rated among the first ten causes for one or more years during 1962-64 for practically all the countries in Table 3.13; the exceptions are England and Wales, Ireland, and Finland, with no ranked data available for the Union of South Africa and Spain. The condition held fourth rank in France, higher than for any other country, a situation that may be associated with the high per capita consumption of alcohol in that country. Actually, recorded deaths are hardly indicative of the health problem occasioned by cirrhosis of the liver, since the quality of its certification is uncertain and the condition may be regarded as contributory to another cause where others are cited on the death certificate.[21,22]

Suicide

The problem of suicide becomes particularly important rather early in life among the countries of the Western world.[23] At ages 15-44, it ranked either third or fourth among the causes of death for most countries listed in Table 3.13 during 1962-64; it ranked fifth in the United States, sixth in Portugal and Italy, and tenth (in 1963) in Ireland.

The suicide rate during 1962-65 was over 15 per 100,000 in the block of countries comprising France, Switzerland, West Germany, and Denmark; also at that high level were Sweden, Finland, and the Union of South Africa. On the other hand, rates of less than 8 per 100,000 were reported by Canada, Ireland, the Netherlands, Norway, Italy, and Spain. Among the English-speaking countries, only the United States and Canada showed relatively little variation in their suicide rate during 1950 to 1965. The trend was markedly upward in Scotland, Australia, and the Union of South Africa, while England and Wales showed a moderate rise. On the other hand, New Zealand was favored by a downward trend. Other countries in Table 3.13 showing a decrease in suicide rates from 1950 to 1965 include Switzerland and Denmark—at relatively higher rates overall—and Ireland, Portugal, Italy, and Spain—which have low rates overall. A detailed analysis, including the findings of Dürkheim, appears in another volume of this series.[23]

Table 3.13 Crude death rates from cirrhosis of the liver and suicide: selected countries of low mortality, 1950 to 1965

Country	Average annual death rate per 100,000				Percent change			
	1962 -65	1958 -61	1954 -57	1950 -53	1958-61 to 1962-65	1954-57 to 1958-61	1950-53 to 1954-57	1950-53 to 1962-65
Cirrhosis of the liver								
United States	12.1	11.1	10.6	9.9	+9.0	+4.7	+7.1	+22.2
Canada	6.1	5.9	5.2	4.6	+3.4	+13.5	+13.0	+32.6
England and Wales	2.8	2.8	2.6	2.5	0	+7.7	+4.0	+12.0
Scotland	4.7	4.3	3.9	3.2	+9.3	+10.3	+21.9	+46.9
Australia	4.9	4.8	4.7	4.7	+2.1	+2.1	0	+4.3
New Zealand	2.7	2.3	3.1	3.0	+17.4	-25.8	+3.3	-10.0
Union of So. Africa[a]	6.0[b]	6.1	6.0	7.5	-1.6	+1.7	-20.0	-20.0
Ireland	2.8	2.2	2.1	2.0	+27.3	+4.8	+5.0	+40.0
Netherlands	3.6	3.8	3.4	2.9	-5.3	+11.8	+17.2	+24.1
Belgium	10.1	9.1	8.2	6.0[c]	+11.0	+11.0	+36.7	+68.3
France	32.5	28.0	30.4	21.7	+16.1	-7.9	+40.1	+49.8
Switzerland	14.8	12.4	13.4	11.6	+19.4	-7.5	+15.5	+27.6
West Germany	20.4	17.3	13.2	8.7	+17.9	+31.1	+51.7	+134.5
Denmark	7.7	8.1	7.0	5.3	-4.9	+15.7	+32.1	+45.3
Norway	3.9	3.9	3.6	2.9	0	+8.3	+24.1	+34.5
Sweden	5.9	5.3	4.8	3.4	+11.3	+10.4	+41.2	+73.5
Finland	3.5	3.4	3.3	2.3	+2.9	+3.0	+43.5	+52.2
Portugal	26.7	20.5	23.7	18.7[c]	+30.2	-13.5	+26.7	+42.8
Italy	17.8	16.7	14.6	12.7	+6.6	+14.4	+15.0	+40.2
Spain	17.1[c]	14.8	13.6	10.4	+15.5	+8.8	+30.8	+64.4
Suicide								
United States	11.0	10.6	10.0	10.5	+3.8	+6.0	-4.8	+4.8
Canada	7.9	7.5	7.3	7.4	+5.3	+2.7	-1.4	+6.8
England and Wales	11.7	11.4	11.6	10.3	+2.6	-1.7	+12.6	+13.6
Scotland	8.5	8.2	7.4	5.4	+3.7	+10.8	+37.0	+57.4
Australia	14.7	11.5	11.0	10.1	+27.8	+4.5	+8.9	+45.5
New Zealand	8.8	9.1	9.1	9.8	-3.3	0	-7.1	-10.2
Union of So. Africa[a]	16.9[b]	14.1	11.4	10.2	+19.9	+23.7	+11.8	+65.7
Ireland	2.0	2.9	2.4	2.4	-31.0	+20.8	0	-16.7
Netherlands	6.6	6.8	6.2	6.1	-2.9	+9.7	+1.6	+8.2
Belgium	14.2	14.3	14.2	13.3	-0.7	+0.7	+6.8	+6.8
France	15.1	16.3	16.5	15.3	-7.4	-1.2	+7.8	-1.3
Switzerland	17.5	19.4	21.7	22.0	-9.8	-10.6	-1.4	-20.5
West Germany	18.8	18.8	18.9	18.4	0	-0.5	+2.7	+2.2
Denmark	19.6	19.9	22.8	23.5	-1.5	-12.7	-3.0	-16.6
Norway	7.7	7.0	7.4	7.1	+10.0	-5.4	+4.2	+8.5
Sweden	18.9	17.4	18.7	16.6	+8.6	-7.0	+12.7	+13.9
Finland	20.2	20.6	20.8	16.6	-1.9	-1.0	+25.3	+21.7
Portugal	9.2	8.8	9.1[d]	10.0[e]	+4.5	-3.3	-9.0	-8.0
Italy	5.4	6.2	6.6	6.6	-12.9	-6.1	0	-18.2
Spain	4.9[f]	5.2	5.5	5.9	-5.8	-5.5	-6.8	-17.0

[a]White only.
[b]1962 only.
[c]Average for 1952-1953.
[d]Average for 1955-57.
[e]Average for 1950-51.
[f]Average for 1962-63.

Motor Vehicle Accidents

With few exceptions, which include the United States, the countries in Table 3.14 present a record of continual rise in the incidence
of motor vehicle fatalities from 1950 to 1965. Whereas the death
rate from this cause for the United States was higher than for any
other country in 1950-53, by 1962-65 there were many approaching
or above its level, a reflection of the more widespread use of the
automobile during the prosperous postwar period. Not only has the
number of drivers been increasing, but their proportion in the total
population has risen as well. Moreover, with the large number of
young people reaching driving age because of the "baby boom"
beginning in the forties and with the cultural emphasis on having a
car, the proportion of young drivers has been increasing, at least in
the United States. These factors contribute to the rise in motor
vehicle mortality, although driver attitudes, road conditions, enforce-
ment of driving regulations, and alcoholism also play substantial
roles. These factors, as well as the influence of the number of motor
vehicles and vehicle-miles traveled in the several countries, are
discussed in the volume of this series dealing more thoroughly with
the subject.[24]

All Other Accidents

Accidents of all forms, including motor vehicle mishaps, take a
high death toll in the economically developed areas of the world.
During one or more years from 1962 to 1964, they ranked first
among the causes of death at ages 1-44 years in practically all
countries listed in Table 3.14. At ages 45-64 they were generally
fourth in rank, and at ages 65 and over they were usually fifth among
the causes of death. Accidents not involving motor vehicles include
industrial and home mishaps. The trend of death rates from these
other forms of accidents was, for the most part, downward during
1950 to 1965. In view of the contrary trends for these two classes of
accidental death, it is evident that injuries other than those sustained
by motor vehicles are playing a diminishing role in the total accident
mortality picture.[24]

Discussion

In the developed countries, including the United States, since
about 1850, mortality and longevity naturally have run essentially

Table 3.14   Crude death rates from motor vehicle accidents and all other accidents: selected countries of low mortality, 1950 to 1965

Country	Average annual death rate per 100,000				Percent change			
	1962 -65	1958 -61	1954 -57	1950 -53	1958-61 to 1962-65	1954-57 to 1958-61	1950-53 to 1954-57	1950-53 to 1962-65
Motor vehicle accidents								
United States	23.8	21.1	23.0	23.9	+12.8	-8.3	-3.8	-0.4
Canada	24.5	20.9	20.7	19.3	+17.2	+1.0	+7.3	+26.9
England and Wales	14.5	13.6	10.9	9.8	+6.6	+24.8	+11.2	+48.0
Scotland	14.5	12.6	10.9	9.8	+15.1	+15.6	+11.2	+48.0
Australia	25.9	24.4	23.6	23.3	+6.1	+3.4	+1.3	+11.2
New Zealand	17.9	16.3	16.2	13.6	+9.8	+0.6	+19.1	+31.6
Union of So. Africa[a]	25.5[b]	27.7	20.4	17.7	-7.9	+35.8	+15.3	+44.1
Ireland	10.2	9.0	7.5	5.8	+13.3	+20.0	+29.3	+75.9
Netherlands	18.4	15.5	13.8	9.4	+18.7	+12.3	+46.8	+95.7
Belgium	20.9	17.5	12.5	11.5[c]	+19.4	+40.0	+8.7	+81.7
France	22.8	18.7	18.6	9.7	+21.9	+0.5	+91.8	+135.1
Switzerland	22.6	21.9	19.1	14.8	+3.2	+14.7	+29.1	+52.7
West Germany	26.3	24.4	23.0	15.5	+7.8	+6.1	+48.4	+69.7
Denmark	19.5	17.0	14.8	9.9	+14.7	+14.9	+49.5	+97.0
Norway	11.1	8.9	7.5	5.0	+24.7	+18.7	+50.0	+122.0
Sweden	17.0	14.3	13.0	10.5	+18.9	+10.0	+23.8	+61.9
Finland	21.0	15.3	11.0	8.3[d]	+37.3	+39.1	+32.5	+153.0
Portugal	12.3	9.3	6.9[e]	9.1[f]	+32.3	+34.8	-63.9	-35.6
Italy	21.8	17.6	16.1	10.3	+23.9	+9.3	+56.3	+111.7
Spain	9.1[g]	7.4	5.3	2.9	+23.0	+39.6	+82.8	+213.8
All other accidents								
United States	30.2	30.6	33.4	37.4	-1.3	-8.4	-10.7	-19.3
Canada	30.4	32.4	36.2	38.3	-6.2	-10.5	-5.5	-20.6
England and Wales	24.7	24.7	24.9	23.3	0	-0.8	+6.9	+6.0
Scotland	34.2	34.0	34.7	35.1	+0.6	-2.0	-1.1	-2.6
Australia	26.4	27.6	31.6	33.2	-4.3	-12.7	-4.8	-20.5
New Zealand	29.6	30.2	32.2	29.0	-2.0	-6.2	+11.0	+2.1
Union of so. Africa[a]	34.2[b]	30.1	29.4	30.5	+13.6	+2.4	-3.6	+12.1
Ireland	24.5	22.2	23.6	22.5	+10.4	-5.9	+4.9	+8.9
Netherlands	23.5	21.1	21.2	25.1	+11.4	-0.5	-15.5	-6.4
Belgium	35.1	36.0	40.2	29.9[d]	-2.5	-10.4	+34.4	+17.4
France	44.6	41.5	42.7	47.5	+7.5	-2.8	-10.1	-6.1
Switzerland	39.1	38.1	37.6	40.7	+2.6	+1.3	-7.6	-3.9
West Germany	32.7	31.7	34.2	33.7	+3.2	-7.3	+1.5	-3.0
Denmark	30.8	28.3	29.3	31.8	+8.8	-3.4	-7.9	-3.1
Norway	37.8	37.2	38.3	38.6	+1.6	-2.9	-0.8	-2.1
Sweden	27.6	28.5	26.8	28.1	-3.2	+6.3	-4.6	-1.8
Finland	35.2	36.2	38.9	47.1[c]	-2.8	-6.9	-17.4	-25.3
Portugal	29.6	28.1	32.3[e]	---	+5.3	-13.0	---	---
Italy	24.3	23.2	21.3	22.1	+4.7	+8.9	-3.6	+10.0
Spain	24.0[g]	21.7	22.5	24.3	+10.6	-3.6	-7.4	-1.2

[a]White only.
[b]1962 only.
[c]Average for 1951-53.
[d]Average for 1952-53.
[e]Average for 1955-57.
[f]1952 only.
[g]Average for 1962-63.

reciprocal courses. The most rapid improvements in both occurred during the first half of this century. Basically, the record of improvement in these countries is the product of gradually evolving scientific, social, and economic factors.[25,26] Although it is a record that the advanced countries can hardly expect to repeat, the possibility of its achievement is present for the developing nations. For many of these countries, mortality and longevity around 1960-65 is at the same level as the major English-speaking and Scandinavian countries at the beginning of the century or earlier. However, for many of the developing countries the influences that have produced mortality reductions and longevity improvements lie outside their traditional social and economic structures. Changes in these structures may have to be fostered to ensure the permanence of the health gains produced with assistance from other countries.

For specific causes of death the position of the United States has retrogressed over the past 30 years, especially at ages 15-24 for males, a factor to which high motor vehicle fatalities contribute markedly. At younger ages, the United States is more favorably situated, but at the middle ages it again shows a relative disadvantage Most countries show long-term increases in mortality from cardiovascular diseases, malignant neoplasms (but not of all sites), diabetes mellitus, and cirrhosis of the liver. For tuberculosis the trend is generally downward and for influenza and pneumonia the picture is mixed.

Suicide is an important cause of death during early adult years. A few countries appear to have experienced a rise in suicide rates, but most have remained stable or declined somewhat. The record of many countries appears to be approaching the relatively high rate of the United States for motor vehicle accidents, while the trend for other accidents has been generally downward.

4 / MORBIDITY IN THE UNITED STATES

Philip Cole

Through the first third of the present century a population's mortality rate was accepted as a measure of its ill-health. Although this was appropriate then, since most serious illnesses resulted from fatal diseases of relatively short duration, mortality data alone do not provide a complete picture of disease. They do not, for example, reflect the ill-health resulting from many significant nonfatal conditions such as arthritis, mental illness, and impairment of limbs and sensory organs. Nor do they reflect fully a population's experience even with some fatal diseases of long average duration, such as the more indolent malignancies. Now, with increasing numbers of older persons in our population and the decrease in acute disease mortality, the limitations of mortality data are such that they must be supplemented with other measures of health.

The problems associated with efforts to gain a more inclusive picture of illness are apparent. Unlike death, the onset of illness usually is not obvious; also, while cause of death usually is ascertainable, the specific nature of illness often is not. A particular insufficiency is that whereas deaths must be reported to a central agency, most illnesses need not. Efforts to overcome these problems have included both ongoing and ad hoc morbidity studies. A review of the development of morbidity measurements is presented in MacMahon and Pugh's *Epidemiology: Principles and Methods.*[1] This chapter is concerned only with the more general aspects of morbidity in the United States. Many of the data presented are derived from reports of the National Center for Health Statistics and are subject to their limitations.[2, 3, 4] It is emphasized that these data refer to the civilian noninstitutional population only. Geographic variations are discussed in Chapter 5.

Problems in Definition

"Morbidity" as a general term is applied to measures of both incidence and prevalence of disease. A major difficulty is encountered in attempting to define morbidity precisely, however, because the range of illness is so great. One extreme of this range is represented by clearly recognizable conditions that limit activity or lead to death. The other extreme is nebulous and is represented only by vague symptoms. Some persons may disregard such symptoms and not consider themselves ill; others, similarly or even less affected, may for a variety of motives exaggerate symptoms.[5] Nonetheless, some operable definition of morbidity, however arbitrary, must be adopted before any attempt at measurement can be made.

The National Health Interview Survey (NHIS), a continuous weekly series of interviews with members of households representative of the United States, has used the following concept:

Morbidity is basically a departure from a state of physical or mental well-being, resulting from disease or injury, of which the individual affected is aware. Awareness connotes a degree of measurable impact on the individual or his family in terms of the restrictions and disabilities caused by the morbidity. Morbidity includes not only active or progressive disease but also impairments, that is, chronic or permanent defects that are static in nature, resulting from disease, injury, or congenital malformations.[6]

There are major difficulties in trying to measure morbidity with the above as the underlying concept. For example, morbid conditions are not necessarily permanent, or of constant severity. During remission, some conditions may not be regarded as illness by the person affected and therefore are not reported to the interviewer unless probing questions are asked. Even the most probing interviews, however, yield an underestimate of morbidity, since examination often reveals conditions of which the individual is unaware. Although the NHIS definition would exclude these discovered conditions, there are several arguments in favor of including them: the conditions do exist after all; and whether the affected person is aware of it or not, there may be an associated disability.

Difficulties in defining and assessing morbidity notwithstanding, the division of morbid conditions into chronic and acute categories has been especially useful. The value of this distinction derives from focusing attention on measures of prevalence with respect to chronic conditions, and measures of incidence with respect to acute conditions. Checklists of conditions and impairments were prepared especially for use in the health interviews. As employed in the Health Interview Survey,

A condition is considered to be chronic if (1) it is described by the respondent in terms of one of the chronic diseases on the "Check List of Chronic Conditions" or in terms of one of the types of impairments on the "Check List of

Impairments" . . . or (2) the condition is described by the respondent as having been first noticed more than 3 months before the week of the interview.

On the other hand, "An acute condition is defined as a condition which has lasted less than 3 months and which has involved either medical attention or restricted activity." Obstetric deliveries and diseases associated with pregnancy are included with the acute conditions.[6]

Important in assessing the impact of both chronic and acute conditions is the concept of disability. This has been defined in many different ways. In 1966, for a national study of disability in the noninstitutionalized civilian adult population, the Social Security Administration defined disability "as a limitation in the kind or amount of work (or housework) resulting from a chronic health condition or impairment lasting 3 or more months."[7] Although the definition was commensurate with the objectives of that particular study, the criteria of work limitation and extended duration to define disability are more specific and restrictive than those used by the National Health Interview Survey. Categories of disability used in the NHIS include and specify work-loss days, restricted-activity days, and bed-disability days as well as major activity limitation. The relatively unrestricted definition of the NHIS is, "Disability is a general term used to describe any temporary or long-term reduction of a person's activity as a result of illness or injury."[6]

Deficiencies of Data

No concept or definition of morbidity is completely satisfactory and it is necessary therefore to have some appreciation of the limitations of morbidity data. These deficiencies vary with the uses the data are to serve, the severity of the illnesses studied, the ease and precision of diagnosis, and the efforts made to collect data systematically.

The use to which the data are put determines the type and quality of data required. Morbidity data are usually gathered for etiologic research, surveillance for alterations in disease frequency, and administrative decision-making with respect to needs, costs, and quality of health care.

For etiologic investigations, incidence data are almost always required. Prevalence data are less acceptable for this purpose, since prevalence necessarily reflects those factors related to duration of illness and survival as well as to onset of illness. An etiologic study usually will require incidence data that are, furthermore, nearly complete for a designated period and a designated population. Finally, in such studies it is usually important to assess the amount of unavailable or missing information and the extent to which the data are unrepresentative.

Information collected for surveillance usually will relate also to incidence, especially for acute conditions. For chronic conditions, prevalence data are generally acceptable. More important than the type of data or its completeness, for purposes of surveillance, is the emphasis that must be placed on comparability and uniformity of ascertainment.

For administrative purposes, both prevalence and incidence data may be useful, although only crude estimates of needs result unless severity of impairment and average duration of illness can be estimated.

In general, the data from the National Center for Health Statistics are ascertained with a high degree of uniformity and completeness and thus are well suited for surveillance. When supplemented with information from ad hoc studies, the data probably also serve the needs of planners very well.

Acute Conditions

Variation by Age and Sex

The incidence rates of many acute conditions vary considerably from year to year because short-term epidemics are common. To provide a representative picture, therefore, Table 4.1 shows the average annual experience during the four years ending June 1968.

As age increases, the incidence rates of acute conditions decrease for both sexes and for all conditions. The phenomenon is very striking for some conditions, such as upper respiratory, and much less so for others, such as injuries. It is also of interest that the incidence rates for males and females are similar in the youngest age groups, but above age 16 rates are higher for women. The excess for women aged 17-44 persists even when the residual category of "other acute" conditions—which includes deliveries and diseases associated with pregnancy—is subtracted from the total. The higher incidence rates of acute diseases among women, like their higher prevalence rates of chronic conditions, are in contrast with their lower mortality from the same conditions.

Table 4.1 Average annual incidence of acute conditions and associated disability reported in interviews per 100 persons by age and sex according to specified condition groups: United States, June 1965 - June 1968 (civilian noninstitutional population)

Condition group	Male					Female				
	All ages	Under 6	6-16	17-44	45 & over	All ages	Under 6	6-16	17-44	45 & over
	Annual incidence per 100 persons									
All acute	194	359	244	158	118	208	341	244	204	136
Infective and parasitic	24	60	39	14	7	25	54	39	20	10
Respiratory	107	208	132	84	69	119	208	146	110	76
Upper respiratory	68	153	85	48	40	75	156	97	62	45
Influenza	35	43	43	32	26	39	42	46	44	27
Other	4	12	4	3	3	4	11	3	4	3
Digestive system	9	15	10	8	8	10	13	11	11	8
Injuries	34	39	40	38	21	23	29	23	22	21
Other acute	19	38	23	14	14	31	37	25	41	21
	Days of restricted activity per 100 persons per year									
All acute	722	970	814	597	682	851	910	802	827	892
Infective and parasitic	96	224	169	47	37	102	192	179	70	53
Respiratory	331	558	389	226	306	384	542	417	320	377
Upper respiratory	171	367	226	104	117	195	353	244	146	159
Influenza	125	128	140	101	140	154	134	151	146	175
Other	35	63	22	21	49	34	56	21	28	44
Digestive system	34	37	26	26	49	41	30	25	47	51
Injuries	189	53	162	251	198	153	54	98	139	245
Other	72	97	70	48	91	171	91	84	252	166
	Days of bed disability per 100 persons per year									
All acute	296	413	349	245	259	377	392	393	381	353
Infective and parasitic	47	93	83	28	17	52	84	91	40	27
Respiratory	160	245	201	122	132	189	229	232	165	171
Upper respiratory	71	134	103	53	39	82	122	120	65	60
Influenza	69	67	86	59	68	87	70	100	84	87
Other	19	44	11	10	25	20	36	12	15	24
Digestive system	17	17	14	13	24	19	9	12	23	24
Injuries	46	17	30	66	49	44	21	26	41	70
Other	27	40	21	16	38	72	49	33	112	62

Source: National Center for Health Statistics, Series 10, Tables 5, 6, and 7 of nos. 26, 38, 44, and 54, Washington, December 1965 to June 1969.

Note: Incidence excludes conditions involving neither restricted activity nor medical attention.

Disability

Several concepts are used by the Health Interview Survey to estimate disability among persons with acute conditions. A day of "restricted activity" is one in which a person substantially reduces the amount of normal activity for that day because of a specific illness or injury. In addition to work, usual activity applies to school attendance or to any other activity usual for that day, such as recreation on a holiday. Further, any day in which more than half the daylight hours are spent in bed because of a specific illness or injury is considered a "bed-disability" day as well as a restricted-activity day. Finally, an "activity-restricting condition" is one that had caused at least one day of restricted activity during the two calendar weeks before the interview week.[6]

For the specified acute conditions, the pattern of restricted activity differs from the incidence pattern in that the low point is established earlier in life: at 17-44 years among males and at 6-16 years among females (Table 4.1). However, as with incidence, the rate of restricted activity is lower for females than for males at ages under 17, but is appreciably higher at older ages. Much of the excess restricted activity in the residual category among women aged 17-44 results from deliveries and diseases associated with pregnancy. However, substantial excess is evident for each acute condition with the exception of injuries. At age 45 and over, the average annual number of days of restricted activity per 100 women, 892, was about one-third higher than that per 100 men.

Females have a higher average annual number of bed-disability days beginning at age 6: below that age, the sexes are nearly equal. Even after the residual category is subtracted, the rate of bed-disability days for women aged 17-44 exceeds that of men by nearly 18 percent. The average annual rate of bed-disability days at ages 45 and over is more than one-third higher for women than for men.

Specific Conditions

Respiratory conditions, principally the common cold, accounted for somewhat more than one-half of all acute conditions reported during the four years ending June 1968 (Table 4.1). Incidence rates for this category decline sharply with advance in age and generally are higher for females than for males: in the 17-44 age group, the rate for women exceeds that for men by nearly one-third. The age-associated decline in the incidence rate of respiratory conditions results largely from the declining rates for upper respiratory conditions. The rates for influenza do not decline until later in life, and the rates for other respiratory conditions are low and stable beyond childhood. During the four-year period encompassed by the data, males were restricted in usual activity because of respiratory conditions at an average annual rate of 3.3 days per man, half of which were bed-disability days. The rate varied from a high of 5.6 days for boys under age 6, to a low of 2.3 days for men at ages 17-44; the range for females was from 5.4 days to 3.2 days for the same age groups.

The second most frequent category of acute conditions among men is injuries, accounting for about 18 percent of the total. The rate is high for the broad age range up to 45, then drops by about 50 percent to a rate of 21 per 100 at older ages. For females, the incidence rate for injuries is about 30 percent lower than the rate for males, with a high of 29 per 100 at ages under 6 and a gradual decline with advance in age. For men, an average of 1.9 days was lost annually from usual activity because of an injury, but the range among age groups was wide: the low of 0.5 day was at ages under 6, and the high of 2.5 days was at ages 17-44. Among females, an annual average of 1.5 days of restricted activity resulted from injuries; at ages under 6, the rate was the same as that for boys, then rose steadily to a peak of 2.5 days at ages 45 and over.

The incidence rate for infective and parasitic conditions is about the same for the two sexes, but this category ranks second for females and third for males. The rates for this cause decline sharply but uniformly for both sexes with advance in age. The associated days of restricted activity also decline sharply with advance in age from about two days annually at ages under 17, to an average of about one-half day at higher ages. Overall, about one-half of the restricted-activity days were bed-disability days.

Only 5 percent of acute conditions were attributed to conditions of the digestive system, among which dental conditions have a prominent role. The incidence rate is nearly identical for men and women, and both sexes show a similar trend of declining rates with advancing age. The pattern of days of restricted activity differed from that of the incidence rates in showing a sharp rise in both sexes for older men and for women in the 17-44, as well as in the 45 and over, age group. For most age-sex groups, bed-disability days accounted for about half the restricted-activity days.

Among the category of "other acute conditions" for females, about one-fifth were reported as genitourinary disorders and one-eighth as deliveries and disorders of pregnancy and the puerperium. Among males, over one-fourth of this residual category was reported as diseases of the ear, one-sixth as diseases of the skin, and about one-tenth as headaches. These conditions were also prominent among females.

Secular Trends

As is true for chronic conditions, trends for acute conditions as a whole for the United States are available only since July 1957 (Table 4.2). During fiscal year 1958, the first full year of record, the highest incidence rates for the period of the survey were observed in every age-sex group. Lowest rates were recorded in 1967 and 1968; this finding too is relatively constant over the age-sex groups. Although highest rates were seen in the earliest years for which data are available, there is no evidence of systematic trend in the incidence of acute conditions during the decade ending June 1969.

It is apparent from Table 4.3 that most fluctuation in the incidence rates of acute conditions is caused by outbreaks of respiratory disease, principally influenza. For most of the years, the rates for the other broad condition groups and even the residual category are quite stable.

This lack of trend in the incidence rate of acute conditions over a short term is quite different from that which would be seen if data were available for a substantially longer period. The high death rates early in this century from conditions such as typhoid fever, diphtheria, poliomyelitis, and others, attest that these now rare conditions once were common.

Relation to Family Income

Incidence rates of acute conditions have a complex relation to family income, one that changes with age. Incidence rates among the young are related directly to family income, but among the elderly the relationship is inverse (Fig. 4.1). However, for several condition groups the association with family income differs from the overall pattern. The most striking of these are conditions of the digestive system—age-adjusted incidence rates among persons with an annual family income of under $2,000 being twice as high as those among persons with a family income of over $7,000. Influenza also shows an inverse association with family income, while the category of "other respiratory conditions" shows no variation among family income groups.

It is quite difficult to separate the effects of the two major factors that contribute to the data: the real differences in disease experience,

Table 4.2   Annual incidence of acute conditions reported in interviews
per 100 persons by age and sex: United States, each fiscal
year ending June 1958 to June 1969
(civilian noninstitutional population)

Sex; fiscal year ending June	All ages	Under 5	5-14	15-24	25-44	45-64	65 & over
Male							
1969	202	333	274	206	173	137	94
1968	183	348	249	175	146	114	85
1967	185	350	251	172	146	121	93
1966	203	362	271	189	172	124	123
1965	203	394	274	179	146	134	124
1964	200	368	274	191	152	128	103
1963	204	371	269	183	163	135	117
1962	208	383	286	183	159	133	119
1961	194	374	259	169	146	124	112
1960	190	364	238	168	152	129	115
1959	205	372	295	164	159	136	105
1958	248	406	347	251	194	157	155
Female							
1969	211	320	273	239	206	142	106
1968	196	319	240	224	183	136	106
1967	195	330	237	217	183	128	111
1966	220	361	273	229	208	152	131
1965	222	370	275	230	200	157	139
1964	216	366	270	222	197	151	124
1963	233	366	267	236	222	182	151
1962	236	350	302	238	226	169	135
1961	210	372	252	207	195	143	124
1960	216	357	272	207	197	151	143
1959	224	333	296	230	207	149	158
1958	272	402	355	291	247	194	169

Source: National Center for Health Statistics, Series 10, Table 17
of nos. 15, 26, 38, 44, 54, and 69; no. 10, Table 20; no. 1, Table 25;
Series B, no. 34, Table 1; no. 24, Table 3, and no. 29, Table 19; no. 18,
Table 3; and no. 6, Table 8, Washington, December 1958 to June 1969.

Note: Excluded are conditions involving neither restricted activity nor medical attention.

and the availability of and willingness to use medical services. The
latter cannot be discounted. But it is true that the overall association
of incidence rates with family income applies to acute conditions of
varying degrees of severity. This suggests that real differences in
disease experience are well reflected by Fig. 4.1.[8]

Table 4.3   Annual incidence of acute conditions and associated disability
            reported in interviews per 100 persons according to specified
            condition groups: United States, each fiscal year ending
            June 1958 to June 1969
                 (civilian noninstitutional population)

Measure; fiscal year ending June	Condition group					
	Total	Infective and parasitic	Respiratory	Digestive	Injuries	All other
Incidence per 100 persons per year						
1969	207	23	122	10	24	28
1968	189	22	106	9	29	24
1967	190	24	104	9	28	25
1966	212	25	126	10	25	25
1965	213	28	116	11	30	28
1964	209	30	110	11	30	28
1963	219	24	127	11	28	28
1962	222	27	128	12	29	26
1961	202	28	110	13	28	23
1960	203	24	119	11	26	23
1959	215	26	126	12	29	22
1958	260	23	169	14	28	26
Days of bed-disability per 100 persons per year						
1969	419	47	250	21	47	55
1968	337	44	185	18	44	47
1967	297	45	147	16	45	44
1966	366	54	196	20	47	48
1965	349	55	170	18	45	61
1964	346	60	157	20	52	57
1963	380	54	206	20	43	57
1962	381	57	202	19	44	59
1961	332	61	150	19	47	55
1960	369	56	197	20	41	55
1959	360	53	190	17	49	51
1958	519	53	352	20	43	50

Source: National Center for Health Statistics, Series 10, Tables 5 and 7
of nos. 10, 15, 26, 38, 44, and 54; no. 1, Tables 9 and 11; no. 69, Tables 1
and 3; Series B, no. 34, Tables 4 and 6; no. 24, Tables 1 and 9, and no. 29,
Table 19; no. 18, Tables 3 and 15; and no. 6, Tables 8 and 20, Washington,
December 1958 to June 1969.

Note: Excluded are conditions involving neither restricted activity nor
medical attention.

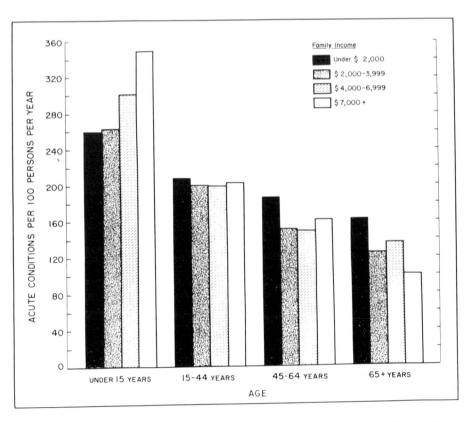

Figure 4.1 Incidence of acute conditions per 100 persons per year, by family income and age: United States, July 1962–June 1963 (excludes all conditions involving neither restricted activity nor medical attention) (Source: National Center for Health Statistics, Pub. Health Service Publ. 1000, Series 10, No. 9, Part VII, Fig. 1, May 1964)

Chronic Conditions

Variation by Age and Sex

In recent years, about 50 percent of the civilian noninstitutional population of the United States has been reported in the Health Interview Survey as having one or more chronic conditions (Table 4.4). Even at ages under 17, one or more chronic conditions were reported for nearly 25 percent of males and more than 20 percent of females. This is the only age group in which the prevalence rate for males exceeds that for females. The increased prevalence rate of

Table 4.4 Percent of persons with one or more chronic conditions by activity limitation status and mobility limitation status reported in interviews, according to sex and age: United States, July 1965 - June 1966

(civilian noninstitutional population)

Limitation	Male					Female				
	All ages	Under 17	17-44	45-64	65 & over	All ages	Under 17	17-44	45-64	65 & over
One or more chronic conditions	47.7	23.8	52.4	68.6	83.5	50.4	20.9	55.2	72.4	86.5
With limitation of activity	11.7	1.9	7.8	20.1	51.2	10.8	1.8	6.9	17.7	40.3
Not in major activity[a]	2.4	1.0	2.4	4.3	4.0	3.3	1.0	2.7	5.7	7.9
In amount or kind of major activity	6.3	0.7	4.5	11.4	26.4	6.3	0.7	3.8	10.8	24.6
Unable to carry on major activity	3.0	0.2	0.9	4.4	20.8	1.2	b	0.4	1.2	7.8
With limitation of mobility	3.0	0.4	1.3	5.1	17.2	3.3	0.3	1.1	4.3	19.3
Has trouble getting around alone	1.5	b	0.8	3.0	6.7	1.5	b	0.7	2.4	7.5
Needs help in getting around										
Special aid	0.7	b	0.3	1.0	5.1	0.6	b	0.2	0.5	4.1
Another person	0.2	b	b	b	1.3	0.4	b		0.4	2.5
Confined to the house										
Not confined to bed	0.4	b	0.2	0.6	2.7	0.6	b	0.2	0.7	4.0
Confined to bed	0.2	b		0.3	1.4	0.2	b	b	b	1.2

Source: National Center for Health Statistics, Series 10, no. 45, Tables 1 and 2, Washington, May 1968.

aMajor activity refers to ability to work, keep house, or engage in school or preschool activities.

bFigure does not meet standards of reliability or precision.

chronic conditions with advance in age is striking. More than 50 percent of persons of both sexes in the 17-44 age group are afflicted, as are about 70 percent of persons aged 45-64, and about 85 percent of persons aged 65 and over.

Along with increasing prevalence rates of persons affected with a chronic condition, advancing age is accompanied by an increasing frequency of multiple chronic conditions. In the Health Interview Survey for July 1957 to June 1958, the prevalence rate of persons reporting three or more chronic conditions was less than 1 percent at ages under 15 years but was about 30 percent among persons 65 and older.[9]

Disability

Disability is assessed in terms of limitation of activity or of mobility. Although a larger proportion of females than males generally reported having one or more chronic conditions, a smaller proportion reported some limitation of activity. During the interval July 1965 to June 1966, 1.2 percent of females and 3.0 percent of males were reported to be disabled to the extent that they could not carry on their major activity; that is, gainfully employed persons were unable to work, housewives could not do housework, school-age children could not attend school, and preschool children were unable to play with others (Table 4.4). Overall, 6.3 percent of persons of both sexes were limited in some way with respect to the amount or kind of their major activity. The prevalence rate of persons limited in some way with respect to their major activity rises steadily with age, but the differences between the sexes are slight. However, the prevalence rate of persons unable to carry on their major activity is higher for men than for women in every age group. Of course, this may reflect the heavier work usually done by men rather than any real difference in the health of the two sexes.

Measures of mobility limitation are more amenable to valid interpretation than are measures of activity limitation. Differences in prevalence rates of mobility limitation are slight between the sexes, while differences among age groups are great. Indeed, the apparent slight excess mobility limitation of women over men may simply reflect the fact that within the oldest age group the average age of women, because of their longevity, is higher than that of men. The prevalence of mobility limitation to some extent parallels the prevalence patterns of activity limitation. During the year ending

June 1966, almost 15 percent of persons with some limitation of activity, other than in their major activity, were also limited in mobility. This figure was 22 percent among persons with some limitation of their major activity, and 61 percent among persons unable to carry on their major activity.[10]

Specific Conditions

Turning from general measures of the impact of chronic diseases, such as activity limitation, to estimates of relatively specific conditions, some striking differences exist between the illness experiences of the two sexes as well as among the different age groups.

For persons under age 45, by far the most prevalent specific condition is orthopedic impairment, excluding paralysis and absence of parts (Table 4.5). However, the rate for males, nearly 80 per 1,000, is greater than that for females, 57 per 1,000. For both sexes, about 17 percent of those afflicted have some limitation of activity. In the under-45 age group, both sexes have the same second-ranking condition, digestive conditions, which limited activity of about 10 percent of afflicted persons. The third-ranking condition for females in this age group is arthritis and rheumatism with a prevalence rate of 21 percent, about double the rate for males. However, the proportion of afflicted women with activity limitation is less than the comparable figure for men. It is unknown whether this disparity is a result of (a) women actually having a higher prevalence of milder disease, (b) the fact that most interviews are conducted with women, who generally act as proxies for their spouses, (c) the reluctance of men to report less severe conditions, or (d) some combination of these factors.

Among men under age 45, the third-ranking condition is hearing impairments; however, this condition apparently limited the activity of only about 6 percent of afflicted persons. About 10 percent of persons in this age group reported visual impairments—conditions that limited the activity of 17 percent of afflicted men, but only 10 percent of afflicted women. Finally, among men in this youngest age group, diseases of the cardiovascular system have a prevalence rate of 16 percent, as compared with a figure of about 22 percent for women. In both sexes, about 40 percent of those reporting a heart condition and 10 percent of those reporting high blood pressure also reported some associated activity limitation.

During the middle years, 45-64, orthopedic impairments and

Table 4.5   Prevalence rates per 1,000 population for selected chronic conditions
reported in interviews and percent causing activity limitation by age
and sex: United States, July 1963 - June 1965
(civilian noninstitutional population)

Sex; condition	Rate per 1,000 population			Percent causing activity limitation		
	Under 45 years	45-64 years	65 years and over	Under 45 years	45-64 years	65 years and over
Male						
Heart conditions	6.9	67.3	168.7	40.6	62.4	70.1
High blood pressure	9.1	57.2	94.4	9.0	13.0	29.9
Arthritis and rheumatism	10.2	113.4	251.6	20.2	23.0	33.7
Digestive conditions	38.5	136.0	223.3	9.3	18.9	22.7
Vascular lesions of central nervous system	a	8.0	40.0	a	66.0	71.3
Visual impairments	11.1	38.9	127.1	16.9	24.6	32.7
Hearing impairments	19.0	87.1	259.0	5.2	4.3	6.2
Orthopedic impairments (excluding paralysis or absence)	79.6	163.4	173.7	16.8	26.8	35.3
Female						
Heart conditions	7.8	53.5	171.1	38.7	58.5	58.5
High blood pressure	13.9	118.8	219.2	10.5	16.3	23.2
Arthritis and rheumatism	21.0	205.8	388.5	15.6	21.2	31.0
Digestive conditions	29.7	115.1	198.1	11.1	17.4	19.1
Vascular lesions of central nervous system	.5	6.8	33.0	a	63.9	69.6
Visual impairments	10.0	40.2	160.3	10.2	16.0	31.2
Hearing impairments	13.9	55.1	182.7	6.8	4.3	5.6
Orthopedic impairments (excluding paralysis or absence)	57.0	130.7	196.5	17.6	25.2	32.7

Source: National Center for Health Statistics, Series 10, no. 32, Tables 21 and
26, Washington, June 1966.
ᵃFigure does not meet standards of reliability or precision.

digestive conditions continue to rank first and second among men,
while third rank is taken by arthritis and rheumatism. For women,
the picture is markedly different: the arthritis and rheumatism
category assumes first rank, orthopedic impairments are second,
while high blood pressure and digestive conditions rank third and
fourth. In moving from the younger to these middle years, particularly striking increases in prevalence rates (about ten-fold) are seen
among both sexes for arthritis and rheumatism and for cardiovascular
conditions. For other conditions, increases were only two- to
five-fold. Not only do the prevalence rates of the chronic conditions
increase markedly with age, but the proportion of afflicted persons
who suffer activity limitation is also increased. This is true for all
conditions with the exception of hearing impairments.

At ages 65 and over, as at younger ages, the prevalence rates of
high blood pressure and arthritis and rheumatism are far greater

among women than among men. Orthopedic and visual impairments are also more frequent among elderly women than among elderly men. In this age group, 25 percent of men and nearly 40 percent of women are afflicted with arthritis and rheumatism. The prevalence rate of high blood pressure is more than twice as high among women (22 percent) as among men (9 percent). However, heart conditions have nearly equal prevalence rates, about 17 percent, in both sexes.

A review of the prevalence rates of chronic conditions does not adequately convey the impact of these diseases among the elderly, especially elderly men. Compared with younger persons afflicted with a chronic condition, the proportion of elderly persons with some activity limitation was increased for every condition in both sexes, except for heart conditions among women. In general, the prevalence rates of persons having some activity limitation as a result of one of the specified conditions are three to four times as high among the elderly as among those in the middle age range. For example, among men the prevalence rate for limitation of activity resulting from vascular lesions of the central nervous system soared from 5 per 1,000 (66.0 percent of a rate of 8.0 per 1,000) at ages 45-64 to 30 per 1,000 (71.3 percent of a rate of 40.0 per 1,000) at ages 65 and over.

Secular Trends

Information on trends in the prevalence rates of chronic conditions in the United States is available for the period since the start of the Health Interview Survey in July 1957 (Table 4.6). The most notable feature of the data is the consistent rise, after the first year of the survey, in the prevalence rate of persons of both sexes reporting one or more chronic conditions. Indeed, this consistent rise is seen within each age group. Overall, during the decade spanned by the data, the rate increased among men from 39 to 49 percent, among women more slowly from 44 to 51 percent.

The trends shown in Table 4.6 may have several explanations apart from a genuine rise in the prevalence rates of chronic conditions. As experience with the survey was gained, it is likely that the quality of reporting improved. Apparent increase may have resulted from changes in interviewing technique, in the checklists used to ascertain chronic conditions, and in the rules for coding medical terms. Notable increases resulted from a change in the method of data elicitation in 1966 and 1967. Since 1957, diagnostic techniques have

Table 4.6 Percent of persons with one or more chronic conditions reported in interviews: United States, each fiscal year ending June 1958 to June 1967 (civilian noninstitutional population)

Fiscal year ending June	Male						Female					
	All ages	Under 17	17-24	25-44	45-64	65 & over	All ages	Under 17	17-24	25-44	45-64	65 & over
1967	48.7	24.6	44.4	57.1	70.4	85.2	51.0	21.8	44.8	61.1	72.6	86.6
1966	47.7	23.8	42.3	57.3	68.6	83.5	50.4	20.9	43.9	60.9	72.4	86.5
1965	44.6	22.7	37.6	52.2	64.0	81.9	48.0	20.0	41.1	58.0	68.2	84.6
1964	43.5	22.0	37.0	50.0	63.2	80.2	46.9	19.2	40.3	56.0	67.5	83.9
1963	43.2	21.6	35.9	50.1	62.6	79.9	45.7	18.6	39.2	54.6	65.9	82.2
1962	41.9	21.1		43.9	61.9	79.0	45.4	18.2		49.7	65.7	82.4
1961	41.2	---	---	---	---	---	44.0	---	---	---	---	---
1960	39.9	---	---	---	---	---	42.3	---	---	---	---	---
1959	38.9	---	---	---	---	---	42.0	---	---	---	---	---
1958	39.1	18.8[a]		39.0[b]	57.6	75.2	43.5	16.0[a]		45.3[b]	63.3	80.6

Source: National Center for Health Statistics, Series B, no. 11 (Table 10); Series B, no. 36 (Table 10); Series 10, no. 5 (Table 8), no. 13 (Table 8), no. 25 (Table 9), no. 37 (Table 9), no. 43 (Table 9); and unpublished data. Data for July 1961-June 1962 estimated from Series 10, no. 17 (Table 1) and no. 5 (Table 8), using population from no. 4 (Tables 18 and 22).

a Ages under 15.   b Ages 15-44.

advanced and screening procedures have become widespread so that the average duration of some conditions, and hence their prevalence rates, have increased. Increased survival as a result of improved treatment methods may also have increased the prevalence rate of persons afflicted with chronic conditions. Finally, it must be remembered that the age groups used to display the data are broad, and during the ten-year period there have been changes in the age structure of the population within these groups. For example, in 1960, among men aged 65 and over, only 31.8 percent were 75 or older. However, by 1970, the proportion had risen to 35.4 percent.

Available data do not permit evaluation of the relative importance of the factors that could explain the apparent rise in the prevalence rates of chronic conditions. It may be, however, that most of the rise after 1965 is artifactual. Much of it may have resulted from increased reporting of less serious conditions. Thus, while the proportion of the population with some activity limitation did rise gradually, the proportion of the population unable to carry on major activity because of a chronic condition increased only from 2.1 to 2.3 percent during the ten-year period from July 1957 to June 1966.[10]

The effects of procedural changes in data elicitation on the reported prevalence rates of chronic conditions are shown in Table 4.7. The rates for three successive two-year periods show substantial increases in reported frequencies of high blood pressure and arthritis and rheumatism. Most of the increases resulted from the use of more searching probe-questions to uncover the presence of these conditions. Other conditions show slight and inconsistent changes.

Finally, since these data relate to noninstitutional persons, the rates for most conditions, especially among the aged, underestimate the prevalence of ill-health in our population. The health problems of the aged are described more fully in Chapter 6 of this monograph.

Relation to Family Income

As with acute conditions, the frequency of chronic conditions has a complex relation to family income. Table 4.8 shows the overall inverse relation of the prevalence rate of chronic conditions to family income. The pattern for chronic conditions differs from acute conditions in that it changes relatively little with age. There is only one suggestion of a direct relation between prevalence rates and family income—in the under-15 age group—but it is neither strong nor consistent. Figure 4.2 gives considerable insight into the cause of

Table 4.7   Prevalence rates per 1,000 population for selected chronic conditions
reported in interviews by age: United States, fiscal years ending
June 1962 to June 1967
(civilian nonsitutional population)

Condition	Fiscal year ending June					
	1962 - 63	1964 - 65	1966 - 67	1962 - 63	1964 - 65	1966 - 67
	All ages			Ages under 45		
Heart conditions	32.3	33.0	39.8	8.6	7.4	11.2
High blood pressure	35.9	41.2	60.6b	9.8	11.5	21.0b
Arthritis and rheumatism	69.6	73.8	86.2b	15.2	15.7	19.2b
Digestive conditions	65.7	68.5	67.6	34.0	34.0	34.1
Vascular lesions of central nervous system	4.7	5.1	7.6	a	0.4	0.6
Visual impairments	26.1	28.8	29.7	9.3	10.5	11.3
Hearing impairments	42.2	45.7	45.3	15.4	16.4	17.0
Orthopedic impairments (excluding paralysis or absence)	84.7	94.8	100.6	59.6	68.1	72.8
	Ages 45-64			Ages 65 and over		
Heart conditions	58.9	60.1	71.8	158.6	170.0	186.9
High blood pressure	77.3	89.1	128.5b	147.8	164.1	213.2b
Arthritis and rheumatism	154.7	161.2	192.2b	304.4	328.1	362.8b
Digestive conditions	120.0	125.2	121.8	191.2	209.3	203.4
Vascular lesions of central nervous system	7.1	7.4	11.7	33.5	36.1	51.5
Visual impairments	35.3	39.6	39.3	136.6	145.6	148.6
Hearing impairments	63.8	70.5	69.4	203.4	216.3	208.0
Orthopedic impairments (excluding paralysis or absence)	133.9	146.4	158.6	170.5	186.4	185.2

Source: National Center for Health Statistics, unpublished data.
[a]Figure does not meet standards of reliability or precision.
[b]Increase in prevalence primarily due to revised probe questions.

the inverse association that generally prevails. Whereas the association is strong and consistent for severe conditions (with activity
limitation), it is weak and actually reversed for milder conditions.
This provides some evidence that the chronic illnesses are themselves
responsible for the inverse relation of prevalence rates to family
income. Presumably, activity-limiting conditions also limit the affected individual's income-earning capacity.

Utilization of Medical Care

The data presented thus far are drawn primarily from a continuous
survey of the population with the major disadvantages that responses
are dependent on memory and that interpretations of interview

Table 4.8   Percent of the population with one or more chronic
             conditions, by family income and age: United States,
             July 1962-June 1963

Age	Family income				
	All incomes[a]	Under $2,000	$2,000-3,999	$4,000-6,999	$7,000 and over
All ages	44.5	57.6	46.5	40.6	42.9
Under 15	19.5	19.2	19.4	18.8	20.8
15-44	46.0	48.3	45.3	46.2	46.6
45-64	64.3	76.8	68.3	62.3	61.1
65 and over	81.2	86.4	81.4	77.2	76.2

Source: National Center for Health Statistics, Series 10,
Table 1 in Part VI of no. 9, Washington, May 1964.

[a] Includes persons with unknown incomes.

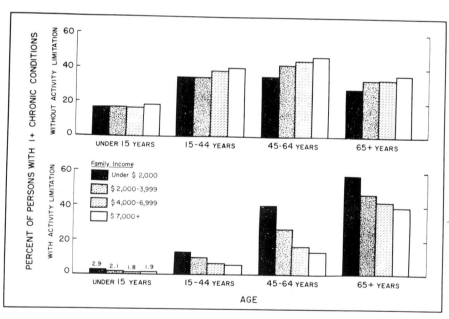

Figure 4.2 Percentage of persons with one or more chronic conditions, with and without activity limitation, by age and family income: United States, July 1962–June 1963 (Source: National Center for Health Statistics, Pub. Health Service Publ. 1000, Series 10, No. 9, Part VI, Fig. 2, May 1964)

questions are subjective. To some extent these deficiencies may be overcome by employing other indexes of morbidity, such as rates of physician visits and of utilization of hospitals. Rates of hospital utilization have the advantage of objectively documenting an episode of ill-health, with the duration of hospitalization as an indicator of its severity. However, major difficulties with such data include the changing indications for hospitalization with time, and the different use of hospitals by various subgroups of the population.

Available data on hospital utilization come from the Hospital Discharge Survey, a continuing nationwide survey conducted by the National Center for Health Statistics. Estimates are based on information transcribed from the medical records of a sample of noninstitutional, short-stay general and special hospitals in the United States. Excluded from these are military and Veterans Administration hospitals and discharges of well newborn infants.

Hospital Discharge Rate

Table 4.9 shows the annual rate of hospital discharges according to age and sex for the United States in 1967. The rate for females, 171.0 per 1,000, is about 40 percent higher than that for males at 120.1. However, if discharges following obstetric deliveries are excluded, the rate for females becomes 135.5, or only about 13 percent higher than the male rate. It is apparent, however, that even excluding deliveries, women are more frequently hospitalized than men during the ages 15-44. The rates for females during this middle period are generally about 18 percent higher than those for men. Yet both from the time of birth through age 14 and from age 65 on, women exhibit lower hospitalization rates than men. Since men have higher mortality rates than women (and higher incidence rates as well, for those conditions on which such data are available), it is unclear why hospitalization rates for men would be lower than those for women at any age.

It is apparent that hospitalization rates, in addition to varying with sex, rise sharply with advancing age: the *rate of rise* also increases with advance in age. An exception to this is women aged 55-64 who show a rate no higher than women aged 45-54. Although not evident from the table, about 45 percent of discharges under age 1 for both sexes are ill newborn.[11]

Table 4.9 Number and annual rate of discharges from short-stay hospitals per 1,000 population by age and sex: United States, 1967

Age	Both sexes			Male		Female		
	Numbers	Rates Including deliveries	Rates Excluding deliveries	Numbers	Rates	Numbers	Rates Including deliveries	Rates Excluding deliveries
All ages	28,417	146.9	128.5	11,202	120.1	17,140	171.0	135.5
Under 15	4,474	74.8	74.6	2,497	82.1	1,960	66.7	66.4
Under 1	1,015	287.4		571	316.7	439	254.0	
1-4	1,185	75.9		670	84.0	512	66.9	
5-14	2,274	56.0		1,257	60.9	1,009	50.5	
15-44	12,279	161.6	114.9	3,323	92.2	8,934	223.6	134.8
15-24	4,846	158.9		1,157	81.1	3,681	227.0	
25-34	4,011	181.3		953	90.2	3,052	263.8	
35-44	3,423	146.3		1,213	108.2	2,202	180.9	
45-64	6,386	161.1	160.9	2,998	158.1	3,370	163.0	162.7
45-54	3,328	149.2		1,452	135.3	1,869	161.5	
55-64	3,057	176.3		1,546	187.8	1,501	164.8	
65 and over	5,215	289.1	289.1	2,352	300.7	2,846	278.5	278.5
65-74	2,818	246.6		1,332	262.1	1,478	232.9	
75 and over	2,397	362.4		1,020	372.0	1,368	353.4	
Not stated	62	-		31	-	30	-	

Source: National Center for Health Statistics, Series 13, Tables 1, 3 and 4 of no. 9, Washington, May 1972.

Note: Figures for both sexes include those for whom sex was not stated. Detailed figures do not always add to totals and sub-totals in original publication.

Table 4.10   Average length of hospital stay in days by age and sex: United States, 1967

Age	Both sexes	Male	Female	
			Including deliveries	Excluding deliveries
All ages	8.4	9.0	8.1	9.0
Under 15	5.5	5.5	5.5	5.5
15-44	6.2	7.3	5.8	6.5
45-64	10.1	10.2	10.1	10.1
65 and over	14.1	13.5	14.7	14.7

Source: National Center for Health Statistics, Series 13, Table 10 of no. 9, Washington, May 1972.

Length of Stay

For both sexes, as with the discharge rate, there is a steady increase in length of hospital stay with advancing age (Table 4.10). In comparison of the sexes the only discrepancy appears for the age group 15-44 in which the average length of stay for men, 7.3 days, is about 12 percent higher than the average for women. This is of interest in that, within the same age group, the hospital discharge rate for women was appreciably higher than that for men. In fact, the annual rate of days of care in this age group reflects the combined effects of these two measures; for women aged 15-44 the annual rate of days of care was 879.1 per 1,000 (excluding deliveries) compared to 675.8 for men, an excess of 30 percent.[11]

Physician Visits

The number of physician visits per person per year, according to age and sex, is shown in Table 4.11. Overall, there is a steady rise in physician visits with advancing age. This trend is less spectacular but more consistent among males. As compared to females of the same age, males under 17 have a higher frequency of physician visits, but this is completely and strikingly reversed in the next age group. In all age groups over 17, women have a higher frequency of visits than men. The pattern for adult women is somewhat unexpected in showing no trend from the 17-44 to the 45-64 age groups. Since women in the 17-44 age group have about one visit per woman per

Table 4.11   Number of physician visits per person per year by age and
sex: United States, 1969

Sex	All ages	Under 17	17-44	45-64	65 & over
Both sexes	4.3	3.6	4.2	4.7	6.1
Male	3.7	3.7	3.1	4.1	5.5
Female	4.7	3.4	5.1	5.2	6.6

Source: National Center for Health Statistics, Series 10,
Table 9 of no. 70, Washington, April 1972.

year for antepartum and postpartum care, the figure given in Table 4.11 for this age group should be reduced to 4.1 for purposes of comparison with the figure for men.[8] Even so, women in this age group would have about 30 percent more visits than men. This discrepancy between the sexes declines steadily with advancing age. Thus, in the 65 and over age group, although women do have a higher frequency of physician visits than men, the number is only about 20 percent higher. The higher figure for women is in compliance with their higher reported frequency of both chronic and acute conditions. However, the possibility that these visits are for relatively minor conditions is suggested by the facts that hospital discharge rates for men and women are more similar and, as is well known, mortality rates for women are lower (at given ages) than those for men.

Relation to Family Income

As was apparent from interview data, family income is related to both the incidence rate of acute conditions and the prevalence rate of chronic conditions. It would thus seem likely to be associated with utilization of medical care. Table 4.12 shows the association of family income with several measures of use of medical care. As might be anticipated, the relationships are complex, especially in the variation among age groups.

Overall, there is an inverse association of discharge rate with family income, rates for the lowest income group being about 75 percent greater than for the highest. However, while the same general pattern is seen in all age groups up to age 75, the trend is strongest for an intermediate group aged 17-44. The trend is moderately strong in the under-17 age group and the 45-64 group, but barely perceptible at ages 65-74, and is reversed for persons aged 75 and over. Data on length of stay tend to be similar to those on discharges and thus to reinforce the overall trend of less hospital use with increasing family income. However, among persons aged 65 and over—the major consumers of hospital services—no strong associations of length of stay with income are apparent.

The data on physician visits show relatively consistent associations with family income over age groups. In the youngest age group,

Table 4.12   Discharges from short-stay hospitals per 1,000 population, average length of hospital stay for discharges,
and percent of population with one or more physician
visits within a year, by age and family income:
United States, 1968-69

Age and family income	Discharges per 1,000 population	Average length of stay	Physician visits per 100 population
All ages			
All incomes[a]	125.6	9.1	69.4
Under $3,000	174.4	12.3	66.2
$3,000-$3,999	151.1	11.1	65.9
$4,000-$6,999	133.5	8.7	68.0
$7,000-$9,999	116.5	7.7	69.5
$10,000-$14,999	106.9	7.3	71.8
$15,000 and over	101.2	8.0	74.5
Under 17 years			
All incomes	62.6	5.6	68.5
Under $3,000	79.8	7.5	56.8
$3,000-$3,999	74.3	6.6	59.4
$4,000-$6,999	64.7	5.6	65.2
$7,000-$9,999	61.3	5.1	69.3
$10,000-$14,999	58.9	4.8	72.7
$15,000 and over	49.7	6.1	77.2
17-44 years			
All incomes	147.4	6.8	70.9
Under $3,000	175.5	7.5	71.3
$3,000-$3,999	194.3	8.5	70.0
$4,000-$6,999	173.1	6.7	70.3
$7,000-$9,999	146.3	6.5	70.5
$10,000-$14,999	127.4	6.2	72.1
$15,000 and over	108.8	5.9	73.7

(Cont.)

Table 4.12   Discharges from short-stay hospitals per 1,000 population, average length of hospital stay for discharges,
and percent of population with one or more physician
visits within a year, by age and family income:
United States, 1968-69 (Cont.)

Age and family income	Discharges per 1,000 population	Average length of stay	Physician visits per 100 population
45-64 years			
All incomes	143.1	11.3	67.4
Under $3,000	189.6	14.4	65.7
$3,000-$3,999	133.6	14.2	64.8
$4,000-$6,999	149.7	11.1	66.3
$7,000-$9,999	140.5	10.1	67.2
$10,000-$14,999	137.2	9.8	69.0
$15,000 and over	127.0	9.5	71.9
65-74 years[b]			
All incomes	209.2	14.5	71.3
Under $3,000	225.4	14.0	69.1
$3,000-$3,999	205.9	13.8	70.9
$4,000-$6,999	195.4	15.1	73.6
$7,000-$9,999	222.9	16.3	72.7
$10,000-$14,999	214.0	11.0	75.4
$15,000 and over	209.6	13.3	78.7
75 years and over			
All incomes	271.7	16.4	
Under $3,000	247.5	17.2	
$3,000-$3,999	282.5	16.2	
$4,000-$6,999	262.7	16.0	
$7,000-$9,999	337.3	14.1	
$10,000-$14,999	242.1	17.4	
$15,000 and over	406.6	15.3	

Source: National Center for Health Statistics, Series 10,
Tables 3 and 15 of no. 70, Washington, April 1972.

[a] Includes unknown income.
[b] Data for "physician visits" apply to ages 65 and over.

under 17, there is a consistent positive association. For young adults,
17-44, the association is positive but weak. For persons aged 45-64,
the association is once again distinct and in the oldest age group, 65
and over, the association with family income is yet stronger.[1][2]

Mental Illness

The difficulties in estimating morbidity caused by physical illness are of even greater significance with respect to mental illness. In addition, a considerable stigma remains attached to mental illness and interview data are particularly unreliable. Partially for these reasons, perhaps, meaningful data on mental illness are scarce. Nonetheless, certain patterns do emerge in the description of mental illness. Because of this and because of the tremendous social and economic impact of these conditions, they are considered here. A separate monograph in this series is concerned in detail with mental disorders,[13] and Chapter 7 of this volume discusses variations by marital status.

Symptom Data

The National Health Examination Survey (NHES) of 1960-67 examined a sample of the adult civilian noninstitutional population of the United States to obtain information on the health status of Americans. Between October 1959 and December 1962, 6,672 members of the sample population filled out a health questionnaire and were examined in connection with the first cycle of the NHES. The questionnaire included 12 symptom items which had been used in several prior studies of "psychological distress." The detailed data and an explanation of their limitations have been published.[14]

Table 4.13 shows the percentage of persons of each age and sex who responded with a "yes" to the 12 questions on psychological distress. There is no constant overall relation of the prevalence of these symptoms to age, and each symptom must be evaluated individually. However, in general, older persons had higher rates than younger persons for nervous breakdown, insomnia, dizziness, and heart palpitations. Curvilinear relationships with age were seen for impending nervous breakdown, nervousness, and headaches. Age appears unrelated to inertia, trembling hands, nightmares, or fainting.

In Table 4.13 is given also what is perhaps a more meaningful summary measure of psychological distress than the data for the individual symptoms. For each subject, positive responses to the 12 symptoms were summed to give a score of 0 to 11 (the first two symptoms being combined); this sum is termed the "scale mean value." Among whites, neither sex shows any trend of score with age, but there is a clear difference between the sexes—with women

Table 4.13 Symptoms of psychological distress in adults per 100 population by sex and age, and by sex and color, and scale mean value by sex, color, and age: United States, 1960–62

Symptom and sex	Age								Color	
	Total, 18-79 years	18-24 years	25-34 years	35-44 years	45-54 years	55-64 years	65-74 years	75-79 years	White	Black
Nervous breakdown										
Male	3.2	1.3	1.8	3.5	3.0	5.4	5.4	1.5	3.2	2.8
Female	6.4	1.0	3.6	5.0	7.3	12.7	10.7	13.1	6.0	10.4
Felt impending nervous breakdown										
Male	7.7	6.9	7.4	8.6	11.7	6.4	3.1	2.2	7.7	8.2
Female	17.5	14.6	21.6	19.3	18.8	14.5	13.8	10.2	17.8	16.1
Nervousness										
Male	45.1	43.5	47.5	51.9	48.1	37.7	36.6	30.2	47.2	31.3
Female	70.6	61.4	74.4	75.0	72.5	72.6	62.9	65.6	73.2	55.2
Inertia										
Male	16.8	17.2	16.1	17.6	16.3	16.9	18.2	12.1	16.9	17.1
Female	32.5	31.0	34.0	35.2	31.1	29.7	31.9	35.6	33.1	29.5
Insomnia										
Male	23.5	20.4	16.7	20.8	26.8	27.0	35.9	26.5	24.1	20.4
Female	40.4	28.0	33.5	33.7	42.8	53.8	59.0	51.0	40.9	38.9
Trembling hands										
Male	7.0	7.6	6.5	5.4	5.7	8.8	10.0	8.5	6.9	7.1
Female	10.9	10.4	12.2	12.1	10.6	9.3	9.2	13.0	10.6	12.3
Nightmares										

Female	12.4	12.8	15.8	14.7	9.9	7.5	11.6	11.8	12.3	14.3
Perspiring hands										
Male	17.0	23.2	24.9	17.7	14.7	11.0	7.9	3.0	17.0	16.8
Female	21.4	28.6	27.7	24.2	19.6	15.0	9.2	5.9	22.2	16.0
Fainting										
Male	16.9	17.6	15.7	15.7	18.1	17.3	17.8	17.2	17.5	13.8
Female	29.1	28.5	33.2	29.9	27.0	26.2	29.7	24.8	30.4	20.5
Headaches										
Male	13.7	13.0	12.8	13.8	15.2	15.6	11.3	10.0	13.8	11.9
Female	27.8	24.0	31.6	29.6	29.5	25.9	24.2	19.3	27.5	30.9
Dizziness										
Male	7.1	6.3	3.0	5.0	7.6	10.7	12.8	14.3	6.9	9.2
Female	10.9	8.4	9.5	8.5	10.1	14.3	16.9	16.6	10.3	15.7
Heart palpitations										
Male	3.7	3.3	2.0	2.1	3.9	7.2	6.4	1.5	3.6	4.8
Female	5.8	1.7	3.1	4.7	6.2	9.7	10.4	14.8	5.7	6.4
Scale Mean Value [a]										
White										
Male	1.70	1.72	1.70	1.72	1.78	1.69	1.66	1.19		
Female	2.88	2.61	3.07	2.93	2.89	2.86	2.82	2.80		
Black										
Male	1.55	1.25	1.03	1.37	1.79	1.87	2.23	2.99		
Female	2.65	1.91	2.61	2.60	2.52	3.27	3.79	2.62		

Source: National Center for Health Statistics, Series 11, Table D of no. 37, Washington, August 1970.
[a]Scale is from 0 to 11.

averaging about one more positive response than men at each age. White women, in fact, had a prevalence rate for each symptom that was nearly double that for men. Among blacks, there is a strong association of increasing mean score with age for men and a weaker, or at least less consistent, trend among women. Among blacks, as among whites, women reported an average of about one more symptom than men at every age except the oldest. Also like whites, black women had higher prevalence rates than men for each symptom; however, the difference between the sexes was less. For nightmares and perspiring hands, there was virtually no sex difference among blacks.

Although patterns differed among symptoms of psychological distress, this survey does allow some generalizations in addition to those that follow from Table 4.13. Symptom prevalence rates were inversely related to education and income level; rates were lower among the never-married and higher among the separated, than among other marital status groups; rates were lower among persons gainfully employed as compared with retired men and housekeeping women; rates were lower in the northeastern part of the country and higher in the southern part as compared with the country as a whole.[14]

Hospitalization

Incidence rates. In the first two columns of Table 4.14 are shown the incidence rates of hospital admissions for psychiatric services, by age and sex, in the United States in 1966. Included are data from mental hospitals (public and private), psychiatric services in general hospitals, and outpatient psychiatric clinics. It is emphasized that these incidence rates are not restricted to new admissions and refer not to the onset of mental illness but to the onset of hospitalization, presumably for mental illness.

In contrast to the interview data from the NHES wherein the responses of women indicated more psychological distress than those of men, Table 4.14 shows that the incidence rates of hospitalizations for mental illness are generally higher for males. Women have a slightly higher rate than men in the 25-34 age group. Overall, the rate for males is about 11 percent higher than that for females, primarily because of the higher rates for males in childhood and young adulthood. In all, the situation is quite similar to that noted for physical disease. There too, women reported higher frequencies of

Table 4.14   Admissions to mental facilities and patients resident in mental facilities per 1,000 population, and estimated average duration of stay, by age and sex: United States, 1966[a]

Age	Incidence rate			Prevalence rate			Average duration[b]		
	Male	Female	Ratio M/F	Male	Female	Ratio M/F	Male	Female	Ratio M/F
All ages	8.4	7.6	1.1	6.7	5.1	1.3	0.80	0.67	1.2
Under 15	4.6	2.3	2.0	3.6	1.7	2.1	0.78	0.74	1.1
15-24	9.7	8.7	1.1	5.8	4.5	1.3	0.60	0.52	1.2
25-34	11.9	13.4	0.9	7.6	6.6	1.2	0.64	0.49	1.3
35-44	13.3	12.7	1.0	9.4	6.7	1.4	0.71	0.53	1.3
45-54	10.4	9.7	1.1	8.6	6.3	1.4	0.83	0.65	1.3
55-64	7.6	7.4	1.0	8.9	7.1	1.3	1.17	0.96	1.2
65 and over	7.1	6.8	1.0	10.4	8.9	1.2	1.46	1.31	1.1

Source: National Institute of Mental Health, Series A, no. 2 (1969); incidence rates from Table B, prevalence rates from Table C.

[a] Includes public and private mental hospitals, psychiatric services in general hospitals, and outpatient psychiatric clinics.

[b] In years.

symptoms despite the fact that their hospitalization and mortality experience were more favorable than those of men. In the case of mental illness as well as physical illness it would seem, then, that women either are afflicted with more of the mild disease forms or are more willing than men to report symptoms of mild illness.

Prevalence rates. Also shown in Table 4.14 are prevalence rates by age and sex of persons hospitalized for psychiatric disorders or on the rolls of outpatient psychiatric clinics. For both sexes, age-prevalence is biphasic with a peak rate in the 35-44 age group and a second and higher peak in later life. In addition, rates for males are higher than those for females at all ages, especially among children. Unlike incidence rates, the prevalence rates show no excess for women in the 25-34 age group.

Prevalence rates, however, are usually quite difficult to interpret since they are the result of two major effects, the incidence rate of the disease in question and its average duration. It is generally quite informative to separate these components. This can be done if the assumptions of "stability"[1] are valid, as they probably are in this case. Under this set of assumptions if the incidence rate and the prevalence rate of a disease are known, the average duration is approximated by the relationship: $D \cong P/I$, where D = the average duration of the disease (in this case, duration of hospital stay), P = prevalence rate, and I = incidence rate.

This equation was used to obtain the estimates of average duration of hospitalization for mental illness shown in Table 4.14. The average at first declines with advancing age, reaching a nadir for males in the 15-24 age group, and for females in the 25-34 age group. The average duration then rises steadily throughout the remainder of life. Clearly this accounts for the increasing prevalence rates after age 45, despite declining incidence rates. It also would seem that the high prevalence rate for boys relative to girls is in fact attributable to their high incidence rates, since in the under-15 age group there is little difference in average duration of hospitalization between the sexes. Generally, durations are longer for males than for females, although the difference is very small in the oldest as well as in the youngest age group. There is the suggestion that the relatively high incidence rate for women aged 25-34 represents an excess of episodes of relatively mild illness, since the average duration of hospitalization is extremely low for this group. On the other hand, this age group includes young mothers, and the short duration may be related to the wish to restore these women to their families. In any case, it is apparent that men tend to have higher incidence rates and longer durations of hospitalization than women. Both factors act together to make the overall prevalence rate for males 31 percent higher than that for females.

As mentioned, the data in Table 4.14 relate to "hospitalizations" in several different kinds of institutions and include outpatients in psychiatric clinics. To supplement these, statistics from the National Health Survey provide estimates of prevalence rates of adults in "long-stay" mental hospitals, that is, institutions with an average patient stay of 30 days or more which specialize in the care of psychiatric patients.[15] The data are of value in permitting comparisons of racial groups and estimates of the burden of severe mental illness. Table 4.15 shows the number of persons in long-stay mental hospitals and prevalence rates by age, color, and sex. There is a steady increase in the prevalence rate with advancing age in each color-sex group. This trend is stronger for women than for men, and for whites than for nonwhites. There is also a higher rate for nonwhites than for whites in every age-sex group. In addition, women have lower rates than men of the same race, a single exception occurring among elderly whites.

Table 4.15   Patients resident in long-stay mental hospitals per 1,000
population 15 years and over, by age, color, and sex:
United States, April-June 1963

Age and color	Number of patients, both sexes	Prevalence rate			Ratio M/F
		Total	Male	Female	
Both color groups					
Total, 15 and over	558,417	4.4	4.9	3.9	1.3
15-44	174,091	2.4	3.1	1.8	1.7
45-54	107,990	5.0	5.6	4.6	1.2
55-64	109,467	6.7	7.0	6.3	1.1
65-74	99,313	8.8	9.7	8.0	1.3
75 and over	67,556	10.8	10.2	11.3	0.9
White					
Total, 15 and over	464,396	4.1	4.4	3.7	1.2
15-44	132,686	2.1	2.6	1.6	1.6
45-54	89,422	4.6	5.0	4.3	1.2
55-64	93,509	6.3	6.5	6.0	1.1
65-74	88,053	8.4	9.3	7.7	1.2
75 and over	60,726	10.5	9.7	11.1	0.9
Nonwhite					
Total, 15 and over	94,021	7.0	8.9	5.3	1.7
15-44	41,405	4.9	6.8	3.2	2.1
45-54	18,568	8.8	11.0	6.9	1.6
55-64	15,958	10.7	12.1	9.4	1.3
65-74	11,260	12.7	14.6	11.1	1.3
75 and over	6,830	14.8	16.1	13.7	1.2

Source: National Center for Health Statistics, Series 12, Tables B
and 1 of no. 3, Washington, December 1965.

Again, it is informative to examine the components of the
prevalence rates. Table 4.16 shows that women have average durations of stay that are quite comparable to those of men at every age
except 65-74. Since the two sexes have similar durations (or possibly,
longer durations for women, as suggested by the median values), it
must be true that the higher prevalence rates seen for men in Table
4.15 are attributable to higher incidence rates for them than for
women.

Table 4.16   Percent distribution of patients 15 years of age and over
             in long-stay mental hospitals, by length of current stay
             and average and median length of stay by sex and age:
             United States, April-June, 1963

| Sex and age | Current length of stay (years) | | | | | Average length of stay (years) | Median length of stay (years) |
	Total	Under 1	1-4	5-9	10+		
Male							
Total, 15 and over	100.0	22.3	24.2	15.1	38.4	10.3	6.1
15-44	100.0	34.1	28.2	15.8	21.9	5.6	3.2
45-54	100.0	20.0	19.4	15.1	45.6	10.8	8.4
55-64	100.0	11.6	18.9	13.4	56.2	14.7	10.4
65-74	100.0	14.3	24.2	16.0	45.6	13.6	8.5
75 and over	100.0	18.1	30.3	13.8	37.8	12.1	5.5
Female							
Total, 15 and over	100.0	22.8	21.7	13.7	41.6	11.0	6.9
15-44	100.0	40.2	22.1	14.1	23.5	5.6	2.7
45-54	100.0	20.1	19.9	12.3	47.7	10.7	9.0
55-64	100.0	13.7	20.6	14.2	51.5	13.3	10.0
65-74	100.0	15.5	19.6	12.2	52.6	15.0	10.2
75 and over	100.0	18.3	27.8	15.6	38.3	12.5	6.1

Source: National Center for Health Statistics, Series 12, Table 4
of no. 3, Washington, December 1965.

It is also of interest to compare these data for long-stay hospitals
with those just presented relating to all hospitalizations for mental
illness (Table 4.14). Presumably the former relate primarily to severe
mental illness, while the latter relate to the totality of mental illness.
This is suggested too by the fact that the durations of stay in
long-stay hospitals are on the order of ten years, while those in all
hospitals are on the order of one year or so. The two sets of data are
consistent in suggesting that incidence rates are higher for men than
for women. However, the sex ratio (excluding the under-15 age
group from Table 4.14) is generally more striking for all hospitalizations than for long-stay hospitalizations. The only apparent "in-
consistency" between the sets of data results from the fact that
among all hospitalizations, men appear to have longer average
durations, while for long-stay hospitals the reverse is true. This
simply reflects the fact that data from the long-stay hospitals

represent the status of only 35 percent of the over-15 persons described by the "all hospitalizations" data.

Finally, it is of interest to compare change with age in the sex ratio of the prevalence rates in the two sets of data. In both there is a tendency for the sex ratio to move toward 1.0 with advance in age, but this is much more striking in the long-stay hospitals. All of this suggests that men have higher incidence rates of both minor and severe mental illness. This appears true throughout the life-span but becomes less apparent for severe illness with advancing age.

Dental Disease

Although dental disease does not convey any appreciable mortality, it has numerous adverse effects. In adolescence and young childhood, active dental disease as well as the effects of prior poor oral hygiene are responsible for halitosis, malocclusions, and other cosmetic deficiencies such as discolored and missing teeth. In adulthood, dental problems, including those of the gingiva, cause expense and inconvenience to many persons who use dentures or other prostheses. Among the elderly, dental disease probably is responsible at least in part for the highly prevalent nutritional problems.

Table 4.17 shows the strong association of age with the probability of having an edentulous jaw arch. At ages 18-24 little more than 1 percent of the population is totally edentulous, but in the very next age group, 25-34, nearly 3 percent of men and 6 percent of women are totally edentulous. The rates continue to rise with age, so that by about age 65 nearly half the population is edentulous. The rates are higher for women than for men at all ages. In addition, for both sexes at virtually every age, the proportion of the white population that is totally edentulous is higher than that of the black population. Overall, only 11.3 percent of blacks as compared to 19.2 percent of whites are totally edentulous.[16]

The proportion of the population that is totally edentulous can be identified readily as having experienced extremely poor dental health. However, a more sensitive index of dental disease is the "DMF score"–the number of individual's permanent teeth that are decayed, missing, filled, or nonfunctional. The count is based on 32 teeth, which includes third molars. In young adulthood, when few

Table 4.17   Percent distribution of adults by number of edentulous
arches, by sex and age: United States, 1960-62

Sex and age	Total	With no arch edentulous	With one arch edentulous	With both arches edentulous
Both sexes				
Total, 18-79	100.0	72.9	9.0	18.1
Male				
Total, 18-79	100.0	75.7	7.9	16.4
18-24	100.0	97.0	1.6	1.3
25-34	100.0	94.7	2.7	2.7
35-44	100.0	88.1	6.0	5.9
45-54	100.0	70.6	9.4	19.9
55-64	100.0	52.1	13.4	34.5
65-74	100.0	38.0	17.0	45.0
75-79	100.0	22.9	21.4	55.7
Female				
Total, 18-79	100.0	70.4	9.9	19.6
18-24	100.0	97.7	0.9	1.4
25-34	100.0	87.3	6.6	6.1
35-44	100.0	80.7	9.3	10.0
45-54	100.0	66.9	13.1	20.0
55-64	100.0	45.8	16.2	38.0
65-74	100.0	31.6	15.5	52.9
75-79	100.0	22.5	12.8	64.8

Source: National Center for Health Statistics, Series 11,
Table 1 of no. 7, Washington, February 1962.

teeth are lost because of periodontal disease, the DMF score is a
measure of the effects of decay. In older adults who lose teeth
because of periodontal disease, the score differences between
adjacent age groups can be interpreted, with some caution, as an
index of periodontal disease.

The National Health Examination Survey found an average of 20.4
DMF teeth per person (17.9 if edentulous persons are excluded). As
shown in Table 4.18, of the 20.4 DMF teeth, 1.2 were classified as
decayed, 13.5 as missing, and 5.7 as filled. At equivalent ages,
women's DMF scores are one or two points higher than men's.
However, the number of decayed teeth is essentially the same for the
two sexes, the disparity resulting primarily from the number of
missing teeth. The overall DMF score rises steadily with advancing

Table 4.18   Average DMF score of adults and average number of decayed, missing, or filled teeth per person by sex and age: United States, 1960-62

Sex and age	DMF	Decayed	Missing	Filled
Both sexes				
Total, 18-79	20.4	1.2	13.5	5.7
Male				
Total, 18-79	19.6	1.2	12.9	5.5
18-24	13.6	2.2	5.0	6.5
25-34	16.2	1.7	6.9	7.6
35-44	18.1	1.2	9.5	7.4
45-54	20.8	1.0	15.2	4.6
55-64	24.5	0.7	20.7	3.0
65-74	26.7	0.4	24.3	1.9
75-79	28.6	0.3	27.4	0.9
Female				
Total, 18-79	21.1	1.1	14.0	6.0
18-24	14.4	2.0	5.3	7.1
25-34	18.4	1.5	9.0	7.9
35-44	20.1	1.2	11.5	7.5
45-54	22.1	0.9	15.6	5.6
55-64	25.7	0.5	21.3	3.9
65-74	27.7	0.3	24.8	2.6
75-79	29.6	0.2	27.9	1.5

Source: National Center for Health Statistics, Series 11, Table 5 of no. 7, Washington, February 1965.

age because of the increased number of missing teeth. Numbers of decayed and filled teeth decline steadily with age as these diseased teeth are extracted or otherwise lost. The data shown in Table 4.18 include edentulous persons; their exclusion reduces the total DMF scores by about one-eighth, but does not affect the age-sex relationships.

The average DMF score for white adults, 21.2, is about 50 percent higher than the score for blacks, 14.5. The higher score for whites results from their excess of filled teeth (6.3 per person as compared to 1.3 for blacks) and, to a lesser extent, to their excess of missing teeth (13.9 for whites and 11.3 for blacks). Blacks, however, did have slightly more decayed teeth than did whites. Nonetheless, it is apparent that dental disease takes a lesser toll among blacks. The overall relationship between the two racial groups was essentially unchanged over the entire age range.[16]

At all ages and in both races DMF scores are higher for women than for men. Overall the difference between the sexes is greater among blacks than among whites. This is largely attributable to differences in the number of teeth missing. The suggestion is that women in fact have poorer dental health than men rather than that women seek more dental attention—in which case their score for missing teeth would be lower and that for filled teeth, higher.

While prevalence rates of dental disease vary between persons of differing age, sex, and color, none of these characteristics provides an understanding of the determinants of dental health, nor can they be modified or favorably altered. Other personal characteristics also are related to prevalence rates of dental disease. One of these—years of education—is apparently a major correlate of dental health, at least as indicated by the proportion of the population that is edentulous. Among men with less than five years of education, the rate of those who are edentulous (40.2 for whites and 15.3 for blacks) is three to four times as high as the rate among men with nine to twelve years of education. Among women, the gradient is even more striking, being about four-fold for whites and five-fold for blacks. However, even within education levels, the previously mentioned differences by sex and color persist—except that no sex difference is evident among whites with nine to twelve years of education.[17]

The association of education with dental health is apparent when DMF scores are used as well as numbers of edentulous persons. With increasing levels of education the mean DMF score among dentulous persons increases. However, this results from a great increase in the number of filled teeth among persons in the upper education levels, since in these same categories there is a decrease in the average number of teeth decayed or missing. In this context, it is especially interesting that education is a better predictor of edentulous status than is family income. For example, at the lowest family income level (under $2,000 annually) as compared with the highest ($10,000 and over) there is slightly more than three-fold difference in the prevalence rate of edentulous white men, from 37.1 per 100 to 11.8.[17] However, the extremes of education are associated with about a five-fold difference in prevalence rates, the rates for white males in the lowest education group (less than five years) being 40.2 and in the highest (thirteen years or more) 7.9.[17] Where data are adequate, similar observations may be made for the other sex-color groups. It may be true that the apparently sharper gradient of dental health with education than with income is an artifact attributable to the comparison of smaller, more extremely divergent groups with respect to education than with respect to income. Available data do not permit resolution of this speculation. However, since the trend of disease with education is sharper over the entire range of the education variable than is the trend of disease with income, the explanation suggested seems unlikely. The data are promising, then, in implying that dental health will improve in the near future as the educational level of older persons rises sharply in the next few decades. For more extensive discussion of dental disease, the reader is referred to the monograph by Pelton and his associates.[18]

Discussion

Most of the information on morbidity currently available in the United States is provided by continuous health interview surveys of the population and is expressed in terms of the incidence rates of acute conditions and the prevalence rates of chronic conditions. The most notable feature of acute conditions, in addition to appreciable fluctuations in incidence rates over time, is the inverse association of incidence rate with age. In general, women have higher incidence rates than men and sustain more resultant disability. Major differences in incidence rates appear between persons with different family incomes; these are especially marked for the digestive conditions, which are nearly twice as frequent among persons with low family income (under $2,000) as among those with higher income (over $7,000).

The chronic conditions also show a striking association with age, but unlike acute conditions the association here is direct. Again, chronic conditions are more frequent among women than among men, but the associated disability is similar for both sexes. There is a strong inverse association of the prevalence of chronic conditions and family income. However, the data suggest that low income levels are themselves an effect, rather than a cause, of chronic conditions.

In addition to these interview data, morbidity can be assessed through information on utilization of medical care. Data on hospital discharge rates, length of hospital stay, and physician visits have been presented, and the patterns that emerge largely corroborate those based on interview data.

From the data on mental illness presented from several sources, it appears that men have higher incidence rates than women of both minor and severe mental illness throughout the life-span, but this sex difference is more apparent among the young than among the elderly. Finally, with respect to dental disease, it appears that women are more severely afflicted than men, and whites more than blacks. Nonetheless, the data suggest that education can be used effectively to improve dental health. Indeed, this general impression of lower disease frequencies among persons with higher levels of education and income suggests that the health inequities that exist in the United States can be diminished further by increases in the over-all standard of living, especially through education.

5 / GEOGRAPHIC VARIATION IN MORTALITY AND MORBIDITY

Herbert I. Sauer

For more than a century, public health statisticians and epidemiologists have been concerned with geographic variation in the incidence of disease and death. In 1846, Shattuck clearly expressed the goal of identifying the geographic differences in disease rates and then searching for factors responsible for these differences.[1,2] More recently, the National Center for Health Statistics and Duffy and Carroll have presented extensive tables showing such differences.[3-6] Woolsey, Enterline, and others have presented analyses of geographic variations.[7-11] Sartwell has emphasized the study of geographic variations in health as a major component of epidemiology.[12]

Variation by Geographic Division

Variations in crude death rates for all causes in 1959-61 are somewhat limited when observed for the nine geographic divisions of the United States, as defined by the Bureau of the Census[13] and shown in Appendix Fig. A.5.1. The division with the highest rate, New England, has a rate 31 percent higher than the division with the lowest rate, the Mountain states (Table 5.1). However, this apparently large difference is the result mainly of variations in the age-sex-color composition of the two divisions; thus, age-adjusted rates for white males are only about 2 percent higher for New England than for the Mountain states, and those for white females only 7 percent higher. For geographic divisions generally, the variations in age-adjusted rates occur independently of the crude-rate variations. As a specific example, the coefficient of correlation between the crude death rates and the age-adjusted rate for all races and both sexes combined, for all nine geographic divisions, is only + 0.17.

These variations, however, are not uniform for the different age-sex-color groups (Appendix Table A.5.1). New England whites under age 45 and nonwhites under age 55 have age-sex-color-specific rates lower than those for the Mountain state residents. Above these ages the age-specific rates for New England residents are somewhat higher, thereby resulting in slightly higher age-adjusted rates.

105

Table 5.1   Crude and age-adjusted death rates per 100,000 population, for all causes by sex and color: United States and each geographic division, 1959-61

Geographic division	Crude rates	Age-adjusted rates				
		Total	White		Nonwhite	
			Male	Female	Male	Female
United States	943.1	751.6	906.3	549.7	1,185.4	878.5
New England	1,049.8	735.3	920.3	569.4	1,127.8	803.8
Middle Atlantic	1,047.1	788.1	946.0	604.6	1,232.4	872.1
E. No. Central	950.4	749.6	908.1	563.2	1,152.1	872.2
W. No. Central	999.1	679.3	839.1	502.6	1,227.7	909.8
S. Atlantic	887.8	796.5	915.7	525.2	1,323.9	957.7
E. So. Central	935.5	782.9	900.8	532.4	1,214.2	933.2
W. So. Central	853.7	723.9	877.2	494.7	1,118.4	841.5
Mountain	798.8	724.0	898.0	529.7	1,095.2	776.4
Pacific	857.1	703.4	887.4	524.0	871.5	624.7

Those concerned with the epidemiologic search for factors other than age, sex, or color that are associated with disease and death obviously need to use sex-color-specific rates that are appropriately age adjusted, and in many instances it will be necessary to use age-specific rates as well. However, those concerned with variations in the risk of dying, regardless of cause, and its relation to the delivery of health care and other services will find even crude rates of value.

Whites

Table 5.1 shows that the lowest age-adjusted rates among whites are for the West Central states, with the West North Central states having slightly lower rates for males and the West South Central states for females. For the West North Central states, crude rates are consistently high because of the high proportion of elderly people in the population. The Middle Atlantic states have the highest age-adjusted death rates among whites, the rate for males being 13 percent higher than that for males in the West North Central states and the rate for females 22 percent higher than that for females in the West South Central states. These differences are definitely more pronounced during, roughly ages 45-74, males having 20 percent higher and females approximately 36 percent higher rates for the Middle Atlantic states than for the geographic divisions with the lowest rates.

In each geographic division the age-adjusted death rates among whites by sex are lower for 1959-61 than for 1949-51 with the most pronounced difference observed for white males of the Pacific states.[14] In spite of this difference between areas, the pattern of variation for 1949-51 is remarkably similar to that for 1959-61; specifically, the age-adjusted rates for the nine geographic divisions have a correlation between the two periods of + 0.87 for white males and + 0.97 for white females.

Nonwhites

For nonwhites, the Pacific and Mountain states have the lowest reported mortality rates. In these geographic divisions substantial portions of the nonwhites are of Oriental and American Indian ancestry. The South Atlantic geographic division has the highest mortality rate for nonwhites; indeed, there is a greater percentage difference between the highest and the lowest-rate divisions for nonwhites than in a similar comparison for whites.

In addition to recognition of the differences in ethnic composition of nonwhites in various parts of the country, two elements of undetermined importance deserve attention: (*a*) uncertainty regarding the quality of demographic data for some American Indian groups, and (*b*) uncertainty regarding accuracy of age determination for nonwhites, particularly in the Southeast.[15-19]

Variation by State

States, as smaller and less heterogeneous units than geographic divisions, constitute a means of identifying geographic variation in greater detail. The state with the highest mortality rate for white males, Nevada (Table A.5.2), has an age-adjusted rate for all causes approximately 36 percent higher than the state with the lowest rates, North Dakota. A similar contrast exists for white females.

For each sex the three states with the lowest age-adjusted rates among whites, arranged in sequence of male rates, are the following:

	Male	*Female*
North Dakota	795.7	
Nebraska	812.0	483.7
Kansas	813.9	
Florida		468.3
Arkansas		477.2

These and several other states all had lower rates than did the geographic division with the lowest rates.

The three states with the highest rates for each sex among whites are as follows:

	Male	*Female*
Nevada	1,082.8	
South Carolina	1,003.1	
Hawaii	991.8	638.2
Pennsylvania		612.2
New York		603.2

In general, most states with high rates for males are in the East, while the high-rate states for females tend to be in or near the Middle Atlantic geographic division; the exceptions are Nevada and Hawaii.

Prior Decades and Migration

The age-adjusted death rates among whites are lower for 1959-61 than for 1949-51 in high-rate as well as low-rate states. Utah is clearly among the group of lowest-rate states for 1959-61, even though in prior periods it was closer to the overall U.S. rate. The other lowest-rate states generally showed less deviation from the U.S. rate than they did in 1949-51 or 1939-41.[5]

Among whites, Florida rates and the rates for California males showed a greater decline from prior periods than did the U.S. rate, but only Florida females fell into the "lowest rate" category. Those born in Florida had age-specific death rates similar to the rates for the United States as a whole, but those of retirement age who had been born in the North had particularly low rates, very strongly suggesting a hypothesis of selective migration.[20] An opposite pattern is apparent for California white males, with those born in California clearly having lower rates than those moving into the state.

For the U.S. as a whole, migration does not appear to affect patterns of mortality greatly. Death rates for all causes, calculated by state of birth for native-born white males aged 45-64, for the 46 states with the largest population showed a coefficient of correlation of + 0.88 with the usual death rates by state of residence.[20]

High-rate states in 1959-61 also tended to show less deviation from the U.S. rates than they did in prior periods. One exception to this generalization is the state of Hawaii, with age-specific rates for ages 45 and over generally tending to be higher in 1959-61 than in 1949-51.

Metropolitan vs Nonmetropolitan Areas

Among whites, by sex, the age-adjusted mortality rates for metropolitan areas are 5 to 6 percent higher than for nonmetropolitan areas (Table A.5.3). This difference is not consistent, however, with the metropolitan areas of the South Atlantic and Mountain states having slightly lower rates than the nonmetropolitan areas, and with white males of New England having nominally lower rates for metropolitan counties than for nonmetropolitan.

As a group, metropolitan counties containing central cities have slightly higher rates than do suburban counties—that is, metropolitan counties without central cities, rates for white males being about 9 percent higher and those for females about 5 percent higher. An exception is the East South Central division with higher rates in the "metropolitan counties without central cities." However, more than two-thirds of the deaths in this category are of residents of two high-rate areas: Russell County (Alabama), and Campbell and Kenton counties (Kentucky). The central cities for each of these areas (Columbus, Georgia, and Cincinnati, Ohio) lie outside the East South Central division. This illustrates the degree of arbitrariness encountered in identifying geographic divisions and other geographic entities.

In general, the rates for whites in the nonmetropolitan counties are similar to those in the suburban counties; for nonwhites there is little difference, on the average, in death rates for metropolitan counties as compared with nonmetropolitan.

Under 45 years of age, death rates tend to be lower for metropolitan areas than for nonmetropolitan areas, the only exception being white females aged 35-44 (Table A.5.4). Among whites under age 45, the suburban counties as a group rather consistently have rates lower than either central-city or nonmetropolitan counties, while for ages 45-84 the suburban counties generally have rates slightly higher than the nonmetropolitan rates.

Variation by State Economic Areas

Areas smaller and more homogeneous than states have already been demonstrated to have greater geographic variation in mortality than do larger, more heterogeneous units.[6,9,21,22] One such geographic classification is state economic areas, as defined by the Bureau of Census. These consist in (a) 206 metropolitan state economic areas, each including one or more counties of a metropolitan area lying wholly within the same state, and (b) 303 nonmetropolitan areas, each usually consisting of six to twenty contiguous counties, within a state, which have similar economic and social characteristics. A map of these state economic areas (SEA's) is presented in Figs. A.5.2 and A.5.3; these figures are adapted from the Bureau of the Census report,[23] which also lists the names of the counties within each SEA.

Age-Specific Rates

Age-specific rates have been shown to be more suitable than age-adjusted rates for all ages in identifying differences in rates between geographic divisions and between metropolitan and non-metropolitan counties, thus supporting the recommendation of a distinguished committee of three decades ago.[24]

The selection of age groups 45-54 and 55-64, combined into a single group of "middle age," focuses attention upon more marked geographic differences. State economic areas had an average of more than a thousand deaths among middle-aged white males during the three-year period 1959-61. Thus, random error or chance fluctuation is generally not a serious problem; moreover, random error may be further reduced by the use of rates for ages 35-74, which consistently show a very close parallel to those for 45-64 (Table A.5.5).

All rates are calculated as ten-year age-specific death rates. For broader age groups, age-specific age-adjusted rates were calculated by the direct method, using as a standard population the total U.S. population for the age group concerned in 1950. The rates for both sexes aged 45-74 were similarly calculated as age-sex-adjusted rates. In this way the results are comparable with those cited in other reports.[9,25-28]

White Males

The 64 state economic areas with the lowest rates for white males, the lowest one-eighth or octile, are located largely in the Great Plains, with several areas in the mid-South and in the Rocky Mountains (Fig. 5.1 and Table A.5.5).*

Many of the areas in the highest octile of death rates for white males are located in the Southeast, but some are also in East Central Pennsylvania, Appalachia, Hawaii, Nevada, and the Gulf Coast. To a very substantial extent the areas in the second highest octile are located close to areas in the highest octile, and areas in the second lowest octile are in reasonable proximity to the areas in the lowest octile.

The two lowest octiles together are obviously comparable to the lowest quartile of other presentations.[8] The "middle half" is simply the second and third quartiles; the range of rates within this middle half is similar to that within the lowest octile, and substantially less than the variation within the highest octile.

Lowest-rate SEA's. A dozen areas had rates for white males of less than 11.0 deaths per 1,000 population. Of these lowest-rates areas, four are in Nebraska, four in Minnesota, two in the Dakotas, one in northern Arkansas, and one in Utah. All of these areas are strictly nonmetropolitan by any standard, except Utah SEA 2, which includes the cities of Provo and Orem.

Highest-rate SEA's. The dozen areas with the highest white male rates, from 18.6 to 22.3 per 1,000 population, are nearly all in the East, the only exceptions being Nevada SEA 1 (including Reno) and the New Orleans metropolitan area. Two of the high-rate areas, Hudson County (including Jersey City, New Jersey) and the District of Columbia, are in essence "center-city" areas and are not really complete metropolitan areas of themselves.

Five of the highest-rate areas are small to moderate-sized metropolitan areas: Scranton and Wilkes-Barre-Hazelton in Pennsylvania, Charleston (South Carolina), Augusta (Georgia), and Russell County, the latter being the Alabama portion of the Columbus (Georgia) metropolitan area.

*Appendix Figs. A.5.2 and A.5.3 identify the location of the nonmetropolitan SEA's with more precision than do the parenthetical descriptions in Table A.5.5.

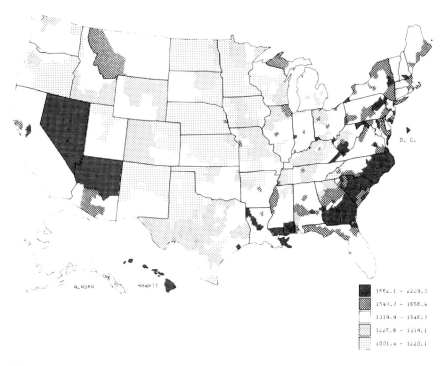

Figure 5.1 Death rates per 100,000 population for all causes among white males aged 45–64 years old by state economic areas: United States, 1959–61

The three nonmetropolitan areas in this highest-rate group are South Carolina SEA 6, in the east central portion of the state, North Carolina SEA 7 (Northeast), and Virginia SEA 9 (Eastern Shore).

White Females

The patterns for white females are somewhat similar to those for white males, but with the lowest-octile areas concentrated to a greater extent in the southern part of the Great Plains and mid-South, and with more of the highest-octile areas located in the Northeast and Chicago and Michigan areas (Fig. 5.2 and Table A.5.5). In most of the Southeast the rates for white females are more or less average, in contrast to the high rates for white males in this section.

Lowest-rate SEA's. The dozen lowest-rate SEA's had rates c f 4.5 to 5.1 deaths per 1,000 population, seven of which were in central Texas, two in the adjacent states of Oklahoma and Arkansas, and the

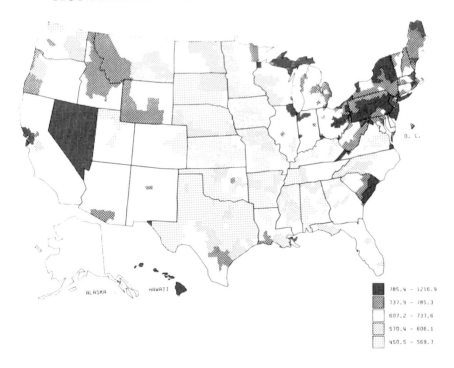

▓ (black)	785.4 - 1216.9
▒	737.9 - 785.3
☐	607.2 - 737.6
▒	570.4 - 606.1
⋯	450.5 - 569.7

Figure 5.2 Death rates per 100,000 population for all causes among white females aged 45–64 years old by state economic areas: United States, 1959–61

others in Missouri, Tennessee, and Utah. The Abilene (Texas) metropolitan area, consisting of Jones and Taylor counties, had the lowest rate; the Denton metropolitan area (Denton County) is also included in this group, but the other areas were all nonmetropolitan. These are obviously less than half the rates for males of the same age group in the lowest-male-rate SEA's.

The lowest-rate areas for one sex consistently have below-average rates for the other sex. For each sex the lowest-rate areas are concentrated in the Great Plains, but the lowest-rate areas for females are in the southern portion and for males in the northern half of this section of the country.

Highest-rate SEA's. Three areas in East Central Pennsylvania and four metropolitan areas in New Jersey were among the dozen with highest rates, from 8.7 to 12.2 per 1,000 population. Two were in Hawaii, two on Lake Superior (one Michigan nonmetropolitan area and Superior, Wisconsin), and El Paso, Texas. Even these highest-rate

SEA's had, with two exceptions, rates *lower* than the rates of the SEA's with lowest rates for white males.

For white females, the highest-rate areas thus are concentrated to a greater extent in the Middle Atlantic States, whereas for males they are more widely distributed from Pennsylvania to Georgia. Areas with the highest rates for white females also generally had high rates for white males: in fact, for all but one of the nine areas with the highest female rates, the male rates were also in the highest quartile. Lackawanna County (including Scranton) and Luzerne County (including Wilkes-Barre and Hazelton) in Pennsylvania, and Hudson County (including Jersey City) in New Jersey, were in the highest-rate groups for each sex.

Age-specific rates for state economic areas provide the opportunity of identifying for further epidemiologic study geographic areas with substantially greater contrasts than do rates for all ages (age adjusted) for states and larger geographic areas. Specifically, the dozen state economic areas with the highest age-specific rates have rates which are 70 to 170 percent higher than any of the dozen areas with the lowest rates. For geographic divisions of the U.S., the extreme range in age-adjusted rates for white males is only 13 percent; for states, it is 36 percent.

Random Error

The effect of the environment and other possible relevant factors upon death rates in middle age is obviously subject to chance fluctuation or random error, which we have measured in several ways, each with limitations.

(*a*) We calculated the standard error, assuming a binomial distribution and using the refinement proposed by Chiang.[29] According to this method, the rates for Nebraska SEA's 4 and 5 are significantly lower than those for Scranton (Pennsylvania) and South Carolina areas 6 and 7, at the 0.001 level. These areas were picked on the basis of their rates in prior studies.

(*b*) We compared rates for several age-specific groups to see if their geographic patterns are similar. The low-rates are consistently low and the high are consistently high, as compared with the United States rate. However, no single area consistently has the highest rate for every age group and, frequently, similar difficulties are encountered in determining from the age-specific rates the area with the lowest overall risk. As a method of measuring random error, this approach assumes that the geographic pattern of risk is the same for each age group, subject only to chance fluctuation; however, restraint must be exercised in using this assumption. The same kind of analysis may be applied to different sex and color groups, with similar limitations applying.

(c) We observed whether or not geographic patterns persisted over time. For example, the geographic pattern shown in Fig. 5.1 is similar to that determined for 1949-51 by slightly different methods.[9] Work presently in progress will permit making such comparisons with greater precision.

(d) By measures of contiguity applied in a prior study, a determination may be made of the extent to which contiguous areas have similar rates.[27,30] This method tests whether the factors affecting death rates, whatever they may be, extend over several adjacent areas.

(e) We measured the homogeneity of rates, county by county, within the multicounty state economic areas with the lowest and highest rates. These results may be summarized as follows, for death rates for all causes in 1959-61 among white males aged 45-64:

	Nebraska SEA 5	South Carolina SEA 6
Death rate per 1,000 population	10.0	19.0
Number of counties	11	11
Standard deviation	0.9	2.3
Death rate in lowest-rate county	8.4	15.6
Death rate in highest-rate county	11.6	24.5

In view of the small populations in some rural counties, substantial chance fluctuation from county to county might be expected. Even so, the lowest county rate in the high-rate area is substantially higher than the highest country rate in the Nebraska area. Such a distribution may be assumed to indicate a statistically significant difference in rates by almost any standard. However, in using this method to measure random error, one is assuming a homogeneity of the forces of mortality within a state economic area. In view of the fact that these are groupings of counties into state economic areas, it scarcely seems reasonable to assume that such a group of counties will necessarily be homogeneous with regard to the unknown factors in the environment that affect the risk of dying in middle age.

Similar shortcomings may be pointed out in the other approaches. The first method proposed above makes assumptions regarding the nature of the distribution. The other methods all seem to assume a homogeneity of risk, and a similarity of relevant environment by age group, sex, color, time periods or years, and area. Present evidence suggests that such assumptions may be sound for a substantial portion of the time but not all the time.

We therefore recognize that we have only begun the study of suitable techniques for measuring random error. For the time being, it seems appropriate to use all of these methods, but to recognize the assumptions being made. It is apparent from this work, that these variations are not randomly scattered in space and are not likely to result from chance.

Persistence over Time

In general, there is a very substantial degree of similarity in the patterns of geographic variation for 1959-61 as compared with 1949-51. The earlier data were tabulated by standard metropolitan areas and the nonmetropolitan portions of economic subregions, a total of 279 areas; in many instances these consisted of two or more state economic areas, thus making precise comparisons difficult. Even with differences in definition of geographic areas, the lowest-rate and highest-rate areas presented in Fig. 5.1 fall generally in the same sections of the country as they did in 1949-51.[9]

The similarity may be described more specifically by considering the dozen state economic areas with the lowest and highest rates in 1959-61, and comparing them with the rates of the economic subregion or metropolitan areas in which the SEA was classified in 1949-51. For white males aged 45-64, all twelve lowest-rate areas in 1959-61 were in economic subregions in the lowest quartile in 1949-51; of the twelve highest-rate SEA's in 1959-61, ten were in metropolitan areas or economic subregions in the highest quartile in 1949-51. For white females aged 45-64, a similar degree of consistency is observed: of the twelve lowest-rate SEA's in 1959-61, ten were in the lowest quartile of areas in 1949-51 and two were in the lower portion of the second quartile. Of the twelve highest-rate SEA's nine were in the highest quartile in 1949-51. For white females the decline in death rates between 1949-51 and 1959-61 was quite substantial, and even in these highest-rate areas, only the two Hawaii areas suggested patterns indicating a clear increase in rates.

Analysis of data for 1940, involving the use of still different methods of classification, produced a pattern with substantial similarity to the patterns for more recent years, particularly in identifying low rates for white males in portions of the West North Central states.[31]

For states with areas having very high or very low death rates, specifically Georgia, North Carolina, Missouri, and Nebraska, deaths have been tabulated and rates calculated for the ten-year period 1950-59 inclusive (1955-60 for Nebraska). Rates by state economic areas and by counties for this longer span of years present patterns very similar to those given in Figs. 5.1 and 5.2 for 1959-61.[27, 32, 33]

The major geographic variations in mortality thus are not transient in time.

Age Relationships

After age 15, the annual risk of dying increases markedly as one becomes older. For all natural causes—that is, for all causes of death combined except accidental and violent causes—from early adult life until age 95, the annual risk of dying for each specific year of age is approximately 10 percent greater than for the preceding year. It has already been shown that this increase is not uniform throughout the United States (Table A.5.1).

The geographic patterns of death rates for ages 65-74 have been shown to be similar to but not identical with patterns for ages 45-64.[21] Whatever factors in the environment affect the risk of dying, it seems reasonable to hypothesize that they do not necessarily affect each age group equally. An exploratory step, then, is to calculate the degree of association of death rates for any specific age group with other age groups. A summary of the coefficients of correlation so derived is presented in Table 5.2. In general, for the 509 SEA's of the United States, the correlation of death rates for any specific age group with an adjacent age group is high. For example, for white males aged 55-64 and 65-74, the correlation is + 0.76. Conversely, for age groups several decades apart, the correlation is likely to be low. Specifically, for ages 35-44 and 75 and over the correlation is only + 0.02. (With $n = 509$, a correlation of 0.12 or larger would ordinarily be considered statistically significant at the 0.01 level.)

The correlations with adjacent age groups of the same sex tend to be slightly higher than the correlations of rates for males with those

Table 5.2   Coefficients of correlation between age-sex-specific death rates for all causes, among whites at specified ages, by sex: United States, 509 state economic areas, 1959-61

Sex and age	45-54	55-64	65-74	75 & over
Male				
35-44	+.53	+.33	+.14	+.02
45-54		+.76	+.62	+.31
55-64			+.76	+.42
65-74				+.56
Female				
35-44	+.40	+.34	+.29	+.12
45-54		+.61	+.57	+.32
55-64			+.80	+.59
65-74				+.67
Male with female of same age	+.38	+.55	+.68	+.68

Note: All coefficients are statistically significant at the .01 level except +.02.

for females in the same age group (Table 5.2). Similar correlations are observed for major cause categories such as cardiovascular-renal diseases and coronary heart disease, correlated separately by geographic areas by age and by sex. These patterns of association seem to lend support to the use of several adjacent age groups to form age-adjusted age-specific death rates, such as ages 45-64 and 35-74. They also suggest the need for caution in the use of age-adjusted death rates for all ages in epidemiologic studies.

Sex Ratios

Death rates already presented by sex clearly indicate that death rates for females tend to parallel those for males, but not perfectly. For all causes of death, for the 509 SEA's of the United States in 1959-61, the coefficient of correlation of whites aged 45-64 by sex is + 0.56 and aged 35-74 by sex is + 0.66. It therefore seems appropriate to describe both similarities and differences by sex in patterns of death rates.

The sex ratio, male rate to female rate, provides a measure for studying such patterns, and for whites aged 45-64 these ratios for state economic areas are presented in Table A.5.5 and in Fig. 5.3. In

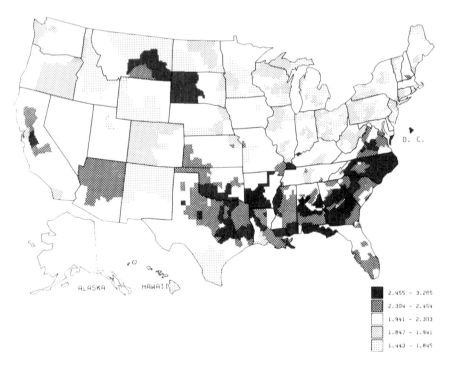

■	2.455 - 3.265
▨	2.304 - 2.454
☐	1.941 - 2.303
▦	1.847 - 1.941
⠿	1.443 - 1.845

Figure 5.3 Ratio of male to female death rates at ages 45–64 years for all causes by state economic areas: United States, 1959–61

the figure the blank portions of the United States are the one-half of the state economic areas with sex ratios closest to the median ratio; that is, the patterns of rates for males are similar to those for females, with male rates double or slightly more than double the female rates. These areas are widely scattered, but a substantial portion of them are located in the central United States. They include some high-rate areas such as Nevada, New York, and other areas north of Chesapeake Bay. They also include some of the low-rate areas of the Great Plains.

The areas in the lowest octile of ratios have rates for males only 40 to 80 percent higher than those for females. These include (a) areas with high female rates, such as in New Jersey, Pennsylvania, and Hawaii, (b) Minnesota and other Great Plains areas with low male rates, and (c) areas with a high proportion of the population having Spanish surnames. The latter is to be expected in view of the extremely low death rates for males born in Mexico, accompanied by an above-average rate for females born in Mexico.[34]

The areas in the highest octile of ratios, those with rates for males

150 to 230 percent higher than those for females, are nearly all located in the South, and the areas in the two highest octiles or the highest quartile are also generally in the South. This suggests the hypothesis that whatever the factors in the South related to the risk of dying are, they affect males more than females. In the Southeast, male rates are particularly high, while the female rates are roughly average. In the Southwest, the male rates are slightly below average and are accompanied by extremely low female rates.

A relatively small area with similar high sex ratios is western South Dakota and southeastern Montana, with adjacent areas to the north having very low ratios. Figure 5.3 thus identifies a section of the country with an unusual pattern of ratios, which may warrant more intensive epidemiologic study than would be inferred from the pattern of rates alone.

The 1949-51 rates for metropolitan areas and economic subregions produce a similar pattern of high ratios in the South and low ratios in areas of the Northeast and northern half of the Great Plains.

Cause Correlations

In the study of geographic variations in death rates, a restriction to all causes of death is obviously too narrow an approach. But the use of cause-specific rates may in some instances assume a greater degree of uniformity from one geographic area to another, in determining the underlying cause of death, than is warranted. A comprehensive summary of factors relevant in this regard is presented in the monographs on cardiovascular diseases and cancer.[35, 36]

A substantial degree of geographic association exists between the death rates for all causes and those for the cardiovascular-renal (CVR) diseases, the product moment coefficient of correlation being in the vicinity of + 0.90 for whites aged 35-74, by sex, for the 509 state economic areas (Tables A.5.6 and A.5.7). Since the CVR diseases are charged with more deaths than all other causes combined, and since this is a correlation of a part with a whole, a positive correlation is to be expected. It is, however, high enough to suggest that in instances in which the death rates for CVR diseases are not available, the death rates for all causes provide a fairly good, but not perfect, basis for estimating the relative levels of the death rates for the CVR diseases. Let us look at a specific illustration. For white persons aged 35-74 we have 1959-61 age-adjusted death rates for all causes and for the CVR diseases for each state economic area; we have currently calculated the death rate for the mid-1960's for all causes (but do not have age-sex-color-specific data for each cause). From the rates for all causes we expect to make fairly good, but not perfect, estimates of the death rates for the CVR diseases for the mid-1960's by assuming that over the short term the 1959-61 relative relationship between the two rates persists.

The cardiovascular-renal diseases also have a high correlation ($r =$ approximately $+0.90$) with coronary heart disease, or more specifically, classification 420 of the International List, Seventh Revision: arteriosclerotic heart disease, including coronary disease. While here again we deal with the correlation of the whole with a part, the relevant point is the same: when coronary heart disease death rates are not available or are in question, CVR death rates are likely to provide a fairly good basis for estimating rates for coronary heart disease.

Death rates for malignant neoplasms have correlations with coronary heart disease by state economic areas that are substantial: for males, $r = +0.63$ and for females, $r = +0.59$. They also have fairly high correlations with the CVR diseases: for each sex separately, $r = +0.55$. In view of evidence implicating cigarette smoking and community air pollution for both lung cancer and coronary heart disease, the hypothesis may be presented that, to some extent, there are common causal factors. Yet the correlations are equally high for "malignant neoplasms other than lung cancer" and coronary heart disease (Tables A.5.6 and A.5.7). These correlations do not appreciably result from the fact that both malignant neoplasms and coronary heart disease death rates tend to be higher in metropolitan areas, because the correlations are almost as high when calculated separately for the group of 206 metropolitan areas and 303 nonmetropolitan areas (Table A.5.8).

Chronic respiratory diseases death rates appear to fluctuate by geographic area independently of the patterns of any other cause category thus far studied. The category of "accidental and violent deaths" combined also has very little similarity in geographic patterns to other cause categories; this generalization is similarly applicable, for the most part, to the category of rheumatic heart disease and rheumatic fever.

"All other" as a residual category includes diabetes, influenza, pneumonia, infectious diseases, cirrhosis of the liver, and all diseases not included elsewhere. The rates for this "all other" category have moderately low correlations with CVR diseases and malignant neoplasms for white males and a somewhat higher correlation for white females (Tables A.5.6 and A.5.7). It has already been demonstrated that the geographic patterns of all causes of death and of causes other than the cardiovascular diseases tend to parallel the geographic patterns of the cardiovascular diseases.[37,38] While this correlation is not extremely high, it persists sufficiently through time and through different geographic classifications (by states, by metropolitan areas, and by SEA's) to propose that whatever the factors may be that are causing geographic variations in death rates, they are not strictly cause-specific within the framework of the present classification of causes.

The parallel in death rates for the CVR diseases and malignant neoplasms is particularly suggestive for further study in specific areas. For example, the age-adjusted death rates of 1959-61 for white males aged 35-74 in many areas fall in the lowest octile of rates for both disease categories: areas in several Great Plain states, including Nebraska; in Mountain states such as Colorado, New Mexico, Utah, and Idaho; and also the Southern Blue Ridge SEA of western North Carolina. At the same time there are a number of areas in the East, in Louisiana, and the Nevada SEA that includes Reno, where the rates are in the highest octile for both categories. These parallels are suggested as providing a setting for testing various etiologic hypotheses: an example is the evidence already presented implicating cigarette smoking as an independent variable associated geographically with both lung cancer and coronary heart disease death rates.[39]

Associated Factors

Both low levels of smoking and large proportions of population engaged in farming have been demonstrated to be associated with low age-specific death rates.[21,39] These associations may very well explain some of the geographic variations in death rates, in view of the low rates reported for farmers of middle age and the high rates for smokers.[40,41] Many other factors have been identified as associated with statistically significant (0.01 level) geographic variations in age-specific death rates; these include characteristics of the drinking water, specifically low levels of total solids, hardness, calcium, magnesium, and sodium, as well as other factors such as low elevation above sea level, relative humidity, small average daily changes in January temperature, proportion of women working, and health manpower available.[10,11,21,22,26,27,38] The evidence pertaining to these and many other variables is, however, so inconclusive at present that it constitutes no more than leads for further study.

If the factors responsible for the experience of the areas with the lowest death rates could be identified, and if these factors could be applied to the United States as a whole, the question then arises: How many fewer deaths per year would occur? The lowest-rate areas for 1949-51 with a population of more than a million whites were selected and, in order to hold chance fluctuations and other factors to a minimum, calculations were made with the rates for a decade later, 1959-61. If the rates of the areas with the lowest rates replaced the U.S. actual rates, there would be approximately 160,000 fewer deaths per year under age 75.[22]

In view of such a potential for longer life, emphasis is being placed upon improving demographic and epidemiologic methods for further study. Currently available knowledge provides a very limited theoretical basis for explaining the known geographic variations. Still, the differences are of sufficient magnitude to be of major interest to health planners and others concerned with the delivery of health services. Table A.5.5 therefore gives death rates for specific areas, for use by administrators as well as by investigators who may wish to test hypotheses related to the risk of dying in middle age.

Morbidity

Morbidity prevalence also varies from one geographic region to another, although information on this subject is much more limited and difficult to collect than is information on mortality. The problems in this regard have been presented elsewhere.[42]

Incidence—that is, new cases of chronic diseases per year—may be more meaningful for measuring the impact of the environment upon the population. Such data are not generally available, and the intensive prospective investigations, such as the Framingham (Massachusetts) study of cardiovascular diseases are designed primarily for testing research hypotheses rather than for studying geographic variations.

Health Examination Survey

In the Health Examination Survey of the National Center for Health Statistics, prevalence data from an actual sample of the population of the United States provide estimates of physiological and medical characteristics of the population of the entire country and for three broad geographic regions: the Northeast, South, and West, as defined by Gordon.[43] As an example, white adults in the South have mean systolic blood pressures 5.0 mm Hg lower than those in the Northeast, whereas on the basis of the disparity in age-sex distributions the expected difference should definitely be less than half as large.[43] No appreciable differences, however, were noted by size of metropolitan area, or for rural areas. In this study most of the North Central states are classified as part of the West.

Health Interview Survey

Another approach to morbidity is the study of the proportion of the population having one or more chronic conditions, as obtained by the Health Interview Survey of the National Center for Health Statistics and presented in Table 5.3 for four geographic regions of the United States;[44,45] these regions are shown in Fig. A.5.1. In interpreting these rates it should be recognized that they are for all races combined.

Both for ages 45-64 and 65 and over, the Northeast region, consisting of the New England and Middle Atlantic divisions, rather consistently presents a pattern of a lower proportion of the population with one or more chronic conditions than the other regions; correspondingly, the Northeast also has a higher percentage of those reporting no chronic conditions. On the other hand, the South, including the South Atlantic, East South Central, and West South Central divisions, appears to have a higher proportion with one or more chronic conditions.

When the definition of "chronic conditions" is restricted to those involving activity limitations, the percentages are all reduced but the geographic pattern persists. This generalization holds even further when the definition is restricted to chronic conditions that limit the amount or kind of major activity.

The chronic conditions appear to be not only more prevalent but more severe in the South than in the Northeast.[44] Specifically, those aged 65 and over with one or more chronic conditions had 24.2 days of bed disability per person per year in the South, whereas in the Northeast they had only 13.5 days. Middle-aged individuals (45-64) in the South reported a nominally greater number of bed days' disability than did those aged 65 and over in the Northeast, in spite of the usual increase in disability with age. The rigid specification of

Table 5.3   Percent of persons with one or more chronic conditions and percent hospitalized, age 45-64 and age 65 and over: United States by geographic region, specified periods, 1957-62

Age and region	July 1957-June 1961		July 1960-June 1962
	With one or more chronic conditions	With activity limitation	Hospitalized
45-64			
United States	60.6	17.4	9.5
Northeast	55.2	14.1	8.6
North Central	61.3	16.8	9.8
South	63.3	20.5	10.1
West	64.3	18.5	9.2
65 & over			
United States	78.0	43.7	11.2
Northeast	73.8	38.3	9.8
North Central	77.6	43.1	11.6
South	81.8	50.1	12.2
West	79.7	43.0	11.0

Source: Wilder, C.S., Bed disability among the chronically limited, United States, July 1957 - June 1961. National Center for Health Statistics, Series 10, No. 12 (1964); Bollo, L.E. and Gleeson, G.A., Persons hospitalized by number of hospital episodes and days in year, United States, July 1960 - June 1962. National Center for Health Statistics, Series 10, No. 20 (1965).

persons aged 65 and over confined to the house with one or more chronic conditions provides an average of 137.8 days of bed disability per person in the South, as compared with 95.5 days in the Northeast.

Percent of the population hospitalized constitutes an objective measure of morbidity, but one that may be affected by the availability of beds in the region and the medical care practices involved in using these beds. The pattern for this measure is similar to that already presented: lowest for the Northeast and highest for the South (Table 5.3).

Although the percentages with reports of one or more chronic conditions have tended to increase in more recent years, the geographic pattern persists, lowest in the Northeast and highest in the South.[46] The New York metropolitan area for ages 45-64 and 65 and over, consistently has the lowest percentage "with one or more chronic conditions with activity limitations," while the Southern regions outside of metropolitan areas have the highest percentages.[47] The contrast is greatest for those aged 45-64 "with one or more chronic conditions with activity limitation": 11.6 percent for the New York area and 32.7 percent for the farm population of the South.

The reported incidence of acute conditions also tends in most years to be lowest or among the lowest for the Northeast.[48-53] The highest rates tend to be in the West.

For epidemiologic study, potential shortcomings in such morbidity data may be considered from several viewpoints. These percentages are for persons of all races, and "age 65 and over" is a broad, open-ended group. If it were possible to present more precise age-sex-race-specific rates, by place at which the chronic disease was acquired, the data would undoubtedly be more useful. Further, the data are for noninstitutional populations only; any geographic variations in the placement of patients in chronic disease hospitals or other resident institutions would affect the rates among the individuals at home. For the testing of epidemiologic hypotheses these possible limitations are of unknown magnitude. However, the data do present the variations of reported conditions of the persons living in these areas, which affect their needs for delivery of health care.

Discussion

Morbidity and mortality rates show some variations for the three or four regions, or other large geographic areas of the United States, but these are usually rather limited, particularly when attention is focused upon age-adjusted rates by sex for whites. The Northeast does, however, tend to have below-average morbidity prevalence and above-average mortality rates for ages 45-64, suggesting the possibility of high fatality rates.

For many characteristics that differ geographically and that may be hypothesized to affect the risk of disease and death, large geographic areas such as regions tend to be rather heterogeneous. Thus, in any consideration of the characteristics of both the independent and the dependent variables, regions do not appear to be the best choice as geographic units for testing epidemiologic hypotheses.

States are frequently useful units for study because of the availability of data for many variables, including mortality

rates.[4,8,35-39,54] However, states are basically units of governmental administration and are often rather heterogeneous with
regard to both environmental variables and mortality rates. The
rationale has been presented for the use of smaller, more homogeneous geographic units for describing differences.[42] Such units obviously have greater value in generating and testing epidemiologic
hypotheses than do states with diverse populations and environment.
While the use of counties may provide a greater degree of homogeneity for some characteristics, a substantial majority of the
counties in the United States have such a small population and a
resulting small number of deaths even within a three-year period that
rates thus calculated possess considerable random error.

Of the geographic units readily available, the 509 state economic
areas, as defined by the Bureau of the Census, seem to have
considerable merit.[23] They provide greater homogeneity than states
and generally have large enough populations to produce stable rates.

As units smaller than states are used, the adequacy of classification
of "usual residence" requires attention.[55] The major deficiency thus
far identified is the effect of counting patients in large mental
hospitals and inmates of other resident institutions as residents of the
county in which the institutions are located, while allocating their
deaths to the county from which they were admitted. When this
demographic problem is clearly present, adjustments have been made
in the estimated population at risk. Because of the substantial
difference in the risk of dying closely associated with age, sex, and
color, rates specific for these variables are required.

With the aforementioned refinements, it is evident that for middle-
aged whites geographic variations in the risk of mortality do exist,
which are not likely to result from chance, are not randomly
scattered in space, and are not transient in time. More specifically:

(1) Patterns for 1959-61 are generally similar to those for
1949-51, with low rates in the Great Plains and high rates
along the East Coast, in both periods.

(2) For white males aged 45-64, the highest mortality rates are
for areas in East Central Pennsylvania, the Southeast, and
other eastern areas; these rates are almost double those for
the lowest-rate areas of Nebraska and Minnesota.

(3) For white females aged 45-64, the highest-rate areas are in
New Jersey, Pennsylvania, and Hawaii, the death rates being

approximately twice as high as those in the lowest-rate areas of Texas, Oklahoma, Arkansas, and other states.

(4) For whites aged 45-64, there are many areas, nearly all in the South, with death rates for males about three times as high as those for females, for all causes of death, 1959-61. In portions of the Northeast, the northern half of the Great Plains, Hawaii, and other areas, the male rates are only about one and one-half times the female rates.

While nonwhites also show substantial geographic variation in rates, several demographic problems make it much more difficult to delineate the patterns of these rates in a meaningful way.[25]

Factors responsible for geographic differences may be primarily biological-physiological in nature, or genetic, or the result of differences in the physical environment, or of differences in the cultural environment, or in the interaction of two or more such variables. Whatever the causal nature of these associations, those born in Mexico have been demonstrated to have age-sex-specific rate patterns substantially different from those of other whites.[34]

The role of migration has been studied for its possible effect upon basic demographic analyses and also for its importance as a cultural factor.[20,56] As other factors of importance are clearly identified, further refinements in the specificity of their classifications may be needed.

At present the delineation of morbidity patterns within the South and other major geographic regions is quite limited.[44-53] In view of the marked variations in the risk of dying for various age-sex-color groups for smaller geographic areas, morbidity data for some of these areas may also be of value.

The death rates for the cardiovascular-renal diseases show a definite association with malignant neoplasm rates, for whites aged 35-74, each sex separately, for 509 state economic areas ($r = +0.55$). This and other cause-of-death correlation patterns suggest many potential approaches for further study. One of them is the possibility that some of the present cause categories are not properly defined for facilitating epidemiologic study. As long as the underlying causes of the various chronic diseases are largely unknown, there may be reservations about the appropriateness of present classifications. It is easy enough to be critical about the use of an obsolete diagnostic classification such as "typho-malarial fever," but in so doing, we should be reminded that even now we do not know which, if any, of the present categories of chronic disease might be equally unsound.[55]

Ninety years ago the statement was made:

The term *malaria* indicates the usual belief that it is due to contamination of the atmosphere—bad air; and a multitude of facts support this belief. A brief exposure . . . is often sufficient to produce poisoning of the most serious character; . . . the atmosphere is more highly charged with malaria at night . . . near the ground. . . . The possibility of the absorption of the malarial poison through the skin cannot be denied. . . .[57]

While infected mosquitoes were not yet being accepted as the essential component of the "bad air" that produced malaria, it seems appropriate to ask such questions as: Have we identified factors even as specific as "bad air" (in relation to malaria) that are consistently associated with geographic differences in chronic disease rates? Are we exercising sufficient ingenuity, care, and flexibility in classifying cause of death, in delineating geographic areas, in defining risk factors, and the like?

It is hoped that the specific relationships already described and in the process of being further developed will provide a basis for increasing the efficiency and effectiveness with which hypotheses pertaining to the search for etiologic factors are generated and critically tested.

6 / THE AGED: HEALTH, ILLNESS, DISABILITY, AND USE OF MEDICAL SERVICES

James O. Carpenter
Ray F. McArthur
Ian T. Higgins

During the past few decades there has been an increasing awareness of the medical problems of old people in the United States. This has arisen partly from the larger number and increasing proportion of the aged in the country and partly from the higher prevalence of chronic illness and the greater frequency of disability among them. The high and rising cost of medical care has made their difficulties particularly acute. Since the early 1940's an increasing amount of legislation has been aimed at alleviating the financial predicament of elderly sick persons, culminating in the Kerr-Mills amendment, or Medical Aid to the Aged, in 1960 and the 1965 amendments to the Social Security Act popularly known as Medicare.

For the purpose of this chapter, the elderly are defined as those persons aged 65 years and over. There are roughly 20 million of them; some 12 million aged 65-74, about 6.5 million aged 75-84, and about a million aged 85 and over. The elderly thus comprised about 10 percent of the total population in 1970, whereas in 1900 they constituted about 4 percent. Most of the increase occurred between 1930 and 1950, because of the declining birth rate before 1940 and high immigration until 1930. Since 1950 the ratio of the elderly to the total population has been much more constant. Only a small increase is predicted for the current decade. The average age of the elderly is increasing. In 1950 the median age of those aged 65 years and over was almost 72; in 1969 it was nearly 73. This change reflects an increasing proportion among the elderly of those aged 75-84.

There are some 135 older women to every 100 men aged 65 years and older in the United States, reflecting the lower life expectancy among men. The ratio increases with advancing age from 120 at ages 65-69 to over 160 at age 85 and older. This situation contributes to patterns in marital status among older people. Thus, most older men are married and most older women are widows. There are about four times as many widows as widowers. These facts also bear upon the living arrangements of older men and women: about three times as many older women as men live alone or with nonrelatives, and a higher proportion of older women than men are found in long-term institutions.

Since 1900 life expectancy at birth has increased from 47 to 71 years. At age 65, however, life expectancy is now only a few years more than it was at the beginning of the century. Thus, in 1900, men aged 65 could expect an average of 11.4 more years and women, 12.1; in 1967, the corresponding figures were 13 and 16.4 years respectively. (See also Chapter 1.)

A much higher proportion of these later years are now spent in retirement. A hundred years ago some 5 percent of men aged 65 and over were retired; the corresponding figure today is nearly 70 percent. In 1900 most of a 65-year-old man's remaining years were spent working; in 1960 less than half of them were. Retirement means a reduced and often fixed income, a shift from regular employment to unlimited free time, and a loss of working colleagues. Older families average less than half the incomes of younger families; older persons living alone or with nonrelatives have only two-fifths the income of their younger counterparts. A quarter of the older population lives in households with incomes below the poverty line for that type and size of family.

The economic situation of the elderly should be kept in mind when their health problems are being considered, especially in times of economic inflation. Fear of catastrophic illness, for example, may lead the older person to conserve meager resources. Selection of cheaper foods, particularly carbohydrates, may contribute to poor nutrition. Restricted finances will limit the use of health services. Financial straits often prevent the elderly from leading the full and active life of which they may be physically capable.

Sixty-five percent of elderly persons live in metropolitan areas, often in central cities. They must face all the problems of life in the city with their limited and declining resources. These include poor and often deteriorating housing, inadequate transportation, loneliness, and isolation. The elderly person is a ready victim of crime. Urban redevelopment and condemnation of property may force unwilling removal with the accompanying risks of illness and death.

Health of the Aged

Aging and ill-health are often considered to be synonymous. Shanas has written, "Most people believe that old age begins when health problems become limiting to the individual. People generally believe that most older people are only in 'fair' or 'poor' health."[1] This view is supported neither by the facts nor by the opinions of old people. Suchman and his colleagues, for example, found that older persons often considered their health to be better than their physicians rated it.[2] In fact, 61 percent of those whose health was rated unfavorably by their physician considered themselves to be in favorable health. This may reflect the fact that physicians, like people generally, tend to rate older persons by standards that are appropriate for younger persons. Older persons tend to rate themselves in relation to the activities they need to perform. Shanas summarized the salient facts about the health of old people on the basis of study of a representative sample: 4 percent live in institutions, 8-10 percent are housebound, 25-30 percent are ill at some time during the year, 12 percent enter the hospital for at least one day, 10 percent are seriously handicapped, and another 20 percent are moderately so.[3] Sixty to 70 percent are not ill in bed during the year and have not seen a doctor. Some of the evidence on which these statements are based is shown in Tables 6.1 to 6.3.

Elderly persons are more often confined to the house or to bed than are younger persons. The number of days spent in such confinement is also greater among them. While persons of all ages (0

Table 6.1 Percent of persons aged 65 and over reporting limitation of mobility: United States, 1957-58

Degree of limitation	Percent	
Total		100
No limitation of mobility		79
All limitation of mobility		21
Trouble getting around alone	12	
Unable to get around alone	4	
Confined to house	5	

Source: Bergsten, J.W., *Preliminary Report on Disability, United States, July-September, 1957,* U.S. National Health Survey, Series B, No. 4 (1958).

Table 6.2 Percent of persons aged 65 and over reporting
difficulty with common tasks, by sex:
United States, 1962

Task	Total (2,432)	Male (1,080)	Female (1,352)
Walking stairs	30	24	35
Getting about the house	6	4	8
Washing, bathing	10	7	13
Dressing, putting on shoes	8	7	9
Cutting toenails	19	15	22

Note: Numbers in survey in brackets.

Source: Shanas, E., et al., Old People in Three Industrial
Societies, New York: Atherton Press, 1968.

Table 6.3 Percent of persons aged 65 and over reporting specified
states of disability, by sex: United States, 1962

State	Total (2,432)	Male (1,080)	Female (1,352)
Ill in bed during past year	26	23	29
Hospitalized during past year	13	14	13
Saw doctor during past month	30	28	31
Giddy during past week	16	13	17
Fell during past week	2	2	2

Note: Numbers in survey in brackets.

Source: Shanas, E., et al., Old People in Three Industrial
Societies, New York: Atherton Press, 1968.

years and over) spent, on the average, about 6 days per year confined
to bed and 16 days of restricted activity, persons aged 65 years and
over spent 13 days confined to bed and 34 days of restricted activity
(Table 6.4). The number of days of disability, measured in these
terms, increased with age and was slightly greater among women than
among men.

Acute Conditions among the Elderly

In the National Health Interview Survey, an acute condition is
defined as one with complete duration less than three months,
involving either medical attention or restricted activity, and not
appearing on a specific list of chronic conditions or impairments.

Table 6.4   Average number of days of disability per person per year
by sex, all ages, and 65 and over by age:
United States, 1965-66

Age	Restricted Activity			Bed disability		
	Total	Male	Female	Total	Male	Female
All ages	15.6	14.4	16.7	6.3	5.5	7.0
65 and over	33.9	32.7	34.8	12.7	12.6	12.9
65-74	30.8	30.9	30.7	11.3	11.5	11.1
75 and over	39.5	36.0	41.9	15.4	14.5	16.0

Source: Ahmed, P., Disability Days: United States, July 1965 –
June 1966, National Center for Health Statistics, Series 10, No. 47 (1968).

(See also Chapter 4.) Respiratory disorders are the most common
acute conditions reported. They comprise 58 percent of all acute
conditions in those aged 65 and over, compared with 59 percent in
those of all ages. Injuries are next in frequency accounting for 14
percent in the elderly compared with 12 percent at all ages (Table
6.5).

Table 6.5   Incidence of acute conditions per 1,000 persons,
all ages, and 45 and over by age:
United States, 1965-66

Condition	All ages	45-64	65 and over
Total	2,120.2	1,382.7	1,270.9
Infective and parasitic	251.2	80.8	67.2
Respiratory system	1,258.9	858.9	742.4
Upper	771.0	465.9	472.1
Other	487.9	393.0	270.3
Digestive system	104.4	69.3	92.8
Injuries	253.6	196.4	172.0
Fractures	74.7	78.0	54.2
Open wounds	75.7	36.0	15.2
Contusions	52.6	47.0	78.9
Other	50.6	35.4	23.7
All other	252.2	177.3	196.6

Source: Peerboom, P., Health, Education and Welfare
Trends, 1966-67 Edition, Part I, National Trends,
Washington, D.C.: U.S. Government Printing Office, 1968.

Acute conditions occur less frequently among the aged than at younger ages (Table 6.6). At all ages each person has, on the average, nearly two acute conditions per year; but among those 65 years and over each person has, on the average, one acute condition per year. The duration of incapacity associated with acute conditions tends to be slightly longer among the elderly than among younger persons 45-64 years of age (Table 6.7).

Table 6.6   Average number of acute conditions per person per year, all ages, and 45 and over by age: United States, 1967-68

Age	Total	Male	Female
All ages	1.9	1.8	2.0
45-64	1.3	1.1	1.4
65 and over	1.0	0.9	1.1

Source: Wilder, C. S, Acute Conditions: Incidence and Associated Disability, United States, July 1967 - June 1968, National Center for Health Statistics, Series 10, No. 54 (1969).

Table 6.7   Average number of days of disability from acute conditions per person per year by sex, all ages, and 45 and over by age, United States, 1967-68

Age	Restricted activity			Bed disability		
	Total	Male	Female	Total	Male	Female
All ages	7.9	7.0	8.7	3.4	2.8	3.9
45-64	7.3	6.2	8.4	2.8	2.3	3.3
65 and over	9.2	6.7	11.1	3.8	2.7	4.6

Source: Wilder, C. S., Acute Conditions: Incidence and Associated Disability, United States, July 1967 - June 1968, National Center for Health Statistics, Series 10, No. 54 (1969).

Chronic Conditions among the Elderly

In the National Health Interview Survey, a chronic condition is defined as one that has been noticed by the respondent for three months or more or that is specified on a checklist of diseases and impairments. In 1965-66, 85 percent of persons aged 65 and over reported one or more such chronic conditions, as compared with 49 percent of persons at all ages (Table 6.8). Both proportions have tended to rise during the past ten to fifteen years: in 1957-58 the corresponding rates were 78 percent for the aged and 41 percent at all ages. The frequency of disability is much greater in those aged 65 and over than in persons under 65, but even among the aged less than 15 percent report that they are unable to carry on their major activity. Although the prevalence of all chronic conditions is slightly higher in women than in men, the frequency of disability, at least as

Table 6.8 Percent distribution of persons by reported chronic conditions and limitation of activity by sex, all ages, and 65 and over: United States, 1965-66

Sex, presence of chronic condition, and degree of disability	All ages	65 and over
All persons	100.0	100.0
No chronic conditions	50.9	14.8
One or more chronic conditions	49.1	85.2
No limitation	37.9	40.1
Limitation but not in major activity	2.8	6.2
Limitation in major activity	6.3	25.4
Unable to carry on major activity	2.1	13.5
Male total	100.0	100.0
No chronic conditions	52.3	16.5
One or more chronic conditions	47.7	83.5
No limitation	36.0	32.2
Limitation but not in major activity	2.4	4.0
Limitation in major activity	6.3	26.4
Unable to carry on major activity	3.0	20.8
Female total	100.0	100.0
No chronic conditions	49.6	13.5
One or more chronic conditions	50.4	86.5
No limitation	39.7	46.3
Limitation but not in major activity	3.3	7.9
Limitation in major activity	6.3	24.6
Unable to carry on major activity	1.2	7.8

Source: Wilder, C. S., Limitation of Activity and Mobility Due to Chronic Conditions, United States, July 1965 - June 1966, National Center for Health Statistics, Series 10, No. 45 (1968).

measured by reports of inability to carry on one's major activity, is higher in men.

Multiple chronic conditions are increasingly likely to be found among the aged. Three or more chronic conditions were found nearly four times as often in persons 65 and over as in persons of all ages (Table 6.9).

Table 6.9   Percent of persons with specified number of chronic conditions by sex, all ages, and 65 and over: United States, 1957-58

Number of chronic conditions	Total		Male		Female	
	All ages	65 and over	All ages	65 and over	All ages	65 and over
0	58.6	21.9	60.9	24.8	56.5	19.4
1	23.0	26.6	23.1	26.2	22.8	26.9
2	10.0	20.5	9.3	21.3	10.7	19.9
3 or more	8.4	31.0	6.7	27.7	10.0	33.8

Source: Gleeson, G. A., Limitation of Activity and Mobility Due to Chronic Conditions, United States, July 1957 - June 1958, U.S. National Health Survey, Series B, No. 11 (1969).

Specific Chronic Conditions

Table 6.10 shows the number and percentage frequency of specific chronic conditions that caused limitation of activity as reported in the National Health Interview Survey in 1963-64. Heart conditions and arthritis and rheumatism were the most important at all ages and particularly in those aged 65 and over. Visual impairment and hypertension without heart involvement also occurred appreciably more often among the elderly. On the other hand, mental and nervous conditions, impairments of the lower extremities and hips, and asthma/hay fever were less often reported by the elderly than by all persons.

The National Health Examination Survey carried out in 1960-62 confirmed the very high prevalence of heart disease, hypertension, and osteoarthritis among older men and women (Tables 6.11 and 6.12). Approximately 40 percent of persons aged 65-79 were reported to have definite heart disease and in a further 20 to 25

Table 6.10 Number and percent distribution of persons with specified chronic conditions causing limitations of activity, by sex, all ages, and 65 and over: United States, 1963-64

Conditions	Total				Male				Female			
	All ages		65 and over		All ages		65 and over		All ages		65 and over	
	Number	Percent	Number	Percent	Number	Percent	Number	Percent	Number	Percent	Number	Percent
All persons limited in activity	22,583	100.0	8,378	100.0	10,837	100.0	4,040	100.0	11,746	100.0	4,338	100.0
Heart conditions	3,619	16.0	1,854	22.1	1,884	17.0	896	22.2	1,775	15.1	958	22.1
Arthritis & rheumatism	3,481	15.4	1,797	21.4	1,252	11.6	643	15.9	2,229	19.0	1,154	26.6
Visual impairment	1,285	5.7	794	9.5	611	5.6	315	7.8	674	5.7	479	11.0
Hypertension without heart involvement	1,369	6.1	701	8.4	402	3.7	214	5.3	967	8.2	488	11.2
Mental & nervous	1,767	7.8	504	6.0	637	5.9	169	4.2	1,130	9.6	334	7.7
Impairments (excluding paralysis & absence) of lower extremities & hips	1,325	5.9	445	5.3	701	6.5	177	4.4	624	5.3	268	6.2
Impairment, back & spine	1,769	7.8	369	4.4	903	8.3	177	4.4	866	7.4	192	4.4
Paralysis, complete or partial	923	4.1	344	4.1	489	4.5	175	4.3	434	3.7	169	3.9
Conditions of genito-urinary system	1,071	4.7	369	3.9	369	3.4	189	4.7	702	6.0	135	3.1
Asthma/hay fever	1,152	5.1	272	3.2	666	6.1	188	4.7	486	4.1	84	1.9
Diabetes	571	2.5	262	3.1	228	2.1	110	2.7	342	2.9	151	3.5
Hernia	566	2.5	236	2.8	377	3.5	164	4.1	179	1.5	72	1.7
Hearing impairment	461	2.0	219	2.6	253	2.3	122	3.0	207	1.8	98	2.3
Malignant neoplasms	260	1.2	115	1.4	120	1.1	62	1.5	140	1.2	53	1.2

Source: Peerboom, P., Health, Education and Welfare Trends, 1966-67 Edition, Part I, National Trends, Washington, D.C.: U.S. Government Printing Office, 1968.

Table 6.11   Percent of persons aged 65 to 79 with specified chronic conditions: United States, 1960-62

Condition	Total		Male		Female	
	65-74	75-79	65-74	75-79	65-74	75-79
Definite heart disease	39.9	42.3	33.2	38.8	45.2	45.8
Suspect heart disease	20.7	25.2	25.3	27.1	17.1	23.3
Definite hypertension	38.5	38.8	27.1	32.4	47.6	45.1
Osteoarthritis	80.7	85.3	75.8	80.9	84.7	89.8
Rheumatoid arthritis	9.2	18.8	3.1	14.1	14.1	23.5
Diabetes	4.8	4.7	3.2	2.7	6.1	6.7
Visual impairment (20/70 or worse[a])	10.1	19.1	10.4	13.0	9.9	24.9
Hearing impairment (+16 dB or higher)	28.2	48.0	30.5	48.7	26.2	47.4
Edentulous	----	----	45.1	55.7	53.0	65.6
Periodontal disease	----		94.4	93.7	84.8	89.1

[a] For "corrected" distance vision.

Source: Gordon, T., Heart Disease in Adults, United States, 1960-1962, National Center for Health Statistics, Series 11, No. 6 (1964); Gordon, T., Hypertension and Hypertensive Heart Disease in Adults, United States, 1960-1962, Ibid., Series 11, No. 13 (1966); Engel, A. and Burch, T., Osteoarthritis in Adults by Selected Demographic Characteristics, United States, 1960-1962, Ibid., Series 11, No. 20 (1966); Engel, A. and Burch, T., Rheumatoid Arthritis in Adults, United States 1960-1962, Ibid., Series 11, No. 17 (1966); Gordon, T., Glucose Tolerance of Adults, United States, 1960-1962, Ibid., Series 11, No. 2 (1964); Roberts, J., Binocular Visual Acuity of Adults, United States, 1960-1962, Ibid., Series 11, No. 3 (1964); Roberts, J., Hearing Status and Ear Examination Findings Among Adults, United States, 1960-1962, Ibid., Series 11, No. 32 (1968); Kelly, J. E., Van Kirk, L. and Garst, C., Total Loss of Teeth in Adults, United States, 1960-1962, Ibid., Series 11, No. 27 (1967); Johnson, E., Kelly, J. and Van Kirk, L., Selected Dental Findings in Adults by Age, Race and Sex, United States, 1960-1962, Ibid., Series 11, No. 7 (1965).

percent heart disease was suspected. Nearly 40 percent of this age group had definite hypertension. Over 80 percent had radiological evidence of osteoarthritis. Ten percent of those aged 65-74 and nearly 20 percent of those aged 75-79 had moderate impairment of vision. Nearly 30 percent of those aged 65-74 and nearly 50 percent of 75-79 year olds had some degree of hearing impairment. Periodontal disease was noted in about 90 percent of those elderly persons who still retained any teeth; these comprised a little less than half of the total. The Health Examination Survey also confirmed the higher prevalence of hypertensive heart disease among nonwhites. Definite hypertensive heart disease was much more frequent and suspect

Table 6.12   Percent of persons aged 65 to 79 with specified chronic diseases by sex, age, and color: United States, 1960-62

Condition	Color	Male		Female	
		65-74	75-79	65-74	75-79
Heart disease					
Definite	White	31.3	39.3	43.5	70.1
	Nonwhite	56.9	32.3	44.8	69.5
Suspect	White	26.4	11.9	17.3	16.2
	Nonwhite	25.3	50.3	16.2	14.2
Coronary heart disease					
Definite	White	12.2	9.8	8.2	5.1
	Nonwhite	3.4	---	5.1	---
Suspect	White	5.1	4.1	6.2	8.5
	Nonwhite	7.5	---	9.0	---
Hypertensive heart disease					
Definite	White	16.3	24.0	37.5	37.1
	Nonwhite	50.2	32.3	66.4	69.5
Suspect	White	13.8	15.7	8.4	10.7
	Nonwhite	----	21.4	10.3	14.2

Source: Gordon, T., *Heart Disease in Adults, United States, 1960-1962*, National Center for Health Statistics, Series 11, No. 6 (1964).

hypertensive heart disease was slightly more frequent among the nonwhites in both age groups and in both sexes. The somewhat higher prevalence of definite coronary heart disease among whites is harder to interpret, since the prevalence of suspect coronary disease was higher among nonwhites.

The Elderly in Institutions

Over a million persons aged 20 years and over in the United States live in nursing homes, chronic disease hospitals, or mental hospitals. The majority are aged 65 and over. Roughly 2.5 percent of the elderly are in nursing and personal care homes, 0.3 percent in geriatric and chronic disease hospitals, and 1 percent in long-stay mental hospitals. The proportion increases with age, particularly in nursing homes and geriatric and chronic disease hospitals (Table 6.13). Thus, under 1 percent of those aged 65-74, but almost 15 percent of those aged 85 and over, are in nursing and personal care homes. There is less of an age gradient in long-stay mental hospitals. The proportion of women in nursing homes is higher than that of

Table 6.13 Number of persons per 1,000 population living in long-stay institutions by type of institution, age, sex, and color: United States, 1963

Type of institution	Age	Total			White			Nonwhite		
		Total	Male	Female	Total	Male	Female	Total	Male	Female
Nursing and personal care homes	20 & over	4.5	3.2	5.6	4.8	3.4	6.0	1.7	1.8	1.7
	65-74	7.9	6.8	8.8	8.1	6.9	9.1	5.9	6.2	5.6
	75-84	39.6	29.1	47.5	41.7	30.5	49.9	13.8	12.4	15.0
	85 & over	148.4	105.6	175.1	157.7	111.9	185.8	41.8	40.4	42.9
Geriatric and chronic disease hospitals	20 & over	0.7	0.8	0.6	0.7	0.8	0.6	0.6	0.8	0.5
	65-74	1.7	2.5	1.1	1.6	2.4	1.0	2.3	3.3	1.5
	75-84	4.4	4.5	4.4	4.5	4.5	4.5	3.5	4.6	2.6
	85 & over	13.6	12.4	14.3	14.2	13.2	14.8	6.7	4.7	8.2
Long-stay mental hospitals	All ages	4.4	4.9	3.9	4.1	4.4	3.7	7.0	8.9	5.3
	65-74	8.8	9.7	8.0	8.4	9.3	7.7	12.7	14.6	11.1
	75 & over	10.8	10.2	11.3	10.5	9.7	11.1	14.8	16.1	13.7

Source: Wunderlich, G., Characteristics of Residents in Institutions for the Aged and Chronically Ill, United States, April - June 1963, National Center for Health Statistics, Series 12, No. 2 (1965); Taube, C., Characteristics of Patients in Mental Hospitals, United States, April - June 1963, Series 12, No. 3 (1965).

men, rising to 18 percent compared with 11 percent of those aged 85 years and over, but there are no consistent differences by sex in other types of institutions. There is a lower proportion of nonwhites, both male and female, in nursing homes and in geriatric and chronic disease hospitals. But the proportion of nonwhites in long-stay mental hospitals is slightly higher than the proportion of whites.

The extent of disability as indicated by certain daily activities among residents of nursing and personal care homes is shown in Table 6.14. Nearly 15 percent of all male and 20 percent of all female residents are confined to bed. Similar proportions are incontinent and confused most of the time. About 16 percent of both sexes are hard of hearing or deaf and nearly 20 percent of them have a serious visual problem or are blind. The pattern is similar for each activity, the proportion incapacitated increasing sharply with age, especially for vision and hearing difficulties—each of which affects nearly 30 percent of those aged 85 and over. As can be seen from the number of residents shown in the table, 88 percent (80 percent of males and 92 percent of females) are aged 65 years and over. The picture is similar for residents of geriatric and chronic disease hospitals.

In some ways older persons in mental hospitals are in better physical health than residents of homes for the aged. Thus, 81 percent of those aged 65 and over in mental institutions are able to walk unassisted compared with only 55 percent of those in homes for the aged. The vast majority of those in long-stay institutions are there because of chronic conditions (Table 6.15). Vascular lesions of the nervous system, heart diseases, arthritis and rheumatism, and hearing and visual impairments are the major causes of disability among the residents. As indicated earlier, multiple conditions are also frequent and increase with age. The proportion of persons with five or more chronic conditions more than doubles between nursing home residents under 65 years (11.5 percent) and those aged 65 and over (25.5 percent).

Use of Medical Services

Overall Picture

Expenditure for medical care is significantly higher among the aged than among younger persons. In 1969 the average annual medical bill

Table 6.14 Percent distribution of residents in nursing and personal care homes by extent of disability in selected health characteristics by sex and age: United States, 1963

Characteristic and extent of disability	Male					Female				
	All ages	Under 65	65-74	75-84	85+	All ages	Under 65	65-74	75-84	85+
Bed status										
Out of bed	61.3	75.4	64.8	58.4	51.8	55.0	63.0	58.2	57.6	47.9
In bed part of time	24.3	13.9	22.8	26.5	30.4	26.6	19.7	25.4	26.0	29.7
In bed most of time	14.4	10.7	12.5	15.1	17.8	18.5	17.3	16.5	16.5	22.4
Walking status										
Walks unassisted	65.1	73.2	66.7	63.6	59.6	54.3	58.3	57.0	58.1	46.8
Walks with assistance	16.4	12.9	16.1	16.7	19.1	19.1	15.6	18.1	17.9	22.2
Never walks	18.5	13.9	17.2	19.7	21.3	26.6	26.1	24.9	24.0	30.9
Continence status										
Continent	75.3	85.4	77.8	72.3	70.0	72.1	77.1	76.4	73.3	67.0
Partially continent	8.3	4.7	7.8	9.0	10.2	7.5	5.7	7.0	7.2	8.7
Incontinent	16.4	9.9	14.3	18.6	19.8	20.4	17.1	16.6	19.4	24.4
Mental status										
Always aware	53.8	66.1	56.7	50.8	46.4	48.4	56.5	53.9	49.4	42.1
Confused part of time	30.9	23.7	30.1	32.5	34.8	32.8	31.0	31.0	31.6	35.8
Confused most of time	15.2	10.2	13.2	16.7	18.7	18.8	12.5	15.1	19.0	22.1
Hearing status										
No serious problem	83.8	94.5	89.7	83.6	70.8	84.2	94.0	91.3	86.6	74.9
Serious problem or deaf	16.2	5.5	10.3	16.4	29.2	15.8	6.0	8.7	13.4	25.1
Vision status										
No serious problem	82.5	91.1	87.4	81.9	72.5	79.7	88.2	85.8	82.1	71.2
Serious problem	14.1	6.9	9.9	14.8	22.3	17.0	8.7	11.8	15.3	24.0
Blind	3.4	2.0	2.7	3.3	5.2	3.3	3.1	2.4	2.6	4.9
Number of residents	173,063	32,021	35,147	65,233	40,662	332,179	27,657	54,472	142,010	108,040

Source: Wunderlich, G., Characteristics of Residents in Institutions for the Aged and Chronically Ill, United States, April - June 1963, National Center for Health Statistics, Series 12, No. 2 (1965).

Table 6.15 Number of specified chronic conditions and impairments per 1,000 residents of nursing and personal care homes by sex and age: United States, May - June 1964

Chronic conditions and impairments	Male					Female				
	All ages[1]	Under 65	65-74	75-84	85+	All ages[1]	Under 65	65-74	75-84	85+
Malignant neoplasms	42.6	14.0	33.1	46.7	50.0	30.5	30.0	34.6	32.6	25.4
Benign and unspecified neoplasms	13.4	9.7	19.9	13.5	10.6	11.7	14.8	4.7	13.2	12.8
Asthma	38.6	33.2	14.7	42.4	31.0	25.0	26.9	22.7	21.3	30.9
Diabetes mellitus	67.4	48.5	94.2	74.0	47.4	86.6	89.1	119.7	94.9	54.7
Advanced senility	208.0	28.9	130.8	229.7	271.2	238.6	55.6	154.0	246.4	327.0
Senility, not psychotic	47.8	8.4	44.0	54.6	51.2	53.0	20.2	39.5	55.2	66.8
Other mental disorders	165.6	461.9	261.8	123.3	88.8	167.9	487.4	232.9	135.8	88.4
Vascular lesions affecting central nervous system	335.6	176.1	357.5	368.1	200.0	350.4	201.9	347.3	359.7	379.5
Parkinson's disease	20.2	28.1	23.7	23.9	10.7	23.1	40.9	35.8	22.2	12.1
Epilepsy	18.5	71.7	38.2	9.0	6.0	18.5	96.8	25.3	11.3	3.3
Chronic diseases of the eye	53.2	36.1	39.3	59.7	56.8	68.9	28.5	54.3	68.3	89.5
Diseases of the heart	307.3	119.5	238.0	324.7	374.3	284.3	114.0	238.2	307.6	324.6
Hypertension without mention of heart	51.8	35.2	41.9	61.7	47.8	70.7	46.1	77.4	75.6	66.4
General arteriosclerosis	88.7	19.8	67.3	89.0	119.7	118.6	28.7	52.5	81.0	104.1
Varicose veins	38.4	29.5	38.8	43.5	33.4	29.0	11.3	21.4	34.1	31.0
Hemorrhoids	36.0	29.0	30.0	34.0	44.2	40.2	25.0	31.8	40.3	49.0
Bronchitis and emphysema	67.9	82.3	56.5	65.9	73.6	24.9	24.1	24.3	23.3	27.7
Sinus and other respiratory conditions	21.9	30.6	20.2	21.8	20.7	17.6	23.7	21.2	15.0	17.5
Ulcer of stomach and duodenum	28.6	24.0	22.8	30.2	30.8	12.3	11.8	11.1	13.6	11.1
Hernia of abdominal cavity	72.0	43.3	48.3	77.4	85.9	18.6	6.6	12.4	20.7	22.4

	1	2	3	4	5	6	7	8	9	10
Other chronic conditions of the digestive system	165.1	119.5	129.4	113.8	134.6	123.9	22.4	73.0	84.6	110.9
Diseases of urinary system	57.0	53.0	59.0	64.6	56.3	74.9	69.0	56.3	37.9	65.9
Diseases of prostate and other male genital organs	...	...	...	...	...	103.7	110.0	77.1	25.0	95.2
Arthritis and rheumatism	299.4	259.2	214.6	120.1	251.9	229.3	182.5	121.1	90.8	178.2
Fracture, femur (old)	52.6	36.4	30.7	5.4	37.7	32.6	19.1	17.5	2.9	21.6
All other chronic conditions	136.1	142.4	166.6	198.5	149.5	123.2	129.7	177.7	177.3	140.2
Visual impairment: inability to read newspaper with glasses	186.1	113.5	92.6	69.1	128.1	166.2	113.4	79.3	51.2	118.2
Other visual impairments	62.1	68.2	45.4	41.6	60.1	57.8	78.7	42.2	47.3	63.3
Hearing impairments	296.9	167.1	89.5	77.7	185.3	351.0	195.2	125.7	69.4	219.7
Speech impairments, all types	56.9	77.0	102.8	206.4	86.2	46.1	102.0	171.7	195.3	105.2
Paralysis, palsy due to stroke	91.0	111.1	172.0	120.8	116.6	72.1	134.0	183.0	115.8	22.4
Paralysis, palsy due to other causes	26.3	35.0	48.1	119.5	41.7	24.4	41.7	53.7	128.0	45.8
Absence, major extremities	5.1	14.0	29.2	11.8	13.8	31.2	29.8	36.8	42.4	32.5
Impairments, limbs, back, trunk	167.9	133.2	117.3	132.5	140.9	145.9	134.2	107.4	108.0	130.8
All other impairments	4.6	10.6	9.5	16.3	9.1	26.8	20.4	25.4	16.9	22.9
Number of residents	109,300	156,800	64,000	30,000	360,200	43,100	74,100	40,400	36,200	193,800

[1]Male rates are adjusted to age distribution of females in nursing and personal care homes, except for diseases of prostate and other male genital organs.

Source: Nelson, A., Prevalence of Chronic Conditions and Impairments Among Residents of Nursing and Personal Care Homes, United States, May - June 1964, National Center for Health Statistics, Series 12, No. 8 (1967).

for those aged 65 and over was $692 compared with $210 for those under 65 (Table 6.16). The largest expenditure was for hospital care, which was nearly four times as great for the aged as for younger persons. Physicians' bills and drug costs were two and three times as high in older compared with younger persons. Although the average out-of-pocket expense for older people has been reduced recently by such programs as Medicare, it is still appreciably higher for those aged 65 and over than for persons under 65. The cost of medical care among the aged is financed mainly out of the public sector: Medicare provides the major cost for hospital and physicians' services, but the aged pay for their drugs largely from personal resources at a time when their income is reduced. Projections of future demands for medical care appear in Chapter 9.

Table 6.16 Average expenditure (dollars) per person per year for medical care by type of care, age, and source of funds: United States, 1969

Type of care	Under 65 years			65 years and over		
	Total	Private	Public	Total	Private	Public
Total	210.30	161.84	48.45	692.22	193.04	499.08
Hospital	86.09	57.19	28.91	335.28	32.89	302.39
Physician services	52.91	47.36	5.55	106.99	21.24	85.75
Other prof. services[a]	24.64	22.93	1.71	27.61	21.86	5.75
Drugs and Sundries	25.45	24.66	.79	79.48	70.25	9.24
Nursing Home Care	1.30	.50	.80	111.40	26.79	84.62
Other Health Services[b]	19.91	9.20	10.71	31.46	20.01	11.44

[a] Includes dental services.
[b] Includes eyeglasses and appliances.

Source: Cooper, B., "Medical Care Outlays for Aged and Nonaged Persons, 1966-69" Social Security Bulletin, Vol. 33, No. 7 (1970), p. 5.

Short-Stay Hospitals

Discharge rates, days of care, and average length of stay in hospital are all higher among the elderly than at all ages (Table 6.17). Discharge rates and average number of days in hospital were higher in 1966-67 than in 1965-66, suggesting that following the introduction of Medicare use of short-stay hospitals by the elderly increased. In the latter period, the discharge rates were largely independent of income, but the number of days of hospitalization was highest in those with a family income of $5,000-$5,999.

Table 6.17 Number and rates per 100 population for discharges and days of care, and average length of stay in acute hospitals, all ages, and 65 and over by age: United States, 1965

Age	Population (1,000's)	Discharges		Days of care		Average length of stay (days)
		Number (1,000's)	Rates	Number (1,000's)	Rates	
All ages	189,787	29,120	15.3	228,398	120.3	7.8
65-74	11,233	2,537	22.6	31,049	276.4	12.2
75 & over	6,201	2,065	33.3	28,986	467.4	14.0

Source: Sirken, M., Utilization of Short-Stay Hospitals: Summary of Nonmedical Statistics, United States, 1965, National Center for Health Statistics, Series 13, No. 2 (1967).

Long-Stay Institutions

An estimated 505,242 persons in 1963 were living in 16,370 nursing and personal care homes (Table 6.14). Eighty-two percent of the homes were proprietary and housed 61 percent of all residents. The average age was approximately 78 years. Women outnumbered men by nearly two to one. Unmarried persons and widows were significantly overrepresented. Other characteristics have been considered earlier in this chapter. With the advent of Medicare, new nursing and personal care homes were developed, so that in 1969 some 845,000 persons were living in 18,850 nursing and personal care facilities.[4]

In 1963 there were 77,067 patients living in 728 geriatric and chronic disease hospitals and in 557 chronic disease wards and nursing home units of general hospitals. Seventy-three percent of the residents were 65 or older. The average age for residents of these hospitals was 71 years compared to 78 years among residents of nursing and personal care homes. Only 15 percent of the geriatric and chronic disease hospitals were proprietary; such hospitals housed only 5 percent of all patients. Sixty percent of all patients were in hospitals with 300 or more beds.

At the same time, it is estimated that 558,000 persons were living in 414 long-stay mental hospitals. Almost 30 percent of them were aged 65 and over. This high proportion of the aged is composed of some patients who have grown old within the institutional walls and others who have been admitted in later life. Forty percent of all residents in mental hospitals in 1963 had been there for ten years or more. This proportion was much higher in federal, state, and county institutions than in nongovernmental facilities.

Use of Personal Services by the Aged

Physician Services

Persons aged 65 and over see a physician more often than younger persons. On the average, in 1966-67 they made six visits each year compared with four visits for persons of all ages (Table 6.18). Physician visits were more frequent among whites than nonwhites and slightly more frequent among women than men. In men the number of visits tended to increase with increasing family income, but in women visits were not consistently related to income. In neither sex were visits clearly related to level of formal education. As would be expected, the frequency of visits was greater among those with chronic conditions (6.2 visits per person per year) than among those without (2.5 per person per year). The frequency was also clearly directly related to the amount of physical limitation associated with the chronic condition (Table 6.19). Persons with chronic conditions but no limitation reported an average of 5.3 visits per person per year. The rate was nearly double (10.4) among those unable to carry on their major activity. It is also interesting to note the low rate of visits among persons 55-74 years reporting no chronic conditions. This may be attributable in part to the lower incidence of acute conditions at these ages.

Table 6.18   Average number of physician visits per person per year, all ages, and 55 and over by age, by color and sex: United States, 1966-67

Age	Total			White			Nonwhite		
	Total	Male	Female	Total	Male	Female	Total	Male	Female
All ages	4.3	3.8	4.8	4.5	4.0	5.0	3.1	2.7	3.5
55-64	5.1	4.9	5.2	5.2	5.0	5.4	3.7	3.8	3.7
65-74	6.0	5.6	6.3	6.1	5.7	6.4	5.0	3.8	6.0
75 & over	6.0	5.1	6.7	6.1	5.1	6.8	4.7	4.9	4.6

Source: Wilder, C., Volume of Physician Visits, United States, July 1966 - June 1967, National Center for Health Statistics, Series 10, No. 49 (1968).

Table 6.19 Annual number of physician visits per person per year for persons with and without chronic conditions, all ages, and 55 and over by age, by activity limitation: United States, 1966-67

Age and sex	Persons with no chronic conditions	Persons with one or more chronic conditions				
		Total	No limitation of activity	With limitation not in major activity	Limitation of major activity	Unable to carry on major activity
All ages						
Total	2.5	6.2	5.3	8.4	8.6	10.4
Male	2.3	5.4	4.6	6.8	6.9	9.6
Female	2.6	6.9	5.9	9.6	10.3	12.4
55-64						
Total	1.3	6.3	4.7	8.0	9.3	12.8
Male	1.4	6.0	4.3	6.8	8.6	12.1
Female	1.2	6.4	5.0	8.7	10.0	15.8
65-74						
Total	1.3	6.9	4.9	8.0	9.2	9.6
Male	1.5	6.4	4.4	8.3	7.0	8.9
Female	1.2	7.3	5.2	7.8	11.4	12.2
75 & over						
Total	---	6.5	5.2	6.5	6.8	8.1
Male	---	5.6	4.2	---	5.4	6.9
Female	---	7.2	5.6	7.3	7.7	9.9

Source: Wilder, C., Volume of Physician Visits, United States, July 1966 - June 1967, National Center for Health Statistics, Series 10, No. 49 (1968).

Table 6.20 shows the type of physician visit by age of the patient. Approximately 72 percent of visits at all ages are made to the physician's office; only 3 percent are made in the home. Among the elderly, a higher percentage of visits are made in the home (8 percent at ages 65-74 and 15 percent at ages 75 and over). A lower percentage of visits is made in hospitals or clinics (roughly 6 percent at ages 65 and over compared with 9 percent at all ages). Company or industrial clinics, which account for nearly 1 percent of physician visits at all ages, are no longer appropriate to the great majority of elderly persons. During the decade 1957-67 physician visits in the home declined strikingly. In 1957 they comprised 10 percent of all visits; in 1966-67, only 3 percent. Among the elderly, home visits accounted for 23 percent of all physician visits in 1957 and only 11 percent in 1966-67.

Table 6.20 Percent distribution of physician visits by type of visit, all ages, and 55 and over by age: United States, 1966-67

Type of visit	All ages	55-64	65-74	75 & over
Total	100.0	100.0	100.0	100.0
Office incl. prepaid	71.8	77.4	76.4	69.3
Home	3.3	4.2	8.0	14.9
Hospital or clinic	9.3	7.4	6.2	5.6
Company/industrial health unit	0.8	1.5	---	---
Telephone	11.3	6.8	6.9	9.2
Other/unknown	3.4	2.6	2.3	---

Source: Wilder, C., Volume of Physician Visits, United States, July 1966 - June 1967, National Center for Health Statistics, Series 10, No. 49 (1968).

Dental Visits

Dental services are used less often by the elderly: they pay 0.8 visit per person per year compared with 1.6 visits for persons of all ages (Table 6.21). The frequency of visits varies with income level. Among those aged 65 and over, those with incomes of $10,000 per year or greater report more than twice as many visits as those with lower incomes. This suggests that an appreciable proportion of the elderly may not receive the dental care they need, perhaps partly

Table 6.21   Average number of dental visits per person
per year and percent of visits involving
specified type of service, all ages, and
65 and over: United States, 1963-64

Type of service	All ages		65 and over	
	Number	Percent	Number	Percent
Total[a]	1.6	100.0	0.8	100.0
Fillings	0.6	37.8	0.2	20.3
Extractions and other surgery	0.2	15.0	0.1	17.0
Cleaning teeth	0.2	13.6	0.1	11.7
Examination	0.3	21.1	0.1	13.2
Straightening	0.1	5.8	---	---
Gum treatment	0.1	3.6	0.0	3.7
Denture work	0.2	13.2	0.3	41.5

Source: Alderman, A., Volume of Dental Visits,
United States, July 1963 - June 1964, National Center for
Health Statistics, Series 10, No. 23 (1965).

[a]Includes other and unknown types of service; more
than one type of service may be performed during
a single visit.

because of the failure of medical insurance and Medicare to cover
dental care. Most dental visits among the elderly are for denture
work, fillings, and other surgery. Only a minority are for examination and cleaning.

Other Personal Services

Older people are more likely than their younger counterparts to
visit selected specialists, including the ophthalmologist, optometrist,
and podiatrist (Table 6.22). Visits are also more common among
women than men. Income influences the use of specialists at all ages.
For instance, three times as many older people with incomes of
$10,000 or more report visits to the podiatrist than do older people
with incomes below $3,000. Moreover, more white than nonwhite
persons report visits to specialists.

Table 6.22 Percent of persons of all ages and persons aged 65 years and over with one or more visits to specified specialists and practitioners by sex, by color, and by family income: United States, 1963-64

Characteristic	Ortho-pedist	Derma-tologist	Otolaryn-gologist	Ophthal-mologist	Optome-trist	Chiro-practor	Podia-trist
Persons of all ages	1.8	1.5	2.5	6.2	8.7	2.3	1.6
Sex							
Male	1.9	1.4	2.3	5.4	7.7	2.4	1.1
Female	1.7	1.7	2.6	6.9	9.7	2.2	2.2
Color							
White	1.9	1.6	2.6	6.6	9.2	2.6	1.8
Nonwhite	0.9	0.8	1.3	3.2	5.3	0.3	0.7
Family income							
Under $2,000	1.3	1.1	2.0	5.2	7.5	2.0	1.3
$2,000-3,999	1.2	1.0	1.8	4.3	7.6	2.4	1.3
$4,000-6,999	1.6	1.2	2.3	5.0	8.3	2.2	1.4
$7,000-9,999	2.1	1.8	2.9	6.8	9.5	2.5	1.7
$10,000 and over	2.9	3.0	3.6	11.0	11.2	2.4	2.7
Persons aged 65 and over	1.4	1.4	2.5	9.9	9.9	2.9	4.5
Sex							
Male	0.9	1.5	2.4	8.0	9.2	3.0	2.2
Female	1.7	1.3	2.6	11.5	10.5	2.8	6.3
Color							
White	1.5	1.4	2.6	10.1	10.1	3.1	4.6
Nonwhite	0.4	0.4	1.2	7.1	7.5	0.3	2.6
Family income							
Under $3,000	1.0	1.3	2.0	8.7	9.7	3.0	3.0
$3,000-3,999	1.3	1.4	2.2	9.8	9.7	3.7	4.4
$4,000-6,999	1.5	1.7	3.1	10.4	9.4	2.8	5.4
$7,000-9,999	2.4	1.0	3.2	12.1	11.6	2.9	7.0
$10,000 and over	2.7	1.8	3.7	14.3	12.1	2.1	9.4

Source: Adapted from Hannaford, M.M., Characteristics of Patients of Selected Types of Medical Specialists and Practitioners, United States, July 1963-June 1964, National Center for Health Statistics, Series 10, No. 28 (1966) and Gleeson, G., Age Patterns in Medical Care, Illness, and Disability, United States, July 1963-June 1965, National Center for Health Statistics, Series 10, No. 32 (1966).

Prescription Drugs

Expenditure on prescription drugs is more than three times as high among the elderly as among persons under 65. Moreover, the aged pay 88 percent of such drug expenses themselves. Table 6.23 compares the average costs of prescribed drugs among those aged 65 and over with those of persons of all ages. The higher drug costs for most chronic conditions and the very much higher cost for hypertension and heart disease are clear. The cost of nonprescribed medicines is also higher for persons aged 65 and over than for younger persons.

Table 6.23　Average expenditure (dollars) on prescribed medicine per person per year by condition for which prescribed, all ages and age 65 and over: United States, 1964-65

Condition	All ages	65 and over
Total	15.40	41.40
Heart conditions (with or without high blood pressure)	1.00	5.70
High blood pressure	1.40	7.10
Other circulatory disorders	0.40	2.10
Arthritis and other disorders of bones and joints	0.60	2.60
Mental illness and epilepsy	1.20	2.50
Diabetes	0.60	2.60
Peptic ulcer	0.30	0.60
Other digestive system	0.70	2.30
Respiratory system	2.80	3.00
Genito-urinary system	0.90	1.70
Skin	0.50	0.60
All other	5.00	10.60

Source: Alderman, A., Prescribed and Nonprescribed Medicines: Type and Use of Medicines, United States, July 1964 - June 1965, National Center for Health Statistics, Series 10, No. 39 (1967).

Home Care

On the basis of the National Health Interview Survey 1,747,000 persons aged 55 years and over were estimated to be receiving home care annually in 1966-68. Of them 1,385,000 were 65 and over (Table 6.24). Home care was defined as any personal assistance or personal services received at home as a result of illness, injury, impairment, or advanced age. Care provided by a physician was excluded; but care from all other persons was included irrespective of

Table 6.24   Percent of population aged 55 and
over, by age, receiving home care,
by selected characteristics:
United States, July 1966-June 1968

Selected characteristics	55-64	65-74	75+
Sex			
Both sexes	2.1	4.4	13.4
Male	2.1	4.2	11.3
Female	2.1	4.5	14.9
Income			
Under $5,000	3.4	4.6	12.1
5,000 or more	1.3	4.1	16.8
Color			
White	1.9	4.2	13.1
Nonwhite	4.0	6.6	17.2
Residence			
SMSA	1.9	3.8	12.4
Outside SMSA	2.4	5.2	14.8

Note: The estimated numbers of persons
receiving home care in the respective age groups
were 363,000, 499,000, and 886,000.

Source: Adapted from Wilder, M.H., Home
Care for Persons 55 Years and Over, United States,
July 1966-June 1968, National Center for Health
Statistics, Series 10, No. 73 (1972).

whether it was provided by professional health workers or others (including family members), or was paid for or free. The type of care included help in moving about, dressing, bathing, eating, and cutting toenails as well as more medical care such as injections, changing bandages, and physical treatment. Family members provided 80 percent of this care. Registered nurses provided care to only 7 percent of all home care recipients. Other persons provided care to about one-third of them. Clearly, home care was often provided by several sources. The proportion of the population receiving home care increased with age from 4 percent of those aged 65-74 to 13 percent of those aged 75 and over. A higher proportion of women than men (15 percent compared with 11 percent in those aged 75 and over), of nonwhites than whites (7 percent compared with 4 percent in the 65-74-year-olds and 17 percent compared with 13 percent in the 75-year-olds and over) and of those with incomes of $5,000 and over (17 percent compared to 12 percent in the 75-year-olds and over) received home care.

In contrast to all forms of home care, medically related home care was more often received by whites than nonwhites aged 55 and over (28 percent compared with 15 percent). One of the effects of Medicare legislation appears to have been an actual reduction in the proportion of the elderly receiving home care. Thus in 1966-67, 5 percent of those aged 65-74 and 14 percent of those aged 75 and over were reported to be receiving home care, whereas in 1967-68 the corresponding percentages were 4 and 13.

Discussion

The elderly are more likely than younger persons to suffer from multiple, chronic, often permanent, and frequently disabling conditions. Their main challenge is to live as fully as possible with such conditions and to adapt to the resulting disability that frequently ensues. In addition, increasing frailty makes it more difficult for them to carry out essential daily activities. Whether an old person can continue to live in the community or must go into an institution of some sort is determined by a number of factors. Some of these are individual preference, support of family and friends, degree of physical or mental incapacity, personal financial resources, and available community resources. The high frequency of women, unmarried persons, and widows in nursing homes indicates clearly the importance of such demographic characteristics. While no estimate can be made of the number of persons in institutions who could have continued to live in the community had more home care services been available, it is reasonable to assume that it would have been considerable. The shortage of nursing care in the home is particularly striking and requires correction. At the same time, competent evaluation of the cost and effectiveness of services in the home should be carried out. Adequate studies of this sort among the elderly have been few, with the notable exception of those carried out at Case Western Reserve University in Cleveland.[5] Recent legislation, by making admission to a nursing home more financially practical, has reduced the proportion of the elderly who receive care in the home. The implications of this trend need to be seriously considered. Careful analyses among older people (and at other times of life) are required to determine where they can live most happily and how this is to be accomplished.

It is clear that family members provide a great deal of support for the elderly. In contrast to the popular conception of the isolated nuclear family and associated disinterest of children in their elders, Shanas and her colleagues have found that family members are of considerable help to older people.[3] Older people without children experience the greatest social isolation.

Many of the chronic conditions from which old persons suffer are punctuated by recurrent exacerbations which result in increased incapacity. Properly treated, some of these episodes may be completely reversible; inadequately managed, they may lead to the patient's becoming bedridden. The concepts embodied in the term rehabilitation are particularly appropriate for illnesses occurring in the aged. As in the case of home services, however, there is a need for sound evaluation of how much physical therapy and the other components of rehabilitation can accomplish among the elderly. Acceptance of the idea that rehabilitation is desirable for the elderly is implicit in the Medicare legislation, which provides for the continuation into the extended care facility of services that were started in the hospital.

It is important that those elderly persons who require institutional management should enter the institution most appropriate to their needs. Evidence suggests that at present this is not the case. In a survey of nursing and personal care homes, a sample of residents was classified according to the type of services that they needed.[6] When these needs were related to the services available to their particular institution, there was a considerable discrepancy. For example, 11 percent of persons who were considered to need neither nursing nor personal care were found in facilities that offered the services of a registered nurse. On the other hand, and clearly more serious, nearly a quarter of those who were considered to need intensive medical care were found in facilities that offered the services of neither a registered nor a licensed practical nurse. Insuring agencies, including Medicare, have tried with varying degrees of success to avoid financial support to persons receiving purely custodial care. In spite of periodic reviews of the services that patients are receiving compared with those medically indicated, custodial care has not been eliminated from institutions concerned primarily with the provision of medical care.

The major concern of the elderly is with the management of well-established or advanced disease. There is a lack of services designed to prevent chronic disease or to diagnose it at an early stage. Yet the silent development of many chronic conditions suggests that such services might be particularly useful among the elderly. The allocation of money for preventive health services clearly will have very low priority among those whose main concern is survival. A negligible proportion of the elderly are covered by prepaid group practice, which generally includes provisions for prevention. Preventive services and measures aimed at promoting and maintaining good health have not been encouraged by the Medicare program, which makes no provision for their payment.

The general measures usually recommended for the maintenance of good health at any age apply to the elderly. In addition to such obvious necessities as an adequate income, sound, safe housing and a sense of purpose and enjoyment of life, other factors are important: a sufficient and varied diet, a reasonable balance of rest and exercise, avoidance of cigarette smoking and overindulgence in alcohol or other drugs. The benefits from these health measures cannot be achieved suddenly, but result from a lifelong practice of sensible living.

Mention should be made of the diseases of deprivation to which the aged are particularly vulnerable. Agate notes the relation between malnutrition and poverty that compels the old person to subsist almost entirely on a diet of cheap carbohydrates.[7] Deficiencies of minerals, notably of iron and calcium, occur more frequently, and of vitamins less often. Restriction of fluid intake is common, either because old people habitually drink too little or because they restrict their intake for fear of incontinence.

Psychological deprivation associated not only with the loss of or separation from friends and relatives and reduced social contacts but with increasing sensory deprivation may contribute to deleterious mental states including depression. Social isolation may also prove a precursor to the onset of dementia. Inadequate transportation entails enforced immobility for many older people, thereby increasing social isolation as well as limiting access to appropriate health services.

Retirement contributes greatly to the problems of old people by its impact on income and social contacts. Loss of regular employment leaves the older person with the problem of finding alternative activities that will give a sense of purpose to life. Whether this is achieved through individual interests or through social or religious activities is immaterial. What is important is that old persons find some creative and satisfying outlet for their energies. Preretirement education is important in preparing people for this major transition from the work role to retirement and in providing tools to cope with their new situation.

Shortcomings in the provision of medical and other services to the elderly, both for those who live in institutions and for the 96 percent who live in the community, have been considered. Financial assistance, a more flexible policy toward retirement, improved transportation, greater attention to preventive measures, especially against accidents and faulty nutrition, greater availability of home care, rehabilitation—these are some of the things that could greatly improve the lot of the elderly in America and enable them to live fuller and happier lives.

7 / VARIATIONS IN MORTALITY, MORBIDITY, AND HEALTH CARE BY MARITAL STATUS

Carl E. Ortmeyer

The prevalence of total disability, measured as inability to work because of chronic health impairments, is about twice as high among widowed and divorced as among married men; the comparison holds even when these marital status groups are adjusted for age. Many similar differences by marital status appear for women as well as men, though often they are not as great.

In 1959-61, the average annual age-adjusted death rate of white men was 2.24 times as high among divorced as among married men; for nonwhite men, the ratio was almost as great (2.05). In the United States in 1968, the estimated percentage (10.3) of divorced and separated men who were hospitalized at least once was only about 10 percent higher than the percentage of married men (9.2); however, the average length of hospitalization for the divorced and separated men (22.7 days) was over 60 percent longer than that for married men (13.0 days). In the same year, 86.5 percent of married men, but only 64.8 percent of divorced and separated men, had insurance covering hospital costs. All of these comparisons are between estimates adjusted to the age distributions of the married groups; they will be discussed in greater detail throughout the chapter.

Death rates of widowed persons, both men and women, in 1959-61 were at least 25 percent above those of married persons of the same color and sex in every age interval from 15-19 years through 60-64 years. In fact, death rates of widowed persons ranged up to 360 percent above the rate of married persons of the same color, sex, and age. Excesses in death rates of the widowed over those of married persons also appeared in most comparisons for 1940 and the period 1949-51. In all three of these periods death rates of divorced and separated persons also exceeded those of married persons of similar color, sex, and age, particularly at older age intervals. Moreover, death rates of single persons also exceeded those of married persons in the same color, sex, and age categories; while these differences were small in the two five-year age intervals from 20 through 29, they increased markedly with advancing age.[1]

Marital status categories and transitions in marital status are not commonly viewed as conditions predisposing the individual to chronic disease and death. Neither will the statistical comparisons presented in this chapter support cause-effect links between marital status and disease phenomena. However, some comparisons indicate significant correlations: a few identify transitions in marital status with consequent increases in mortality, while a few indicate differences in marital status of several years' duration to be correlated with differences in chronic impairment and shortened longevity.

Before we survey the national statistical variations in mortality and chronic impairment by marital status, one other kind of evidence for the significance of many of these statistics should be mentioned. Let us compare the scale of some of these marital status differences with the scale of differences that are more widely accepted as indicative of serious health problems, for example, sex and race.

Male-female sex ratios for age-adjusted mortality rates for all ages, and for infants under one year of age, by color, for the United States in 1960 are shown below:[2]

	All Ages	Infants
Total	1.53	1.30
White	1.56	1.32
Nonwhite	1.34	1.25

Nonwhite-white ratios of these rates, by sex, are as follows:[3]

	All Ages	Infants
Total	1.42	1.89
Male	1.33	1.84
Female	1.55	1.96

Of these six sex ratios by color and six color ratios by sex, only the three color ratios of infant death rates approach the ratios of age-adjusted death rates for divorced-married of 2.05 for nonwhite men and 2.24 for white men, or the widowed-married ratios of age-adjusted death rates of 2.16 for nonwhite men and 1.69 for white men. Detailed inspection of death rates by five-year age intervals from 15-19 years to 85 or over reveals that the male-female ratios are 2.00 or more only at 15-19 years and almost reach 2.00 in the three age groups from 50 through 64. The nonwhite-white ratios are 2.00 or more only at the age intervals 25-29 through 45-49.

Many differences in death rates that are widely accepted as part of the evidence that males have lower vitality than do females, or nonwhites than whites, are no greater than many differences between death rates of married and nonmarried groups. More investigation of individual variations in impairment and longevity among divorced, widowed, and single persons should identify the characteristics and events that account for lowered vitality of persons in these categories.

Chronic Impairment and Mortality by Marital Status

The complexities of the multiple relationships among rates of mortality, prevalence of chronic impairment, and marital status will be simplified for our purposes by proposing a "constructed type" that hypothesizes an ordering of the sizes of these rates. This takes advantage of available data on age, sex, and color as well as marital status. It is an approximation to many of the patterns of relationships actually estimated between marital status and mortality, incapacity, and utilization of health services. However, it is used as a heuristic strategy for describing variations by marital status in large numbers of rates. The following is the ordering of age-standardized measures of mortality, incapacity, and use of health services, according to this construct:

(1) Married persons would have the lowest mortality and incapacity but the highest use of health services and degree of coverage by health insurance.
(2) Divorced and separated persons would have the highest mortality and incapacity but the lowest use of health services and degree of coverage by health insurance.
(3) Single persons and widowed persons would have intermediate levels of mortality and incapacity as well as use of health services.
(4) The ordering specified in this construct would apply to both sexes and to both nonwhites and whites.

To what extent are the data in Tables 7.1 through 7.9 evidence for or against the usefulness of this constructed type? Where the

Table 7.1   Average annual death rates per 100,000 population 15 years of age and older and specified ratios of rates by color, sex, and marital status: United States, 1959-61

Color, sex, and type of estimate	Total	Single	Married	Widowed	Divorced
White					
Male					
Observed rate	1,461.8	759.2	1,286.9[a]	8,932.8	3,186.1
Expected rate[b]	...	1,950.1	1,286.9	2,176.0	2,879.1
Ratio obs./exp.[c]	...	0.39	1.00	4.11	1.11
Ratio exp./stand.[d]	...	1.52	1.00	1.69	2.24
Female					
Observed rate	1,041.5	591.4	533.9	4,487.6	971.9
Expected rate[b]	...	912.3	750.2	997.0	1,048.8
Ratio obs./exp.[c]	...	0.65	0.71	4.50	0.93
Ratio exp./stand.[d]	...	0.72	0.59	0.78	0.82
Nonwhite					
Male					
Observed rate	1,515.5	746.6	1,335.9	7,004.8	2,972.4
Expected rate[b]	...	2,428.1	1,498.0	3,241.5	3,077.3
Ratio obs./exp.[c]	...	0.31	0.89	2.16	0.97
Ratio exp./stand.[d]	...	1.91	1.18	2.54	2.41
Female					
Observed rate	1,114.1	407.5	684.4	3,893.1	1,072.4
Expected rate[b]	...	1,460.8	1,039.2	1,858.4	1,405.9
Ratio obs./exp.[c]	...	0.28	0.66	2.10	0.76
Ratio exp./stand.[d]	...	1.15	0.82	1.46	1.10

[a] Standard rate.

[b] Age distribution of white married men used as standard to compute expected rates by direct method.

[c] Ratio of observed to expected rates; measures effects of age adjustment.

[d] Ratio of expected to standard rates, a measure of differences among rates adjusted for age.

Source: National Center for Health Statistics, Division of Vital Statistics, unpublished tables.

evidence is favorable, what more can be said to explain why this order, rather than some other, was found? Where the constructed type explains little, how might it be revised to describe the existing ordering? What more can be said to account for the usefulness of the revised construct?

Evidence bearing on these questions is presented in the tables in the form of:

(1) Observed rates, proportions, or means computed by established procedures from tabulated data on deaths, morbidities,
injuries, and the like.
(2) Corresponding expected rates, proportions, or means computed using the age distribution of a standard population. In
tables showing data by marital status, sex, and color, this
population is white married males; where color categories are
not shown, it is all married males. For the standard population, the observed and expected figures are equal.
(3) Ratios of expected to standard rates, proportions, or means.
Since the expected and standard age distributions are equal,
this ratio measures the relative amount of excess (greater
than 1.00) or deficit (less than 1.00) in mortality, morbidity,
hospital utilization, and so on, in a specified group compared
to the same characteristic in the standard population.
(4) Ratios of observed to expected rates (shown only in Table
7.1). These indicate the relative extent to which the age
distribution in the observed population was older (greater
than 1.00) or younger (less than 1.00) than the age distribution in the standard population.

As an example of these statistics, the observed death rate of white
single men (Table 7.1) was 759.2 per 100,000 such men 15 years of
age and older. If the age distribution for white single men had
equaled that for white married men (standard), this rate would have
been 1,950.1. The ratio of this expected rate to the observed rate for
white married men was $1,950.1/1,286.9 = 1.52$. Thus the death rate
for white single males was 1.52 times as high as for white married
males (or 52 percent higher) when age distributions in the two
populations were set equal. The ratio of observed to expected for
white single males was $759.2/1,950.1 = 0.39$. Since this ratio would
have been 1.00 if the age distributions of these single and married
males were the same, the ratio measures simply the effect of a
younger or older age distribution of the observed population on
lowering or raising its observed death rate.

These ratios of expected to standard death rates among white men
and women (Table 7.1) fit the specifications of the constructed type
closely. The ratios are highest in each sex for divorced and lowest for
married, while those of other marital status are intermediate. The
excess mortality of white men who are widowed or divorced is
relatively greater than that of white women of similar marital status,

compared to mortality among the married. For example, the ratio for married men, 1.00, is about 69 percent above that for married women, 0.59; but the ratio for divorced men, 2.24, is more than 170 percent above that for divorced women, 0.82. Ratios for nonwhite men and women are higher for widowed than for either divorced or single persons, but are also lowest for married persons. It is the mortality of nonwhite widowed persons that is unusually high relative to that of other persons of the same sex group. The relative excesses in death rates of divorced compared to other groups are more nearly the same magnitude for nonwhites and whites. The data also show that levels of the ratios for men are so much higher than those for women that only the two ratios for married men are less than the highest ratio for any female group (1.46 for nonwhite widowed women).

The ratios of expected to standard death rates by cause are the entries in the four columns of Tables 7.2 and 7.3 for marital status. With the exception of malignant neoplasm of the breast, shown only for women, white married men provided the age distribution used to age-standardize each other rate; they also provided the "standard death rate" over all ages used as the denominator of the ratios shown for each marital status in the two tables.

Death rates for white men are indeed highest for divorced and lowest for married men for all but three of the eleven types of causes shown. In the case of leukemia, the age-standarized rates are about equal for all except divorced men, who have higher rates. The rate for malignant neoplasm of the genital organs is slightly lower among single than among married men. Suicide rates are at least as high among widowed as among divorced men. Perhaps the most unusual feature of these rates is the great size of a few of the differences between married and one or more of the other marital status groups. Tuberculosis death rates are more than six times as high among divorced, and roughly four times as high among single and widowed, as among married white men. Divorced men are victims of homicide at more than seven times, and of cirrhosis of the liver at more than six times, the rates of married men. Suicide rates for both widowed and divorced white men are more than four times those for married white men, and more than two times those for widowed and divorced nonwhite men. Both widowed and divorced white men are the victims of motor vehicle traffic accidents at rates higher than those for widowed and divorced nonwhite men, about four times the

Table 7.2 Observed death rates per 100,000 population and ratios of expected[a] to standard death rates of white persons 15 years of age and older for specified causes of death by sex and marital status: United States, 1959-61

Sex and cause	Observed rate	Ratios by marital status			
		Single	Married	Widowed	Divorced
Male					
All causes	1,461.8	1.52	1.00	1.69	2.24
Tuberculosis, all forms (010-019)	11.0	4.01	1.00	3.83	6.61
Malignant neoplasm of digestive organs and peritoneum (150-159)	83.6	1.27	1.00	1.32	1.54
Leukemia and aleukemia (204)	10.7	0.96	1.00	0.99	1.21
Diabetes mellitus (260)	19.5	1.48	1.00	1.62	1.97
Vascular lesions affecting central nervous system (330-334)	148.2	1.39	1.00	1.46	1.79
Arteriosclerotic heart disease, including coronary disease (420)	531.2	1.31	1.00	1.40	1.76
Cirrhosis of liver (581)	22.3	2.65	1.00	3.97	6.26
Malignant neoplasm of genital organs (171-179)	25.1	0.95	1.00	1.12	1.36
Motor vehicle traffic accidents (E810-E835)	41.1	1.69	1.00	3.76	3.88
Homicide (E964, E980-E985)	4.8	2.05	1.00	3.47	7.23
Suicide (E970-E979)	25.4	1.94	1.00	4.30	4.18
Female					
All causes	1,041.5	0.72	0.59	0.78	0.82
Tuberculosis, all forms (010-019)	3.5	1.35	0.35	0.69	0.83
Malignant neoplasm of digestive organs and peritoneum (150-159)	66.8	0.79	0.70	0.82	0.79
Malignant neoplasm of breast (170)[a]	38.3	1.41	1.00	1.02	1.13
Leukemia and aleukemia (204)	7.2	0.62	0.61	0.66	0.67
Diabetes mellitus (260)	26.5	0.92	1.32	1.57	1.15
Vascular lesions affecting central nervous system (330-334)	155.2	0.91	0.82	1.02	1.07
Arteriosclerotic heart disease, including coronary disease (420)	302.1	0.45	0.41	0.54	0.52
Cirrhosis of liver (581)	10.4	0.48	0.56	1.12	1.47
Malignant neoplasm of genital organs (171-179)	35.2	1.76	1.51	1.99	2.42
Motor vehicle traffic accidents (E810-E835)	13.1	0.33	0.37	0.97	0.86
Homicide (E964, E980-E985)	1.8	0.26	0.43	1.35	1.99
Suicide (E970-E979)	7.4	0.42	0.31	0.63	1.01

[a]Age distribution of white married men used as standard to compute expected rates, except for malignant neoplasm of breast for which the age distribution of white married women was used.

Source: National Center for Health Statistics, Division of Vital Statistics, unpublished tables.

Table 7.3 Observed death rates per 100,000 population and ratios of expected[a] to standard death rates of nonwhite persons 15 years of age and older for specified causes of death by sex and marital status: United States, 1959-61

Sex and cause	Observed rate	Ratios by marital status			
		Single	Married	Widowed	Divorced
Male					
All causes	1,515.5	1.90	1.18	2.54	2.41
Tuberculosis, all forms (010-019)	29.1	10.16	3.22	10.99	10.66
Malignant neoplasm of digestive organs and peritoneum (150-159)	85.2	1.66	1.22	2.12	2.16
Leukemia and aleukemia (204)	6.1	0.82	0.66	0.72	0.75
Diabetes mellitus (260)	21.0	1.91	1.30	2.33	2.41
Vascular lesions affecting central nervous system (330-334)	187.4	2.07	1.65	3.16	2.69
Arteriosclerotic heart disease, including coronary disease (420)	309.3	2.11	0.66	1.29	1.14
Cirrhosis of liver (581)	20.3	3.04	0.94	2.98	4.01
Malignant neoplasm of genital organs (171-179)	31.5	1.50	1.61	2.48	2.44
Motor vehicle traffic accidents (E810-E835)	48.6	2.21	1.25	2.97	3.02
Homicide (E964, E980-E985)	54.1	21.14	10.41	37.26	33.68
Suicide (E970-E979)	12.2	0.91	0.46	1.77	1.15
Female					
All causes	1,114.1	1.15	0.82	1.46	1.10
Tuberculosis, all forms (010-019)	12.7	12.98	1.43	2.63	2.75
Malignant neoplasm of digestive organs and peritoneum (150-159)	51.5	0.82	0.66	1.04	0.94
Malignant neoplasm of breast (170)[a]	27.6	1.11	0.82	1.15	1.17
Leukemia and aleukemia (204)	4.3	0.36	0.43	0.59	0.61
Diabetes mellitus (260)	35.5	2.64	2.27	3.34	2.60
Vascular lesions affecting central nervous system (330-334)	189.0	1.78	1.45	2.60	1.73
Arteriosclerotic heart disease, including coronary disease (420)	203.8	0.52	0.38	0.68	0.51
Cirrhosis of liver (581)	12.6	1.34	0.65	1.53	1.49
Malignant neoplasm of genital organs (171-179)	47.1	2.96	2.24	3.79	3.45
Motor vehicle traffic accidents (E810-E835)	12.2	0.44	0.35	0.71	0.59
Homicide (E964, E980-E985)	13.7	4.17	3.07	6.41	5.80
Suicide (E970-E979)	3.0	0.11	0.11	0.28	0.22

[a] Age distribution of nonwhite married men used as standard to compute expected rates, except for malignant neoplasm of breast for which the age distribution of nonwhite married women was used.

Source: National Center for Health Statistics, Division of Vital Statistics, unpublished tables.

rates for married white men, and from four to more than six times those for widowed and divorced women of either color group.

Death rates of white women by cause vary in eight of twelve cases from the constructed type for marital status differences. In two cases, tuberculosis and malignant neoplasm of breast, rates are highest for single, although lowest for married women. In the other six cases, rates for the single are lowest or rates for the widowed are highest or both. While the levels of rates for white women are well below those for men, the relative differences by marital status are greater for the same kinds of causes. The tuberculosis rate for single women is about one-third that for single men, but almost four times that for married women; the rates for widowed and divorced women are also two or more times that for married women. Rates of death from cirrhosis of the liver for widowed are double those for married women; for divorced women, the rates are more than 2.5 times as high. Widowed and divorced women are victims in motor vehicle traffic accidents at more than double the rates of married women; they are victims of homicide at three to five times the rate for married white women (but less than half the rates for widowed and divorced white men); divorced women are suicides at three times the rate for married women.

The ratios of age-standardized death rates for both nonwhite males and females indicate that the expected rates have many small deviations from the constructed type (that is, lowest for married and highest for divorced persons of the same sex). Only four categories of causes of death fit this type for males; only one fits it for females. Most of the deviations consist of higher rates for widowed persons than for divorced persons of the same sex. Several differences between rates for whites and nonwhites are large. For tuberculosis, age-standardized rates of nonwhite males who are single, widowed, or divorced and of single nonwhite females are each more than ten times the rate for white married males. Rates at which nonwhites, especially males, are victims of homicide are exceedingly high, but suicide rates are generally below those for whites. Rates of death in the largest categorical cause of death, arteriosclerotic heart disease, are lower for nonwhite than for white men, except for the "single" status group; for women, these rates are approximately the same regardless of color.

In summary, the greatest likelihood of having age-standardized cause-specific death rates double those of white married males was found among either widowed or divorced males who were nonwhite. On the other hand, the greatest likelihood of having cause-specific death rates at levels less than 75 percent of those for white married males was found among married or single females who were white. Some of the causes for which these contrasts were marked are listed below with the ratios indicating the scale of the differences:

| | Ratios of expected standard rates | | | |
| | White females | | Nonwhite males | |
Cause of death	Single	Married	Widowed	Divorced
Tuberculosis	1.35	0.35	10.99	10.66
Malignant neoplasm of digestive organs and peritoneum	0.79	0.70	2.12	2.16
Diabetes mellitus	0.92	1.32	2.33	2.41
Vascular lesions affecting central nervous system	0.91	0.82	3.16	2.69
Arteriosclerotic heart disease, including coronary disease	0.45	0.41	1.40[b]	1.76[b]
Cirrhosis of liver	0.48	0.56	2.98	4.01
Motor vehicle traffic accidents	0.33	0.37	3.76[b]	3.88[b]
Homicide	0.26	0.43	37.26	33.68
Suicide	0.11[a]	0.11[a]	4.30[b]	4.18[b]

[a]Ratios for nonwhite females, which were less than those for whites.
[b]Ratios for white males, which exceeded those for nonwhites.

The relative differences in rates of death are greatest for deaths attributed to homicide, suicide (with whites exceeding nonwhites), tuberculosis, and motor vehicle traffic accidents (white males exceeding nonwhite). However, the actual numbers of excess deaths indicated by these differences are largest by far for arteriosclerotic heart disease and for vascular lesions affecting the central nervous system. The number of deaths per 100,000 population attributed to all of the first four causes enumerated above was less than the number attributed to "vascular lesions," which in turn was much less than the number attributed to arteriosclerotic heart disease.

The mortality statistics presented in this chapter are based on the coding of only one cause of death, and there may well have been a number of chronic conditions that contributed to mortality, even though they were not judged to be the underlying cause. We can safely conclude that most of the chronic conditions specified among the causes of death were present during the decedent's lifetime for periods of several months to several years. Unfortunately, data on the time sequences of marital status changes and changes in the severity of chronic diseases are difficult to find.

In Table 7.4, the data on proportions of persons reporting one or more chronic conditions indicate that, relative to married men, widowed and divorced or separated women had the highest age-standardized (expected) proportions, with both married women and divorced or separated men also having proportions somewhat above those for married men. However, men of each marital status have higher proportions completely unable to carry on their usual work than any found among women. Highest proportions—those for widowed and for divorced or separated men—are, respectively, 113 and 98 percent above the proportion for married men. Divorced or separated persons, both men and women, along with widowed women, have the highest proportions of work-limiting impairments. Persons who report no chronic health conditions nor any limitations on their usual activities make up higher age-standardized proportions of married men and women and single women than any other marital status groups. In general, chronic impairment is more characteristic of widowed and of divorced or separated persons than of the single and married, even when age differences are controlled by statistical adjustment. One or more chronic conditions and some limitation on work activities were reported about as frequently by women as by men.

Average annual proportions of persons injured, after the data are adjusted for age differences, are lower for widowed men and single women than for any other marital status group (Table 7.5). For all injuries, 31 percent of divorced or separated women, 29 percent of married men, and 25 percent of divorced or separated men had an annual average of at least one injury. Over one-half of the age-adjusted proportions of injured men in each marital status reported injuries at work, whereas approximately one-half of all women injured reported injuries at home. The adjusted proportions of men with work injuries are more than six times the proportions of men injured by moving motor vehicles. The proportions of women (except for the single) injured at home are more than four times as great as the proportions of women injured by moving motor vehicles.

Table 7.4   Average annual proportions of persons 17 years of age and older reporting
one or more chronic conditions and specified limitations on activities,
by sex and marital status: United States, July 1961 - June 1963

Sex, condition, and type of estimate	Total	Marital status				
		Never married	Ever married	Married	Widowed	Divorced/ separated
Male						
1+ chronic conditions						
Observed proportion	0.55	0.40	0.58	0.57[a]	0.75	0.63
Expected proportion[b]	...	0.50	0.58	0.57	0.56	0.62
Ratio expected/standard[c]	...	0.88	1.00	1.00	0.97	1.08
Entirely unable to do usual work						
Observed proportion	0.05	0.03	0.05	0.04[a]	0.24	0.09
Expected proportion[b]	...	0.06	0.05	0.04	0.09	0.08
Ratio expected/standard[c]	...	1.15	1.12	1.00	2.13	1.98
Merely limited in usual work						
Observed proportion	0.10	0.06	0.10	0.10[a]	0.20	0.15
Expected proportion[b]	...	0.11	0.10	0.10	0.11	0.15
Ratio expected/standard[c]	...	1.15	1.02	1.00	1.14	1.50
Limited only in non-work activities						
Observed proportion	0.04	0.02	0.04	0.04[a]	0.04	0.04
Expected proportion[b]	...	0.03	0.04	0.04	0.03	0.03
Ratio expected/standard[c]	...	0.74	0.98	1.00	0.64	0.87
No reported chronic conditions or activity limitation						
Observed proportion	0.82	0.89	0.81	0.82[a]	0.53	0.73
Expected proportion[b]	...	0.80	0.82	0.82	0.77	0.74
Ratio expected/standard[c]	...	0.97	0.99	1.00	0.94	0.90
Female						
1+ chronic conditions						
Observed proportion	0.60	0.43	0.62	0.59	0.77	0.62
Expected proportion[b]	...	0.50	0.62	0.61	0.64	0.64
Ratio expected/standard[c]	...	0.87	1.07	1.06	1.12	1.12
Entirely unable to do usual work						
Observed proportion	0.02	0.02	0.02	0.01	0.09	0.02
Expected proportion[b]	...	0.03	0.02	0.01	0.03	0.03
Ratio expected/standard[c]	...	0.71	0.46	0.27	0.80	0.64
Merely limited in usual work						
Observed proportion	0.10	0.05	0.11	0.08	0.22	0.12
Expected proportion[b]	...	0.07	0.10	0.10	0.13	0.13
Ratio expected/standard[c]	...	0.68	1.06	1.01	1.32	1.32

Table 7.4 Average annual proportions of persons 17 years of age and older reporting one or more chronic conditions and specified limitations on activities, by sex and marital status: United States, July 1961 - June 1963 (cont.)

Sex, condition, and type of estimate	Marital status					
	Total	Never married	Ever married	Married	Widowed	Divorced/ separated
Female						
Limited only in non-work activities						
Observed proportion	0.06	0.03	0.06	0.06	0.08	0.06
Expected proportion[b]	...	0.04	0.06	0.06	0.06	0.06
Ratio expected/standard[c]	...	1.05	1.50	1.52	1.56	1.56
No reported chronic conditions or activity limitation						
Observed proportion	0.83	0.90	0.81	0.85	0.61	0.80
Expected proportion[b]	...	0.86	0.82	0.83	0.78	0.78
Ratio expected/standard[c]	...	1.05	1.00	1.01	0.95	0.95

[a] Standard proportion.
[b] Age distribution of married men used as standard, to compute expected proportions by direct method
[c] Ratio of expected to standard proportions, a measure of differences among proportions adjusted for age.

Source: National Center for Health Statistics, Division of Health Interview Statistics, unpublished tables.

Do users of physician and hospital services increase with higher prevalences of chronic conditions and of mortality attributed to chronic conditions? Results in Tables 7.6 to 7.9 indicate that higher proportions of impairment are far from the only factors in the use of medical services. Proportions of women having one or more hospital stays are higher than for men, except for widowed persons (Table 7.6). Average annual numbers of days spent in hospitals are decidedly higher for single and widowed than for married persons of both sexes; they are also more than 40 percent greater for divorced or separated men than for married men. Despite the high proportions of married and divorced or separated women who are hospitalized one or more times, they have relatively short hospital stays.

Larger proportions of women than of men in each marital status obtain health services by visiting physicians (not counting hospital in-patient visits), and women visit physicians more frequently than do men (Table 7.7). Proportions not visiting physicians are higher for single persons than for other marital statuses of the same sex, but single users report approximately as many visits annually as do persons who are married or widowed. Divorced or separated persons

Table 7.5 Average annual proportions of persons 17 years of age and older injured by type of injury, by sex and marital status: United States, July 1965 - June 1967

Sex, type of injury, and type of estimate	Total	Marital status				
		Never married	Ever married	Married	Widowed	Divorced/ separated
Male						
All types of injuries						
Observed proportion	0.29	0.31	0.28	0.29[a]	0.13	0.25
Expected proportion[b]	...	0.17	0.29	0.29	0.15	0.25
Ratio expected/standard[c]	...	0.58	0.99	1.00	0.51	0.87
Injured by moving motor vehicle					$\overbrace{\qquad\qquad}$	
Observed proportion	0.03	0.04	0.02	0.03[a]	0.02	
Expected proportion[b]	...	0.01	0.03	0.03	0.02	
Ratio expected/standard[c]	...	0.41	1.00	1.00	0.94	
Injured at work						
Observed proportion	0.18	0.13	0.19	0.19[a]	0.14	
Expected proportion[b]	...	0.09	0.19	0.19	0.14	
Ratio expected/standard[c]	...	0.47	0.99	1.00	0.72	
Injured at home						
Observed proportion	0.06	0.06	0.06	0.07[a]	0.06	
Expected proportion[b]	...	0.04	0.07	0.07	0.06	
Ratio expected/standard[c]	...	0.57	1.00	1.00	0.98	
Injured, not at work or at home						
Observed proportion	0.08	0.14	0.06	0.07[a]	0.05	
Expected proportion[b]	...	0.06	0.07	0.07	0.06	
Ratio expected/standard[c]	...	0.97	1.00	1.00	0.88	
Female						
All types of injuries						
Observed proportion	0.19	0.26	0.18	0.17	0.19	0.31
Expected proportion[b]	...	0.15	0.18	0.17	0.18	0.30
Ratio expected/standard[c]	...	0.54	0.63	0.58	0.62	1.05
Injured by moving motor vehicle					$\overbrace{\qquad\qquad}$	
Observed proportion	0.03	0.05	0.02	0.02	0.02	
Expected proportion[b]	...	0.02	0.02	0.02	0.03	
Ratio expected/standard[c]	...	0.70	0.83	0.82	1.27	
Injured at work						
Observed proportion	0.05	0.06	0.05	0.04	0.05	
Expected proportion[b]	...	0.04	0.05	0.04	0.05	
Ratio expected/standard[c]	...	0.19	0.23	0.21	0.28	
Injured at home						
Observed proportion	0.10	0.06	0.11	0.10	0.14	
Expected proportion[b]	...	0.05	0.11	0.10	0.13	
Ratio expected/standard[c]	...	0.71	1.69	1.60	2.08	

Table 7.5   Average annual proportions of persons 17 years of age and older injured
by type of injury, by sex and marital status: United States, July 1965 -
June 1967 (continued)

Sex, type of injury, and type of estimate	Total	Marital status				
		Never married	Ever married	Married	Widowed	Divorced/ separated
Female						
Injured, not at work or at home						
Observed proportion	0.05	0.09	0.04	0.04		0.06
Expected proportion[b]	...	0.07	0.04	0.04		0.08
Ratio expected/standard[c]	...	1.05	0.62	0.54		1.16

[a] Standard proportion.
[b] Age distribution of married men used as standard to compute expected proportions by direct method.
[c] Ratio of expected to standard rates, a measure of differences among rates adjusted for age.
    Source: National Center for Health Statistics, Division of Health Interview Statistics, unpublished tables.

who use physician services visit physicians more frequently than do other persons of the same sex.

Higher proportions of women than of men obtain dental services, and except for those divorced or separated, women users visit dentists more frequently than do men users (Table 7.8). Proportions who use dental services are lower for widowed and divorced or separated persons than for single and married persons of the same sex. However, the frequencies with which users visit dentists are higher for the widowed and divorced or separated.

Insurance coverages, both for hospital and for surgery costs, are more adequate for married men and women than for any nonmarried subpopulation, when adjustment has been made for age differences (Table 7.9). Coverages for single women are higher than for single men, but in every other marital status the men's coverage differs little from the women's. Over all subpopulations and both types of insurance, coverages range from lows of 60-65 percent for divorced or separated persons up to 80-85 percent for married persons.

The "constructed type" proposed at the outset of this review can be used to summarize the data in Tables 7.4 through 7.9:

- Divorced or separated persons show age-adjusted estimates equaling or exceeding those for any other marital status for:
    (1) Men and women reporting one or more chronic conditions

Table 7.6   Proportions of persons 17 years of age and older who were users of hospitals and average number of user days[a] by sex and marital status: United States, 1968

Sex, measure, and type of estimate	Total	Marital status				
		Never married	Ever married	Married	Widowed	Divorced/ separated
Male						
Proportion of users						
Observed	0.09	0.06	0.10	0.09[b]	0.18	0.10
Expected	...	0.08	0.09	0.09	0.13	0.10
Ratio exp./stand.[c]	...	0.84	0.98	1.00	1.38	1.12
Average days per user						
Observed	13.97	12.61	14.18	12.99[b]	22.24	22.68
Expected	...	17.84	14.60	12.99	21.09	18.52
Ratio exp./stand.[c]	...	1.37	1.12	1.00	1.62	1.43
Female						
Proportion of users						
Observed	0.15	0.07	0.16	0.16	0.14	0.15
Expected	...	0.08	0.15	0.15	0.11	0.14
Ratio exp./stand.[c]	...	0.89	1.63	1.64	1.22	1.55
Average days per user						
Observed	9.84	4.70	9.70	7.99	19.34	10.80
Expected	...	15.77	9.70	8.86	16.53	11.19
Ratio exp./stand.[c]	...	1.21	0.75	0.68	1.27	0.86

[a] A hospital episode is any continuous period of stay of one or more nights, any portion of which occurred during calendar year 1968; for each user, all of the hospital episode days falling in 1968 were summed to compute hospital days.

[b] Standard rate.

[c] Ratio of expected to standard rates, a measure of differences among rates adjusted for age.

Source: National Center for Health Statistics, Division of Health Interview Statistics, unpublished tables.

(2) Men and women merely limited in their usual work (partly disabled)

(3) Women suffering all types of injuries

(4) Women with each of four types of injuries shown in Table 7.5 (widowed combined with divorced or separated because of small numbers)

(5) Average annual number of physician visits per user, by men and by women

Table 7.7 Proportions of persons 17 years of age and older who were users of physicians' services and average number of visits[a] by sex and marital status: United States, July 1966 – June 1967

Sex, measure, and type of estimate	Total	Marital status				
		Never married	Ever married	Married	Widowed	Divorced/ separated
Male						
Proportion of users						
Observed	0.63	0.61	0.63	0.63[b]	0.66	0.59
Expected	...	0.51	0.63	0.63	0.63	0.59
Ratio exp./stand.[c]	...	0.81	1.00	1.00	1.00	0.93
Average visits per user						
Observed	6.12	5.11	6.35	6.22[b]	8.01	7.35
Expected	...	6.31	6.28	6.22	6.93	7.43
Ratio exp./stand.[c]	...	1.01	1.01	1.00	1.11	1.20
Female						
Proportion of users						
Observed	0.73	0.67	0.74	0.74	0.73	0.72
Expected	...	0.63	0.73	0.73	0.73	0.72
Ratio exp./stand.[c]	...	1.00	1.16	1.16	1.16	1.14
Average visits per user						
Observed	7.49	6.35	7.67	7.57	7.94	8.22
Expected	...	7.72	7.57	7.60	7.47	8.26
Ratio exp./stand.[c]	...	1.24	1.22	1.22	1.20	1.33

[a] A physician visit is any consultation in person or by telephone, except as a hospital in-patient, with a doctor of medicine or osteopathic physician.

[b] Standard rate.

[c] Ratio of expected to standard rates, a measure of differences among rates adjusted for age.

Source: National Center for Health Statistics, Division of Health Interview Statistics, unpublished tables.

(6) Average annual number of visits to dentists per user by men.

- Widowed persons show age-adjusted estimates equaling or exceeding those for any other marital status for:
    (1) Women reporting one or more chronic conditions
    (2) Men and women entirely unable to do their usual work
    (3) Women merely limited in their usual work
    (4) Women limited only in nonwork activities

Table 7.8   Proportions of persons 17 years of age and older who were
             users of dentists' services and average number of visits[a]
             by sex and marital status: United States, July 1963 -
             June 1964

Sex, measure, and type of estimate	Total	Marital status				
		Never married	Ever married	Married	Widowed	Divorced/ separated
Male						
Proportion of users						
Observed	0.40	0.48	0.38	0.40[b]	0.18	0.27
Expected	...	0.36	0.39	0.40	0.24	0.27
Ratio exp./stand.[c]	...	0.92	0.98	1.00	0.62	0.68
Average visits per user						
Observed	3.75	3.56	3.80	3.73[b]	5.09	5.36
Expected	...	3.94	3.80	3.73	4.58	5.21
Ratio exp./stand.[c]	...	1.06	1.02	1.00	1.23	1.40
Female						
Proportion of users						
Observed	0.44	0.59	0.42	0.46	0.25	0.36
Expected	...	0.51	0.43	0.44	0.36	0.35
Ratio exp./stand.[c]	...	1.28	1.08	1.12	0.90	0.89
Average visits per user						
Observed	4.12	4.18	4.10	4.07	4.28	4.32
Expected	...	4.06	4.15	4.13	4.65	4.39
Ratio exp./stand.[c]	...	1.09	1.11	1.16	1.25	1.18

  [a] A visit to a dentist is any visit to a dentist's office for treatment or advice.
  [b] Standard rate.
  [c] Ratio of expected to standard rates, a measure of differences among
rates adjusted for age.
    Source: National Center for Health Statistics, Division of Health
Interview Statistics, unpublished tables.

(5) Proportion of men with one or more hospital stays

(6) Average number of days in hospital in one year for male and female users

(7) Average annual number of visits to dentists by female users.

• Married persons show age-adjusted estimates equal to or less than any other marital status for:

(1) Males and females entirely unable to do their usual work

(2) Males merely limited in usual work

Table 7.9 Proportions of persons 17 years of age and older who were insured for hospital or surgical costs by sex and marital status: United States, 1968

Sex and type of insurance	Total	Marital status				
		Never married	Ever married	Married	Widowed	Divorced/ separated
Male						
Hospital insurance						
Observed	0.83	0.73	0.85	0.87[a]	0.85	0.65
Expected	...	0.70	0.85	0.87	0.70	0.65
Ratio exp./stand.[b]	...	0.81	0.98	1.00	0.81	0.75
Surgical insurance						
Observed	0.81	0.72	0.84	0.85[a]	0.83	0.64
Expected	...	0.69	0.84	0.85	0.70	0.64
Ratio exp./stand.[b]	...	0.81	0.99	1.00	0.82	0.76
Female						
Hospital insurance						
Observed	0.82	0.77	0.82	0.84	0.86	0.61
Expected	...	0.78	0.82	0.85	0.69	0.64
Ratio exp./stand.[b]	...	0.90	0.95	0.98	0.80	0.74
Surgical insurance						
Observed	0.80	0.76	0.81	0.82	0.84	0.59
Expected	...	0.76	0.80	0.83	0.67	0.62
Ratio exp./stand.[b]	...	0.89	0.95	0.98	0.78	0.73

[a] Standard rate.
[b] Ratio of expected to standard rates, a measure of differences among rates adjusted for age.

Source: National Center for Health Statistics, Division of Health Interview Statistics, unpublished tables.

(3) Females injured at locations other than places of work and home
(4) Average number of hospital days annually for hospitalized males and females
(5) Average annual number of physician (or of dentist) visits by males with at least one such visit.
- Single (never married) persons show age-adjusted estimates equal to or less than any other marital status for:
  (1) Males and females reporting one or more chronic conditions

(2) Females merely limited in usual work
(3) Males and females limited only in nonwork activities
(4) Females with any of four types of injury
(5) Males and females injured by moving motor vehicles, injured at work, and injured at home
(6) Proportions of males and of females hospitalized during a year
(7) Proportions of males and of females using physicians' services during a year
(8) Proportions of females using dentists' services during a year.

- Lowest proportions with no reported chronic conditions or activity limitations were estimated for divorced or separated males and for either widowed or divorced or separated females.
- Lowest proportions reporting any type of injury for males were estimated for the widowed.
- Fewest annual physician visits per user among females were estimated for the widowed.
- Lowest proportions of users of dentists' services were estimated for widowed males and for divorced or separated females.
- The most limited insurance coverages, both for hospital and surgical expenses, were estimated for divorced or separated males and females.

The initial constructed type is useful for describing many of the differences among marital status groups presented in the nine tables. Principal exceptions are the following. In general, estimates of reported chronic conditions, activity limitations, and injuries are higher for either the divorced or separated or the widowed than for either married or single persons of the same sex. This conclusion also holds for proportions having one or more hospital stays and for average annual days spent in hospitals by users, for physicians' visits, and for annual numbers of visits by users to dentists. Higher proportions of married men and women than of any other marital status visited dentists at least once during the reporting year.

Related Studies

This section will review selected studies of the relation between marital status and specific health problems. These studies have been chosen to illustrate investigations of five specific kinds of questions raised by variation according to marital status in the statistics presented in the nine tables of this chapter. The populations studied vary in coverage from those that are localized to a few that are nationwide. Each study presents only partial answers to the questions raised.

(1) If deaths, chronic conditions, and injuries occurring to persons with present or past histories of treatment for behavior disorders were deducted from the deaths of entire populations, would differences among marital status groups in rates of these phenomena be significantly lessened? If the answer were affirmative, what would be the distributions among marital status groups of various behavior disorders such as paranoid delusions, manic-depressive states, or hypochondriacal behavior? Do these distributions correlate with those for disability or mortality? Are these distributions generated by differential selections of marriage partners or by factors in cultural expectations or "ways of life" that differ among marital status groups?

In an extensive review of applications of statistics to mental health planning, Kramer presents classifications by marital status, age, and sex, of hospital admissions for functional psychoses, release rates, recidivism rates, makeup of populations in all mental hospitals, and termination rates of psychiatric patients at outpatient clinics.[4] Age-adjusted first admission rates to state and county mental hospitals in a 13-state reporting area in 1960 varied from 16.0 and 29.0 per 100,000 for married men and women to 109.9 and 124.1 for separated and divorced men and women. Rates for single and widowed were 73.4 and 58.9 for men, 66.7 and 66.2 for women. However, the proportions of first admissions for functional psychoses released within six months varied from about 80 percent for married to only 56 percent for the single, with the other two marital status groups' release rates being intermediate to these figures. Recidivism rates of patients who were released during the first three months after first admission were highest for the single and the separated and divorced, with widowed rates being intermediate and rates for married persons the lowest.

The 1960 census findings on the rates of patients resident in all mental hospitals per 100,000 population in the United States, specific for age by sex and by marital status, indicate that the rates for single, divorced, and separated persons, particularly single men, were above those for married persons of the same sex, with these differences increasing rapidly as age increased. Kramer also presents evidence that all nonmarried groups, especially separated and divorced persons, were overrepresented among outpatients at 493 reporting psychiatric clinics in 23 states. These differences were most marked for persons about 30-40 years of age. They decreased at older ages, possibly because higher proportions of the separated, divorced, and single became residents in mental hospitals, or possibly because survival rates favored the married patients.

In an earlier statistical analysis of first admissions of adults aged 25-54 years to all hospitals for mental diseases in New York and Ohio, Thomas and Locke found that the ratios of age-standardized rates for all admissions in both states were roughly 4 to 1 for widowed or single compared to married men, and 7 to 1 for divorced and separated compared to married men.[5] Corresponding ratios for women were smaller—roughly 2 to 1 and 3.5 to 1, respectively.

Rosen, Anderson, and Bahn estimated age-specific termination rates in 1964 of patients aged 65 years and older at 800 of 1,500 known outpatient psychiatric clinics for adults in the United States.[6] These rates varied less by marital status at 75 years and older than at ages 65-74. In the younger age interval, all nonmarried groups had higher rates than the married of either sex, the differences being most marked for divorced and separated men and women.

One obvious question raised by these statistics is the involvement of psychiatric disorders, and especially hospitalization for such disorders, as a reason for separation and divorce actions. Data on legal grounds for divorce are not helpful since they are affected by the various legal stratagems used to obtain divorce decrees.

Blumenthal reports some interesting localized findings gained as by-products from a survey of a group of 192 families with children with serious problems.[7] One-third of the families surveyed had a phenylketonuric child, one-third had a child with some other form of mental retardation, and one-third had a child with cystic fibrosis. In structured interviews about family relations and indicators of mental health, the parents were queried about previous divorces involving themselves, their parents, and their siblings. An analysis of variance was made for each of seven indexes of behavior disorders and socioeconomic status among the divorced vs never-divorced subjects, with statistical controls for socioeconomic status. The analysis indicated that the factor of hospitalization in a mental hospital placed first as a predictor for divorces among respondents (F-test), second for divorces among siblings, and third for divorces among parents. In this group, as in the larger population, divorce is correlated with hospitalization for mental illness.

One of the largest community surveys of mental health undertaken in the United States gathered protocols for psychiatric evaluation from a sample of adults selected from a central-city population of about 1,400,000 persons.[8] Compared with the nation, the area's people included an overrepresentation of Puerto Ricans, of unmarried adults, and of working wives, with a scarcity of children. One finding pertinent to this review was that nonmarried men had unusually high prevalences of need for psychiatric therapy.

The data in these studies build a strong case for significant associations of the prevalence of behavior disorders with variations in marital status, with such disorders being most prevalent among divorced and separated persons, next among single persons, and least prevalent among married persons. It also seems likely that these differences are greater for men than for women. Very little seems to be known about at least two important subquestions: (a) To what extent are the statistical excesses in mortality or in inability to work also reported for divorced, separated, and single adults preceded or accompanied by behavior disorders? (b) To what extent do persons receiving care for behavior disorders, who change their marital status from single to married or from divorced to remarried, experience remissions in their disorders? In order to design studies to answer the latter question, better empirical estimates are needed of the probabilities of first marriage and of remarriage for adults with diagnosed behavior disorders.

(2) Do disabling conditions that are painful and/or reduce income and/or generate anxieties about increasing disability or death lead to "failures" to perform the usual roles of husband or wife, father or mother? Do marital or parental ties disintegrate more frequently for couples one or both of whom are experiencing increasing disability evidenced as restrictions on their usual work activities?

Only one study was found in the literature in which data were gathered on indications of "failure" experienced in meeting the demands of marital or parental roles. Klein, Dean, and Bogdanoff observed a series of 121 patients, 20-55 years of age, with chronic diseases of six months or more duration, none on welfare, and none being treated for mental illness or alcoholism.[9] They also gathered data from 46 husbands and 27 wives of the patients. Both the patients and their spouses reported that, as the illness developed, they experienced increases in symptoms of psychophysiological distress, in feelings indicating marital tensions, and in such expressed feelings as "fatigue," "feeling weak all over," and "couldn't get going." Role tension items most often noted by patients and their spouses for both themselves and their marriage partners were "jumpy" or "jittery," "angers easily," and "easily depressed"; spouses also frequently noted for themselves "tends to hide feelings." The investigators also noted that the higher a spouse's role tension index, the greater the number of symptoms he reported for the patient.

Categories of problem behavior such as attempted suicide, alcoholism, or sundry behavior or personality disorders are not accepted by this author as evidence, ipso facto, of "failure" in meeting the demands of marital and parental roles. Not all of the behavioral science literature in this area has been covered by the author, but among the many research reports and articles reviewed there were, with the exception noted above, very few investigations of how patients and their spouses, parents, siblings, and children define their roles and evaluate their own and one another's competencies or failures as "family" in situations of increasing disability and perhaps approaching death.

(3) Do persons suffering from chronic, or severe acute, diseases or impairments have markedly lowered probabilities of first marriage or of remarriage after divorce or widowhood?

Statistical evidence was presented previously of marked differences in mortality rates and in proportions of persons with chronic disability between single and married persons, and between divorced or widowed and married persons. No studies were found that estimated age-sex-specific marriage rates of persons with chronic diseases or impairments. Nor were data found for comparing proportions of work-limiting disability or specified chronic diseases in divorced and widowed populations with similar proportions for persons remarried for less than one year after a period of divorce or of widowhood.

Estimating the extent of differential selection for first marriage should be feasible with data already available from the 1970 census. Age-sex-specific first marriage rates of a disabled population could be compared with corresponding age-sex-specific first marriage rates of persons without chronic diseases or impairments. Since it is unlikely that many chronic diseases or impairments would happen to persons simply by virtue of their marrying, this interpretation of differences in marriage rates between disabled and nondisabled populations could be ruled out. Differences between age-sex-specific marriage rates should, then, measure the effect of disability on the probability of first marriage. Data are available from the 1970 census on work-limiting disability of adults and, if ever married, their ages at first marriage. Disability prevalence of persons married for the first time in the year preceding the census could be compared with disability prevalence among never-married persons of similar age, sex, and color. If selection operates in favor of persons without disability, one would expect the differences in prevalence to increase as age increased, with the single always having the higher disability prevalence. An added question in the National Health Interview Survey about age at remarriage and marital status preceding remarriage, combined with the current item on marital status, should permit similar analyses of the effects of several chronic morbidities and impairments on marital selection.

(4) Are certain transitions in marital status—particularly disruptions of marriage by separation, divorce, or death of one's spouse—direct antecedents, for some persons, of impairment or even death?

The studies found in the literature pertain largely to widowhood. Blumenthal's study of the divorces occurring in his localized sample of families with impaired children found that "hospitalization in a mental hospital" (of self or spouse) was a sharp differentiator between never-divorced and divorced persons.[7] This type of study is a beginning, but more data are needed on the correlations of divorce vs no-divorce proceding or during disability, and the duration or outcome of the disability.

MacMahon and Pugh, in a carefully designed investigation of suicide rates among widowed persons, selected a sample of the death certificates of widowed Massachusetts residents who had committed suicide in 1948-52.[10] For each sample death, they selected a matched death certificate of a Massachusetts resident who also had committed suicide and who was in the same sex, color, and five-year-of-age subpopulation as the study subject. Suicide rates of the widowed were above the matched sample rates more often during the first year after death of the spouse, and declined as length of time since bereavement increased.

Parkes found that 30 adult patients admitted for psychiatric care to Bethlehem Royal and Maudsley Hospitals, London, England, in

1949-51 had been widowed within six months of admission.[11] This number of patients was six times the frequency expected from death rates of persons of the same age and sex as their spouses in England and Wales in 1949.

Stein and Susser estimated age-standardized rates of first registration for psychiatric care by marital status for all adults in Salford, England, in the four-year period 1959-63.[12] For 1,945 of these new registrations, the rates of first registration per 100,000 population for widowed men (586) and women (534) were markedly higher than those for married men (214) and women (321). These researchers also selected two patient populations: (a) all adult patients entering psychiatric care for the first time in 1962, and (b) all adult patients entering psychiatric care for the first time during the three-year period 1961-63. They found that persons widowed during the 12-month period preceding first admission made up 18 percent of all widowed men and 12 percent of widowed women in the first population, and 21 percent of widowed men and 12 percent of widowed women in the second population. These percentages compare with 6 percent of the widowed men and 4 percent of the widowed women in a random sample of persons in the community who had been widowed during the 12 months before being interviewed.

In 1969, Parkes and his colleagues published death rates estimated from a nine-year follow-up of 4,486 men widowed in 1955 at ages 55 years and older.[13] Two hundred thirteen died within six months after bereavement, 40 percent above the expected number estimated from death rates for married men of the same age in England and Wales. By socioeconomic level, relative excesses of widowed over married deaths were highest in the top level, Class I (74 percent), and least at the lowest level, Class V (19 percent). The high death rates of men after bereavement were followed by gradual returns to rates equaling those for married men. The principal excesses in deaths by cause were found to be for coronary thrombosis and "other arteriosclerotic and degenerative heart disease."

More cohort studies like this follow-up of widowed men after bereavement should establish the extent of statistical differences in death rates and in proportions of persons with long-term disability among previously widowed or divorced persons by length of time since bereavement or divorce. Comparative studies of series of patients suffering from chronic diseases and behavior disorders with nondisabled populations of similar age, color, and sex would become feasible if patients' medical histories included changes in marital status, and population censuses or sample surveys also obtained such data periodically.

(5) Do the roles of wife and mother in many families include teaching and enforcing health practices and uses of health care for other family members? Do men living separately from women in either role, or families who have lost a wife and mother, show higher prevalences of disability or higher death rates than persons in families that include a woman in the role of wife and mother?

Direct studies of the roles of wives and mothers, or of other family members, as teachers and enforcers of good health practices and uses of health care were not found in the literature that was reviewed. From the two studies analyzed below, one may only note differences in the expected direction when comparing utilization rates of medical services by married and nonmarried adult men.

In a comprehensive compilation of utilization rates of hospital and medical services based on adults covered by Group Health Insurance, Inc., Avnet found a wide-ranging list of services for which utilization rates were markedly higher for married men than for either single or for widowed-divorced-separated men.[14] These included total services, general office visits, preventive care visits, home visits, outpatient diagnostic X-rays, and surgical procedures, both ambulatory and hospital. On the other hand, average lengths of hospitalization and rates of hospitalization for medical (other than surgical) treatments were greatest for persons in the combined widowed-divorced-separated categories, perhaps because of their older age distributions. The data indicate that married men, despite their younger age distributions, visit physicians and hospitals in larger proportions and use more preventive services than do widowed-divorced-separated men. In order to estimate these marital status differences in utilization more accurately, the data need to be age adjusted in each marital status category to an equivalent age distribution. More specific studies are needed of how medical care utilization varies by age, sex, and color for persons in households with and without a wife or mother.

A survey of personal care and nursing home residents in the United States conducted by the National Center for Health Statistics found that 17 percent of married residents needed only "room and board" care when they entered.[15] However, 23 percent of widowed, 24 percent of divorced or separated, and 31 percent of single residents entered nursing homes merely for "room and board" care. These data suggest that elderly married couples provide "room and board" care for each other in their own homes more satisfactorily than such care can be obtained by other elderly persons.

Discussion

Men and women who are single, those who are divorced or separated, and those who are widowed, show higher death rates and proportions with chronic disability or impairment than do married men and women. Most such differences are greater for men than for women. Differences in death rates have been consistent in direction, if not exact magnitude, in nationwide estimates for 1940, 1949-51, and 1959-61. Some evidence indicates that larger proportions of married persons than of nonmarried persons utilize a variety of medical services, including those for preventive care, but hospital stays for nonmarried persons, when they are hospitalized, are generally longer.

Five questions about reasons for these differences are raised and illustrative studies related to each question are summarized. The questions are: (1) To what extent may the differences in death rates and chronic impairment be accounted for by higher prevalences of care for emotional behavior disorders among nonmarried than among married persons? (2) If disabling conditions are painful or reduce income or generate anxieties about increasing disability or death, does this lead to "failure" to perform the usual roles of parent or spouse? (3) Does the presence of a chronic disease or impairment, or of a severe acute condition, markedly lower a person's probability of first marriage, or of remarriage after divorce or widowhood? (4) Are some transitions in marital status, particularly disruptions of marriage by divorce or death of the spouse, direct antecedents of impairment or even death? (5) Is the role of wife-mother crucial to teaching and enforcing good health practices and to obtaining medical care when needed? Do persons habitually living in households without a wife-mother show more evidence of chronic "poor health" combined with infrequent use of medical services?

The studies found in the literature are useful for making these five questions more precise and detailed. They do not, however, provide even partial answers, except in the case of those measuring excess deaths during the first months after deaths of spouses. Data indicate marked excesses in divorced or separated proportions of patients and of first admissions for care for behavior disorders compared to their proportions in the general population. However, one cannot estimate from these data the contributions of mortality or disability of persons receiving care for behavior disorders to variations by marital status in mortality and disability. If disability and any accompanying reductions in income and activity limitations generate feelings in families that the disabled adult is "failing" in responsibilities as a parent or marital partner, this could lead to more separations and divorces following disability. Only one study of a special localized group of parents used data bearing directly on these relationships. One of each of 73 married couples was a chronically ill patient. Feelings of marital tension and personal inadequacy were frequently reported by both the patients and their spouses. Disability, including disabling injuries, may lower probabilities of first marriage or of remarriage after divorce or bereavement. Comparisons of marriage rates, age level by age level, of disabled with nondisabled (or general) populations should directly yield estimates of the extent, if any, to which probabilities of marriage are less for disabled populations.

Except for studies of mortality of bereaved spouses, no studies were found measuring changes in mortality or disability subsequent to changes in marital status.

Some comparisons of utilizations of preventive and other essential medical services by marital status suggest that men who are widowed or divorced have lower utilization rates. No data were found bearing directly on differences in health status, in health practices, or in utilization of medical services including comparisons of households that do and do not include a woman in the role of wife and/or mother. The absence of a woman in this role from the day-to-day living, particularly of males, was suggested as a partial explanation of the excesses in rates of mortality and disability of nonmarried compared to married groups. These differences are greater for males than for females.

Based on several years of working with vital statistics and discussing with colleagues possible reasons for differences such as those presented in this chapter, I have formulated five plausible explanations. It is the concluding contention in this review that these hypotheses, presented earlier in question form, should be testable at least to the extent of computing associations, if any, between the variations in health conditions by marital status and the suggested variables. Brief specific examples of appropriate studies for testing each of the five hypotheses are given:

(1) Test in an inclusive population whether or not removal of mortality and disability data from persons with present or past histories of behavior disorders narrows one or more of the mortality or disability differences among marital status categories.

(2) Test in an inclusive population the extent to which activity-limiting disability precedes separation and divorce. Measure the degree to which rates of separation and divorce are higher in populations where disability onsets preceded separation or divorce than in nondisabled populations.

(3) Measure differences between disabled and nondisabled populations in rates of first marriage and remarriage. If, as age increases, an increasing relative deficiency is found in the rates for the disabled compared to the nondisabled, this is evidence of lowered probabilities for disabled persons.

(4) Measure rates of onset of activity-limiting disabilities and of mortality in persons experiencing separation and divorce compared to persons not recently divorced.

(5) For a sample of a general population and for populations with specified disabilities of interest to the researchers, determine the periods of time during which each person was and was not living in the same household with a wife or mother (or a surrogate). Follow such samples to determine when activity-limiting disability, recovery, and/or death occurs. Compare rates of death and rates at which disability appears among persons in households with a woman in the role of wife and/or mother to the rates in households without such a person. For a sample of a general population and for populations with specified disabilities of interest to the researchers, determine the periods of time during which each person was and was not living in the same household with a wife or mother (or a surrogate). Follow such samples to determine when activity-limiting disability, recovery, and/or death occurs. Compare rates of death and rates at which disability appears among persons in households with a woman in the role of wife and/or mother to the rates in households without such a person.

8 / INFANT MORTALITY IN THE UNITED STATES

Brian MacMahon

Infant mortality is a sensitive indicator of the availability and effectiveness of certain types of medical and social services, and as such deserves special attention. The level of infant mortality in the United States at the present time illustrates a significant accomplishment as well as a serious challenge. The accomplishment is that the infant mortality rate is now only one-fifth of what it was 60 years ago. The challenge lies in the facts that approximately one liveborn infant in 50 dies before his or her first birthday and that some segments of the population manifest rates substantially higher than the national average.

The trend in infant mortality rates in this country since 1915 is shown in Fig. 8.1. Concern was felt at one point regarding the leveling off of the downward trend which occurred in the mid-1950's.[1] This leveling off was manifested in many developed countries, although in several it occurred at a lower level than in the United States.[2,3] In more recent years there has been a resumption of the decline. The recent decrease does not have (and indeed cannot be expected to have) the same absolute magnitude as when rates were much higher. In relative terms, however, the rate of decline, particularly among nonwhites, is comparable to that seen in earlier years.

Historical and international patterns of infant mortality have been discussed in detail by other authors[1-5] and will not be considered further in this chapter. Rather, we shall look at current variation in infant mortality rates in the United States and the extent to which this variation reflects factors that may be modified to reduce further the national level of infant mortality. Particular consideration will be given to national data that have appeared since the detailed review of the subject published in this monograph series.[5]

Sources of Data

The basic continuing sources of national data on infant mortality are the tabulations prepared by the National Center for Health

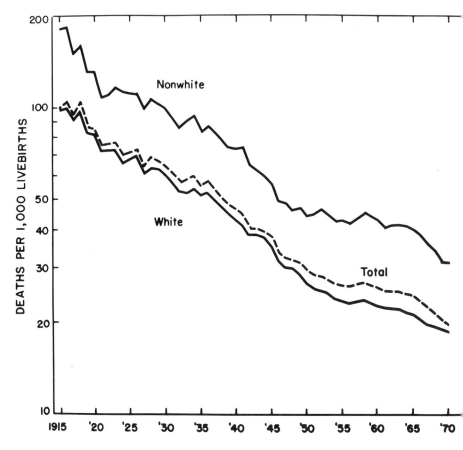

Figure 8.1 Infant Mortality rates per 1,000 live births by color: registration states, 1915–32; United States, 1933–70 (Source: National Center for Health Statistics and predecessor agencies, *Monthly Vital Statistics Report, Births, Deaths, Marriages and Divorces,* and annual volumes, *Vital Statistics in the United States*; and R. D. Grove and A. M. Hetzel, *Vital Statistics Rates in the United States, 1940–1960,* U. S. Govt. Printing Office, Washington, D. C., 1968)

Statistics from copies of certificates of birth or death provided by the individual registration areas.[6,7] Extensive analyses of these data have been published.[4,5,8,9]

The National Office of Vital Statistics undertook a special study of neonatal deaths among infants born during January-March 1950. By matching certificates of birth and death, information was obtained on variables such as birth weight, birth order, and prior fetal loss, which appeared on the birth certificate but not on the death certificate.[10] A similar study of births in 1960 included all deaths in the first year of life.[11-13]

Information not available from routine vital records was collected by the National Center for Health Statistics in the National Natality Survey and the National Infant Mortality Survey of 1964-66.[14,15] For samples representative of all United States births and deaths, information was solicited from hospitals and, by mail questionnaires, from parents. Since similar procedures and instruments were used in the two surveys, estimates of infant mortality rates could be obtained from the national estimates of the distribution of births and deaths. These surveys provide previously unavailable national data on infant mortality rates in relation to socioeconomic status and maternal reproductive history. Illegitimate infants—and for some specified tabulations, infants born of multiple births—are excluded from published analyses of this material.

Age at Death

Table 8.1 shows infant mortality rates by age. Over 40 percent of deaths during the first year of life occur in the first day, 65 percent in the first week, and 70 percent in the first month. Only 6 percent of infant deaths occur in the second half of the first year. The higher rates for males relative to females are seen at all ages within the first

Table 8.1   Infant mortality rates per 1,000 live births by age, color, and sex: United States, 1967

Age	All races			White			Nonwhite		
	Total	Male	Female	Total	Male	Female	Total	Male	Female
<1 year	22.4	25.2	19.6	19.7	22.4	16.9	35.9	39.3	32.5
<7 days	15.0	17.0	12.8	13.7	15.7	11.6	21.1	23.4	18.7
<1 hr.	1.9	2.0	1.8	1.7	1.8	1.6	2.7	3.0	2.4
1-23 hrs.	7.8	8.8	6.6	7.0	8.1	5.9	11.5	12.6	10.3
1-6 days	5.3	6.2	4.4	5.0	5.8	4.1	6.9	7.8	6.0
7-27 days	1.6	1.7	1.4	1.3	1.5	1.2	2.7	2.9	2.5
28 d.-5 mos.	4.5	5.0	4.0	3.5	4.0	3.1	9.3	10.0	8.6
6-11 mos.	1.4	1.5	1.3	1.1	1.2	1.1	2.8	3.0	2.7

Source: U.S. Department of Health, Education and Welfare, National Center for Health Statistics, Vital Statistics of the United States, Vol. II, Part A, Mortality: 1967, Washington, D.C. (1969).

year. As noted below, the proportion of deaths occurring after the first month is greater for nonwhites than for whites.

Demographic Correlates of Infant Mortality

Race

As shown in Fig. 8.1, mortality rates for nonwhite infants in the United States have consistently exceeded those for white infants by a ratio of approximately two to one. Table 8.2, which specifies rates by race, shows the high rate for nonwhites to be a function primarily of the high rates for blacks and for American Indians. A study of infant mortality rates by race in California, based on linkage of birth and death certificates, showed that rates for Indian, Chinese, and Japanese infants are seriously distorted by discrepancies in the reporting of race on birth and death certificates.[16] A substantial proportion of infants reported as Indian, Chinese, or Japanese on their birth certificates are recorded as white on certificates of death. Consequently, conventional mortality rates, using birth certificate information in the denominator and death certificate classification in the numerator, underestimate actual rates in these racial groups. It is likely that a similar phenomenon exists in national data. This suggests that the discrepancy between rates for whites and Indians is

Table 8.2   Infant mortality rates per 1,000 live births by age and specified race: United States, 1967

Race	Under 1 year	Under 28 days	28 days– 11 mos.
All races	22.4	16.5	5.9
White	19.7	15.0	4.7
Black	37.5	25.0	12.5
Indian	30.8	14.9	15.9
Chinese	9.5	7.2	2.2
Japanese	10.7	8.5	2.3
Other	15.9	12.1	3.8

Source: U.S. Department of Health, Education and Welfare, National Center for Health Statistics, Vital Statistics of the United States, Vol. II, Part A, Mortality: 1967, Washington, D.C. (1969).

even larger than that shown in Table 8.2. The magnitude of the effect of this error in California is such as to suggest that, while Chinese and Japanese infants probably do not have higher infant mortality than white infants, their rates are probably not much lower than those for whites—contrary to the impression given by Table 8.2.

The differentials between rates for whites and those for blacks and Indians are greater after the first month than in the neonatal period. The suggestion in the table that death rates under 28 days are no higher in Indians than in whites must be regarded skeptically, not only because of the problem outlined in the previous paragraph, but because of the possibility of underregistration of early deaths. The data for nonwhites as a group do not suggest any deficit of deaths in the first hour or day, such as would be expected if underregistration were a serious problem (Table 8.1). But Indians form only a small proportion of the total nonwhite group, and substantial underregistration among them might not be reflected in data for all nonwhites. Data by specified race are not available for deaths in the first day of life.

Socioeconomic Status

Parental education and family income show strong inverse relations to infant mortality (Table 8.3). The relations with education of father, education of mother, and family income are of approximately equal strength and, although all three variables are strongly correlated, the associations appear to have independent components.[14] The relation with father's education for white infants is illustrated in Fig. 8.2. Between the median and higher socioeconomic groups, encompassing approximately two-thirds of all live births, there is no important variation in infant mortality in relation to socioeconomic status. It would appear that the median group (corresponding to an average family income of $5,000 or completion of twelfth-grade education) has overcome the disadvantages—in terms of infant mortality—associated with low socioeconomic status, and that further increase in socioeconomic level does not lead to further decline in infant mortality risk. The lowest socioeconomic group, however, shows a distinct disadvantage, with rates almost 50 percent higher than those in the higher socioeconomic groups. The rates for black infants shown in Table 8.3 are subject to larger sampling errors than are the rates for white infants, and the trends are not clear. Nevertheless, higher infant mortality rates in the two lowest socio-

Table 8.3   Numbers of live births and infant mortality rates per 1,000 live births for legitimate infants by race and three indices of socioeconomic status: United States, 1964-66

Socioeconomic index	Annual live births (1,000s)			Deaths per 1,000 live births		
	All races	White	Black	All races	White	Black
Father's education						
Grade 8 or less	570	433	124	33.0	30.3	42.4
Grades 9-11	734	604	119	27.4	23.9	44.8
Grade 12	1,263	1,127	121	19.0	17.6	32.2
1-3 yrs. college	422	384	32	20.6	19.0	37.6
4 yrs. college or more	493	468	16	17.4	17.0	*
Mother's education						
Grade 8 or less	423	320	93	35.2	32.0	45.9
Grades 9-11	868	706	148	27.7	24.6	41.7
Grade 12	1,525	1,375	134	19.5	18.0	34.5
1-3 yrs. college	425	391	26	15.9	15.0	32.1
4 yrs. college or more	241	224	12	20.0	19.6	*
Family income ($)						
Under 3,000	691	467	206	32.1	27.3	42.5
3,000-4,999	780	671	97	25.1	22.1	46.8
5,000-6,999	890	811	69	18.1	17.8	22.0
7,000-9,999	716	679	28	19.9	19.2	37.6
10,000+	406	388	12	19.9	19.4	*

* Numbers too small for estimation.

Source: MacMahon, B., Kovar, M.G., and Feldman, J.J., Infant Mortality Rates: Socioeconomic Factors, National Center for Health Statistics, Ser. 22, No. 14, (1972).

economic classes are present for black as well as for white infants. Noteworthy is the fact that half the black infants—in contrast to one-seventh of the white—are in the lowest category of family income.

For white infants in the lowest socioeconomic classes, high mortality rates are seen at all ages during the first year of life. However, the disparity between the lowest and higher groups is considerably greater for deaths after the first week of life than for those in the immediate postnatal period (Fig. 8.3). While most major causes of death show higher rates in the lower socioeconomic groups, accidents, respiratory diseases, and digestive diseases show particularly

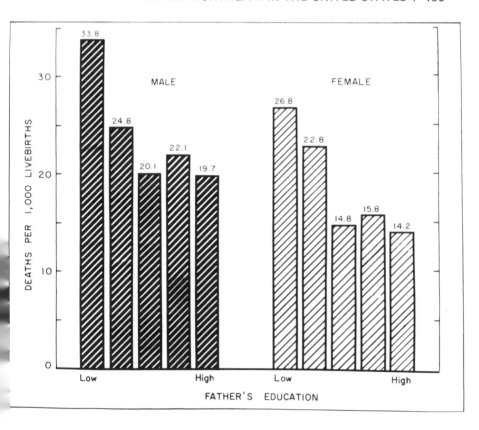

Figure 8.2 Infant mortality rates per 1,000 live births among white, legitimate births by sex and by education of father: United States, 1964–66 (specific educational classes are shown in Table 8.3) (Source: B. MacMahon, M. G. Kovar, and J. J. Feldman, *Infant mortality rates: socioeconomic factors*, Vital and Health Statistics, Series 22, No. 14, National Center for Health Statistics, March 1972)

strong associations (Fig. 8.4). These three categories all comprise pathologic conditions that have their greatest impact after the first week of life.

Region

In the white population, differences in infant mortality rates between geographic regions of the United States are minor (Table 8.4). There are, however, some notable differences for nonwhite infants—particularly in deaths after the first month. In the three southeast divisions, the West North Central division, and the Moun-

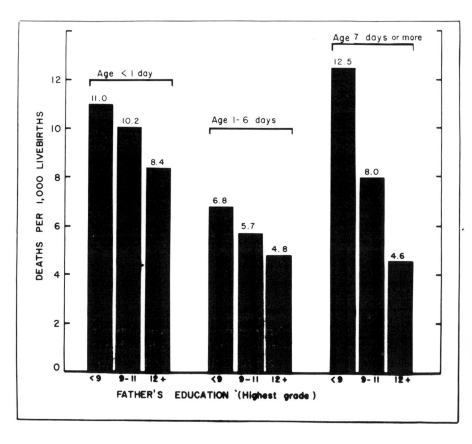

Figure 8.3 Infant mortality rates per 1,000 live births among white, legitimate births by education of father and by age at death: United States, 1964–66 (Source: B. MacMahon, M. G. Kovar, and J. J. Feldman, *Infant mortality rates: socioeconomic factors*, Vital and Health Statistics, Series 22, No. 14, National Center for Health Statistics, March 1972)

tain states, mortality rates for nonwhites between 28 days and 1 year of age are substantially higher than those in the northeast and Pacific divisions. "Nonwhites" in the southeast are, of course, predominantly black and those in the Mountain states, American Indian. The low mortality of nonwhite infants in the Pacific states reflects the (probably spurious) low infant mortality rates referred to earlier in the Chinese and Japanese populations.

There is an interaction of some note between socioeconomic status and geographic region as determinants of infant mortality. Data from the 1964-66 National Infant Mortality Survey permit analysis of this

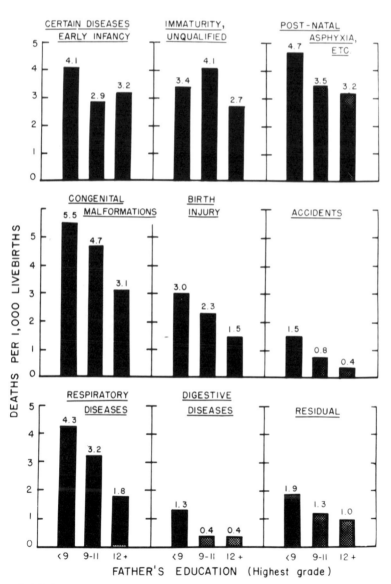

Figure 8.4 Infant mortality rates per 1,000 live births among white, legitimate births by education of father and by underlying cause of death: United States, 1964–66 (Source: B. MacMahon, M. G. Kovar, and J. J. Feldman, *Infant mortality rates: socioeconomic factors*, Vital and Health Statistics, Series 22, No. 14, National Center for Health Statistics, March 1972)

Table 8.4   Infant mortality rates per 1,000 live births by age at death and color:
United States and each geographic region, 1967

Region	Under 1 year			Under 28 days			28 days - 11 mos.		
	Total	White	Non-white	Total	White	Non-white	Total	White	Non-whit
United States	22.4	19.7	35.9	16.5	15.0	23.8	5.9	4.7	12.1
New England	20.1	19.3	33.8	15.3	14.8	25.4	4.8	4.5	8.4
Middle Atlantic	22.1	19.2	37.7	17.1	15.1	28.1	5.0	4.1	9.6
E. North Central	21.8	19.7	35.6	16.4	15.1	25.2	5.4	4.6	10.4
W. North Central	20.6	19.2	38.2	15.7	15.0	24.8	4.9	4.2	13.4
South Atlantic	25.1	20.0	37.4	17.6	15.4	22.9	7.5	4.6	14.5
E. South Central	27.2	21.8	40.9	18.5	16.0	24.8	8.7	5.8	16.1
W. South Central	23.8	20.5	35.5	17.0	15.3	23.0	6.8	5.2	12.5
Mountain	21.8	20.6	33.6	15.7	15.5	17.4	6.1	5.1	16.2
Pacific	19.5	18.7	25.0	14.3	13.8	17.7	5.2	4.9	7.3

Source: U.S. Department of Health, Education and Welfare, National Center for
Health Statistics, Vital Statistics of the United States, Vol. II, Part A, Mortality:
1967, Washington, D.C. (1969).

interaction for white infants only (Fig. 8.5). While overall differences
between regions are small—ranging from 19.1 to 21.7 per 1,000—the
association between socioeconomic status and infant mortality is
stronger in the South than in any other region. There the lowest
socioeconomic category of white infants has a higher mortality, and
the central and upper socioeconomic groups have a lower infant
mortality, than comparable groups in any other region.[14]

Infant Characteristics

Sex

Mortality rates are approximately 25 percent higher for male than
for female infants (Table 8.1). This higher mortality of males is one
of the most consistently observed features of infant mortality and
has prevailed throughout the period of decline in rates in this
country. The sex differential is seen during the entire first year of
life, although it is smaller in the second six months than the first. No
single cause of death is responsible, rates for males being consistently
higher than those for females for all the major causes of infant
death.[4]

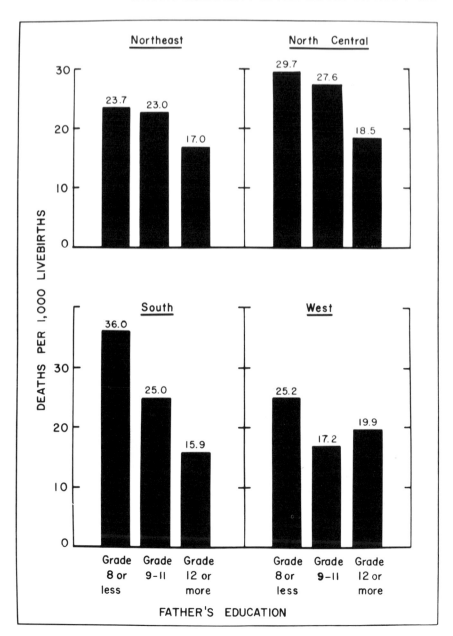

Figure 8.5 Infant mortality rates per 1,000 live births among white, legitimate births by education of father and by geographic region: United States, 1964–66 (Source: B. MacMahon, M. G. Kovar, and J. J. Feldman, *Infant mortality rates: socioeconomic factors*, Vital and Health Statistics, Series 22, No. 14, National Center for Health Statistics, March 1972)

Birth Weight

Apart from actual clinical signs of impending death, birth weight is the strongest single predictor of mortality in infancy. The relation between birth weight and mortality is illustrated by data from the 1960 United States birth cohort (Table 8.5).

The high mortality rate of low birth weight infants is a conse-

Table 8.5   Infant, neonatal, and postneonatal mortality rates by birth weight and color: United States, 1960

Birth weight	Total	White	Nonwhite
	Under 1 year[a]		
Total	25.1	22.2	41.4
1,000 grams or less	919.3	929.3	893.6
1,001-1,500 grams	548.5	575.6	478.1
1,501-2,000 grams	206.6	219.0	171.8
2,001-2,500 grams	58.4	58.2	59.4
2,501-3,000 grams	19.0	17.3	25.3
3,001-3,500 grams	10.1	8.9	17.4
3,501-4,000 grams	8.0	6.9	17.0
4,001-4,500 grams	8.3	7.0	21.0
4,501 grams or more	13.3	11.2	28.1
	Under 28 days[a]		
Total	18.4	16.9	26.7
1,000 grams or less	912.8	924.1	883.7
1,001-1,500 grams	521.5	555.1	434.2
1,501-2,000 grams	180.6	198.4	130.3
2,001-2,500 grams	41.4	45.0	30.7
2,501-3,000 grams	9.9	10.1	9.4
3,001-3,500 grams	4.7	4.4	6.4
3,501-4,000 grams	3.6	3.3	6.6
4,001-4,500 grams	4.2	3.6	10.1
4,501 grams or more	8.7	7.7	16.3
	28 days-11 months[b]		
Total	6.9	5.4	15.1
1,000 grams or less	74.0	67.8	84.4
1,001-1,500 grams	56.5	46.2	77.6
1,501-2,000 grams	31.7	25.6	47.7
2,001-2,500 grams	17.7	13.8	29.5
2,501-3,000 grams	9.2	7.3	16.0
3,001-3,500 grams	5.5	4.5	11.1
3,501-4,000 grams	4.3	3.6	10.5
4,001-4,500 grams	4.1	3.4	11.0
4,501 grams or more	4.6	3.5	11.9

[a] Rate per 1,000 live births.
[b] Rate per 1,000 survivors.

Source: Chase, H.C., Infant Mortality and Weight at Birth: 1960 United States Birth Cohort, Am. J. Pub. Health, 59: 1618 (Sept. 1969).

quence primarily of the high proportion of prematurely born infants among them. Indeed, in the past it has been common to equate low birth weight with premature or preterm birth. It is now recognized that premature delivery is only one of the causes of low birth weight, and that there are causes of low birth weight that are not associated with increased infant mortality risk—for instance, sex of infant, primiparity, and maternal cigarette smoking. These factors generally are not associated with the more extreme levels of low birth weight. Rather, they produce a shift of the overall distribution of births toward the lower weights, so that different proportions of infants fall under any arbitrarily selected "low" birth weight. For example, it is customary to consider as "premature" infants with birth weights under 2,500 grams. For purposes of selecting infants for special care this is a reasonable operational definition, since the disadvantages of treating an infant as premature if it is not are, so far as we know, relatively small. Furthermore, in the prediction of perinatal mortality low birth weight is far more effective than is estimated fetal age.[17]

Recent data permit a separation of the effects of low gestational age (< 37 weeks) and low birth weight (2,500 grams or less) on neonatal mortality and postneonatal mortality, as well as total infant mortality.[12] With respect to all three measures of outcome, infants classified as "high risk" on the basis of low birth weight alone (that is, gestational age 37 weeks or more) manifested substantially higher mortality rates than those classified as high risk on the basis of low gestational age alone. For neonatal mortality, however, rates were very much higher for infants classified as high risk on the basis of both low birth weight and low gestational age (300 per 1,000) than for those satisfying only the low birth weight criterion (43 per 1,000). With respect to postneonatal mortality, death rates were almost as high for those satisfying only the birth weight criterion as for those satisfying both (13.9 and 14.5 per 1,000, respectively).

Conceptually, however, we should recognize that there are children weighing less than 2,500 grams who represent simply the lower tail of the distribution of infants of normal gestational age. The proportion of such children will be higher among female infants, infants of primiparae, and infants whose mothers are smokers. Such children may not experience the high mortality risk of prematurely born infants. One should not assume, therefore, that because a population group has a high proportion of low birth weight infants it will *necessarily* exhibit a high infant mortality rate, although many such groups do.

Maternal Characteristics

Age and Parity

The relation of infant mortality rates to age of mother and birth order of the infant have been studied extensively in local series. However, national data are limited to neonatal deaths in the 1950 and 1960 birth cohorts, and to the 1964-66 National Infant Mortality Survey.[10,13,15] The main features of the association of infant mortality with these two variables are as follows:

(1) Infant mortality rates for legitimate, single-born, white infants are low for first births and high in the higher birth orders (Fig. 8.6). There is little trend between the second and fifth birth orders. Earlier, both in this country and in Britain, first births showed higher infant mortality rates than second births.[10,18] The data in Fig. 8.6 exclude illegitimate births; it must be considered whether this exclusion accounts for the reversal of the relationship of mortality rates in first-born and second-born infants. However, the earlier British series[18] was also limited to single-born legitimate infants, and comparison of neonatal death rates in the 1950 and 1960 U.S. birth cohorts[13]—both of which included legitimate and illegitimate infants—showed the same reversal. It seems likely that first births have experienced a somewhat greater reduction in mortality risk than have infants in second and later birth orders. Table 8.6 shows that, in contrast to the trend for all maternal ages combined, first births to mothers aged 30 and over still show mortality rates higher than those of infants in the later birth orders. This is also true for neonatal deaths in the 1960 birth cohort.[13]

(2) Infants of mothers under 20 years of age have higher mortality rates than those born to mothers in any other age group except the oldest. Particularly striking is the high mortality of infants who are the second children of mothers under 20 (Table 8.6). Neonatal deaths show similar trends with rates for infants of mothers under 20 being 17.3, 26.3, 31.7, 36.1, and 71.5 for infants of first, second, third, fourth, and fifth or more birth orders, respectively.[13]

(3) Infants born to mothers aged 35 and older experience mortality rates comparable to those born to the youngest mothers. The high rates among infants of older mothers are seen particularly for infants at the extremes of the birth order distribution.

The relations between maternal age and parity, between these two variables and infant mortality, and between them and other variables

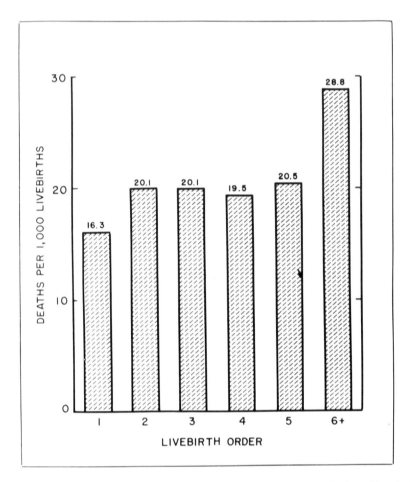

Figure 8.6 Infant mortality rates per 1,000 live births among single, white, legitimate births by livebirth order: United States, 1964–66 (Source: B. MacMahon, M. G. Kovar, and J. J. Feldman, *Infant mortality rates: relationship with mother's reproductive history, United States*, Vital and Health Statistics, Series 22, No. 15, National Center for Health Statistics, April 1973)

related to infant mortality risk (such as socioeconomic status) are complex and so far have defied attempts to isolate their underlying determinants.

Previous Reproductive Loss

Infants of mothers who have had a previous child die in infancy have a mortality rate two and a half times as high as infants of

Table 8.6   Infant mortality rates per 1,000 live births for single, white legitimate births by age of mother and live birth order: United States, 1964-66

Birth order	Age of mother					
	All ages	<20	20-24	25-29	30-34	35+
All orders	19.5	23.6	17.8	17.8	20.3	24.1
First	16.3	20.1	14.1	11.7	25.6	*
Second	20.1	30.5	19.5	16.7	17.3	29.0
Third	20.1	*	21.4	18.7	17.5	17.1
Fourth	19.5	*	22.3	18.8	19.2	16.7
Fifth	20.5	*	*	18.9	18.5	26.4
Sixth or more	28.8	*	*	30.1	26.8	29.2

* Numbers too small for estimation.

Source: MacMahon, B., Kovar, M.G., and Feldman, J.J., Infant Mortality Rates: Relationship with Mother's Reproductive History, United States, National Center for Health Statistics, Series 22, No. 15, April 1973.

mothers without such a history (Fig. 8.7). Among white infants the differential is almost three-fold. History of previous fetal death also is associated with an approximate doubling of infant mortality risk (Fig. 8.8). These relationships are independent of maternal age, birth order, and socioeconomic status.[15] Table 8.7 shows the data by age at death. Mortality rates for infants with a history of previous maternal reproductive loss are higher throughout the first year, but they are particularly high among deaths in the first day. Causes such as hemolytic disease, postnatal asphyxia and atelectasis, immaturity, and other conditions associated with very early death figure prominently in the excess mortality. However, rates for such infants are higher than for those without history of prior loss for nearly all causes, including causes such as accidents that are associated with relatively late infant death.[15]

In New York State the decline in perinatal mortality (fetal deaths after the fifth month of pregnancy plus deaths in the first month of life) over the 30 years 1936-65 has been less for infants of women with a prior child loss (fetal death or death of any previous child prior to the pregnancy under study) than for parous women without such loss. Risk of perinatal death for infants of women with prior child loss, relative to those of women without, was 2.2 in 1936 but 3.0 in 1965-66.[19]

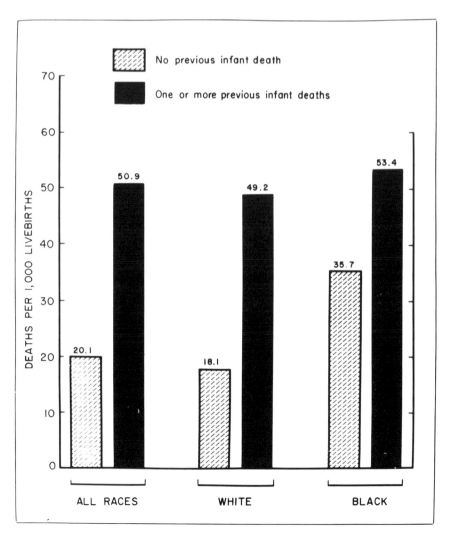

Figure 8.7 Infant mortality rates per 1,000 live births among single, legitimate births according to whether or not the mother had had a previous infant death, by color: United States, 1964–66 (Source: B. MacMahon, M. G. Kovar, and J. J. Feldman, *Infant mortality rates: relationship with mother's reproductive history, United States*, Vital and Health Statistics, Series 22, No. 15, National Center for Health Statistics, April 1973)

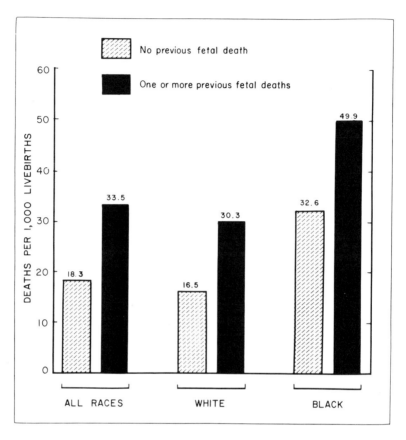

Figure 8.8 Infant mortality rates per 1,000 live births among single, legitimate births according to whether or not the mother had had a previous fetal death, by color: United States 1964–66 (Source: B. MacMahon, M. G. Kovar, and J. J. Feldman, *Infant mortality rates: relationship with mother's reproductive history, United States*, Vital and Health Statistics, Series 22, No. 15, National Center for Health Statistics, April 1973)

Implications

In 1970 the infant mortality rate in the United States was an estimated 19.8 per 1,000 live births.[6] The data presented above allow some assessment of the further reduction that might be anticipated if medical and social resources were more widely or more effectively applied. Two categories of improvement must be distinguished: the discovery and application of new methods of preventing infant death, and the broader application of known preventive measures.

Table 8.7   Infant mortality rates per 1,000 live births for single, white legitimate births by age at death and mother's previous reproductive loss: United States, 1964-66

Age at death	Previous infant death		Previous fetal death		
	None	One or more	None	One	Two or more
Under 1 year	18.1	49.2	16.5	27.4	36.9
Under 1 day	7.5	25.6	6.5	13.4	19.1
1-6 days	4.7	10.6	4.3	6.6	9.1
7-27 days	1.4	2.4	1.3	1.6	2.2
1-5 mos.	3.2	7.4	3.1	4.5	4.3
6-11 mos.	1.4	3.2	1.4	1.2	2.2

Source: MacMahon, B., Kovar, M.G., and Feldman, J.J., Infant Mortality Rates: Relationship with Mother's Reproductive History, United States, National Center for Health Statistics, Series 22, No. 15, April 1973.

Regarding the first category, future trends cannot be predicted with any degree of confidence, since they depend on the acquisition of new scientific knowledge. Foremost among the knowledge required is an understanding of the etiology of premature onset of labor and of congenital malformation. The consistently higher infant mortality for males than females is a characteristic that would also appear to depend on biological mechanisms not currently understood.

What may be expected from the broader application of existing knowledge? One must assume that the most favorable social circumstances and most effective medical care are available to persons in the higher categories of income and education. While this assumption may be open to challenge as a generalization, the consistent historical and current relation between infant mortality risk and socioeconomic status—as measured either by income or by education—makes the assumption a reasonable one in this context. One sees, then, in the data from the 1964-66 surveys evidence that the majority of United States infants are born into an environment which provides practically all that existing medical and social services have to offer in the way of prevention of death in infancy (Table 8.3). The basis of this statement is the fact that infants in the median classes of parental income or education have mortality rates just as low as those in the highest class. In 1964-66, approximately 60 percent of legitimate, single-born infants were born into the upper three categories of socioeconomic status shown in Table 8.3. If father's education is used as the index of socioeconomic status, the infant mortality rate in the highest socioeconomic category was 17.4 per 1,000. That is, presumably, the rate that would have prevailed nationally if all infants had experienced the environment and medical services available to the higher socioeconomic groups.

On the further assumption that socioeconomic status, or its concomitants, can be changed, the deaths occurring in excess of this basic rate may be considered preventable. For all legitimate, single births in 1964-66 the infant mortality rate was 23.0 per 1,000 live births.[14] Thus, the excess rate attributable to the concomitants of low socioeconomic status was 5.6 per 1,000 or about 25 percent of all infant deaths. In the lowest socioeconomic group, comprising about one-sixth of all births, approximately one-half of the infant deaths were attributable in this sense to low socioeconomic status or its consequences. These infant deaths were therefore—at least in theory—preventable.

Of major concern must be the continuing high mortality rates for nonwhite infants, and the fact that the mortality rate for black infants exceeds that for white infants within each category of socioeconomic status (Fig. 8.1 and Table 8.3). Indeed, the relative differential between the rates for black and for white infants is greater in the higher than in the lower socioeconomic groups. The categories used in Table 8.3 are broad and it is likely that within each group, the average socioeconomic status of the families of the black infants is lower than that of the white. However, since the mortality rate for black infants even in the highest socioeconomic categories exceeds that of white infants in the lowest categories, it is clear that a given level of socioeconomic status (as measured by family income or by parental education) does not have the same implications for infant mortality risk among black as among white infants.

In short, if the social circumstances and medical services now enjoyed by persons in the higher socioeconomic categories were to become available to the total population, the consequent reduction in total infant mortality rate would likely be modest. However, within certain subgroups of the population—notably among the economically deprived and among blacks and Indians—the effect would be substantial.

Discussion

The infant mortality rate in the United States has fallen from about 100 per 1,000 live births around 1915 to about 20 per 1,000 at the present time. In recent years deaths in the first week of life have accounted for 65 percent of all deaths in the first year. Infant mortality rates are higher for black infants and American Indians than for white infants, for males than for females, for infants born of parents of low socioeconomic status, for infants of low birth weight, and for infants born to the youngest or oldest mothers, mothers of high parity, or mothers with a history of previous fetal or infant death.

Approximately 25 percent of infant deaths are in excess of the number expected if all infants experienced the rates observed in the most favored socioeconomic classes. Rates in the lowest socioeconomic class, comprising about one-sixth of all births, are approximately double the rates in the highest socioeconomic groups. An implication is that one-half of the deaths of infants in the lowest socioeconomic group are preventable.

9 / PROJECTIONS OF HEALTH SERVICE PERSONNEL AND FACILITIES*

John F. Newman
Odin W. Anderson

Most societies, in a manner particular to each, make provisions for the health and well-being of their members. Since 1945 there has been increasing interest in Western Europe and North America in working out rational resources-need-demand concepts for the structure and operation of health services for immediate and future use. In this chapter we shall attempt such an analysis for the United States.

Whatever new health delivery plans may emerge in the future, manpower and facilities will be required to implement them. It is usually assumed that the traditional ways of providing professional manpower and facilities will continue to operate; that is, medical, dental, and nursing schools, as well as schools of social work and public health, will continue to graduate specialists in several areas, while various government programs and agencies will continue to provide funds for the construction of facilities. Additional programs for paraprofessional personnel may be needed, however.

Concern for future health needs frequently has been based on the assumption of a long-term trend in population growth. Rather than rely on a single estimate of population growth, however, we shall examine materials based on a series of population projections prepared by the United States Bureau of the Census.[1] The projections in turn will be examined with respect to current availability of selected health service personnel and facilities—physicians, dentists, nurses, and hospital beds—in an attempt to specify the relative magnitude of future requirements. Finally, we shall consider the impact of trends in mortality and morbidity, in conjunction with selected measures of utilization and demographic trends.

Since we are concerned with estimates of future trends, a note of caution is in order. Long-term estimates and projections may be

*This contribution was begun while the senior author was Research Associate, Center for Health Administration Studies, University of Chicago, engaged in projects supported in part by Grant HS 00080, National Center for Health Research and Development, Department of Health, Education and Welfare.

subject to considerable error resulting from an inability to predict the complex interaction of demographic and social factors. Our projections and estimates should therefore be viewed with caution. They are made simply to suggest some expectations for the future; like airline timetables, they are subject to change without notice.

Considerations in the Need for Health Services and Facilities

The estimation of a society's need for health services and facilities depends on many factors including morbidity and mortality patterns, organization of the medical care system, demographic processes related to the size and composition of the population, and patterns of health service utilization.

With respect to morbidity and mortality, it is important to know if rates are increasing or decreasing and whether there are changes in the causes of illness and death. Other factors may relate to the incidence or prevalence of morbidity. Such considerations should provide the rationale for redirecting government priorities for research: whether to build short-stay or long-stay facilities or whether to develop programs to produce medical-care specialists in particular areas. Since other sections of this book deal with trends in mortality and morbidity (particularly Chapters 1, 2, and 4), we restrict our comments to a few general observations.

The long-term trend in crude death rates for the United States has been downward, although the rate of decline has slowed considerably in recent years. The crude death rate in 1900 was 17.2 per 1,000 population, and by 1970 it had declined to 9.4.[2,3] However, as pointed out in Chapters 1 and 2 as well as by other authors, the decline has been primarily in deaths from infectious and parasitic diseases.[4-6] Counteracting the downward trend to some extent has been an increase in the rates for cardiovascular disease and malignant neoplasms (Table 9.1). The percentage decreases from 1900 to 1970 for tuberculosis and for influenza and pneumonia were approximately 99 and 85 respectively, while the percentage increases in rates for major cardiovascular-renal diseases and malignant neoplasms were 43 and 153 respectively.

Not only have there been significant changes in the leading causes of death, but there is some indication that there has been a decrease in the incidence of acute conditions in recent years—from a rate of 260.1 per 100 persons per year in 1957-58 to 203.4 per 100 persons per year in 1970, or a decrease of 22 percent[7,8] (see also Chapter 4).

Table 9.1   Selected mortality rates and the percent change
in rates: United States, 1900 to 1970

Cause of death	Rate per 100,000		Percent change
	1900	1970	
Tuberculosis (all forms)	194.4	2.7	-98.6
Influenza and pneumonia	202.2	30.5	-84.9
Major cardiovascular-renal diseases	345.2	494.0	+43.3
Malignant neoplasms	64.0	162.0	+153.1

Source: Bureau of the Census, Historical Statistics of the United States, 1900-1957, Washington, 1958, and Bureau of the Census, Statistical Abstract of the United States, 1972, Washington, 1972.

If we assume that the self-reporting of conditions is accurate, then, on the basis of the overall decline in the mortality rate and a decrease in the incidence of acute conditions, it may be argued that the population of the United States is healthier than in 1900. However, several qualifications should be made. First, the long-term decrease in infectious and parasitic disease was associated with a variety of concomitant influences on disease patterns. These range from such general influences as the effect of improved living standards on tuberculosis, to more specific ones, such as the elimination of poliomyelitis. These factors may not be applicable to the current leading causes of death. Unless new breakthroughs in medicine occur, in view of the aging of the population we face the possibility of higher mortality and morbidity brought about by increases in cardiovascular diseases and malignant neoplasms.

Second, as Sanders[9] has noted, improved health care may also result in a long-term increase in the prevalence of chronic conditions, because of earlier diagnosis and the consequent prolongation of life.

Further, improvements in health care for chronic conditions that decrease mortality at younger ages simply mean that the proportion of persons at older ages who suffer from chronic conditions will increase. Such a postponement of death may mean that, while the crude mortality rate remains relatively constant, age-specific rates will show considerable variation.

The changing pattern of mortality by age and cause of death as related to changes in life expectancy is contained in a United Nations publication.[10] Figure 9.1 depicts the distribution of deaths by five cause-of-death categories for different levels of expectation of life at birth, ranging from 40 to 76 years. The standard population upon

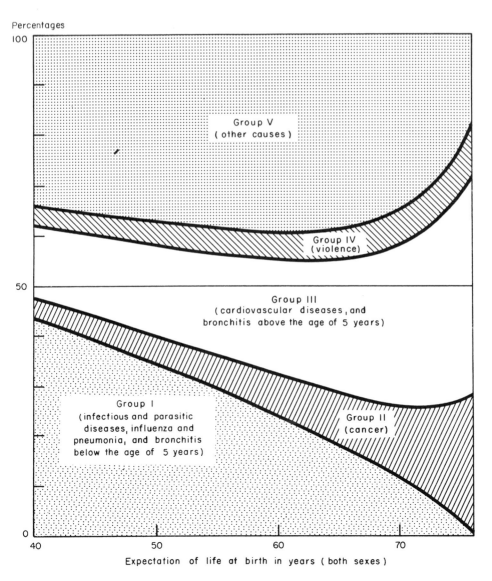

Figure 9.1 Distribution, in a standard population, of deaths (all ages and both sexes) by cause of death groups for different levels of expectation of life at birth ranging from 40 to 76 years (redrawn from *Population Bulletin of the United Nations*, No. 6–1962, p. 110)

which Fig. 9.1 was based corresponds to the world age structure for 1960.

Increases in life expectancy from ages 60 to 70 show a continued decrease in group I, accelerating increases for groups II and III, and almost no change in groups IV and V. Increases in life expectancy above age 70 show the proportion of deaths in group I approaching zero, while groups II and III continue to increase, group IV remains constant, and group V decreases.[10] Figure 9.1 was constructed on the basis of a "young" age structure in which the level of fertility was relatively high. For older age structures, as the United Nations report indicates, the cause-of-death groups with the exception of group IV would experience the general trend shown in this figure.

The impact of these trends in mortality and morbidity on the need for health services is evident. Persons with chronic conditions, particularly older persons, have higher rates of health service utilization, as well as greater needs for long-term care and facilities.[11-13] One of the authors of this chapter has warned of the consequences, in terms of public policy and the allocation of health resources, of attempting to provide long-term care for the chronically ill.[14] Hence it is not unreasonable to assume that demands for a wide range of services and facilities will be made in the future. Such demands will inevitably result in some restructuring and expansion of the health services system, and also in a considerable and continuing increase in expenditures.

While changes in morbidity and mortality patterns may be a consideration in terms of the need for services and facilities, changes in the organization and structure of the medical care system may also be important. Even here a range of models is probably needed for different areas of the country. For example, the continued concentration of physicians and dentists in urban areas may mean that medical care will become even less accessible in rural areas. And it is by no means clear that higher ratios of physicians and dentists to population in urban areas imply that individuals are receiving more or even better medical care. On the contrary, it would appear that, even in urban areas, the economically deprived receive only minimal care.

One of the outgrowths of the concern for the lack of medical care has been the development of neighborhood health centers. Whether such centers are successful in providing care in the long run depends on several factors: the solution of problems related to community participation and/or control, the willingness of trained professionals to take part in such activities, the degree of success in training indigenous and paraprofessional personnel as the requirements for health care increase, and the financial costs that the establishment of such health care centers entail. Indeed, the last may be the single most important factor. Not only must the facilities be established, but funds must be available on a continuing basis for salaries, supplies, and maintenance. In spite of the potential problems related to financing, it seems evident that the proliferation of neighborhood centers would certainly entail a demand for more services and personnel.

An additional factor related to the organization of the health services system is the continuing effect of insurance or prepayment programs that are currently generating discussion, particularly at the national level. Presumably insurance plans would not only facilitate access but would also increase total utilization of the health services system. Although not conclusive, some recent evidence of the effect of Medicare has shown that since its adoption the average length of stay in short-term general hospitals for the over-65 age group has increased by almost one day.[15]

The proportion of the population covered by hospital insurance increased from 51 percent in 1950 to 89 percent in 1971, and the proportion of these covered by surgical insurance increased from 36 to 83 percent in the same period. The increase in dental insurance coverage, on the other hand, is still relatively insignificant.[2] In fact, it has been estimated that in 1967 only 6 percent of the population was covered for dental services. Thus any large-scale increase in the proportion of persons covered by dental insurance, independent of any consideration of the influence of extension of fluoridation on oral disease, could have considerable impact on the need for dentists and related personnel, since there has been a relatively slow rate of increase in the number of dentists.

Another factor that may influence estimates of needs for health services is the assessment of future population growth, crucial for planning of manpower requirements. An absolute increase in population size, holding other factors constant, means that the supply of personnel and facilities should increase at approximately the same rate. Even a relatively small growth rate of 1 percent per year will produce a large increase in absolute numbers if the population base is large. Thus if programs for professional training in the health field do not keep up with population growth, serious shortages and deficiencies may develop.

Population Projections

The Bureau of the Census has prepared population projections according to four different schedules taking into account the possible future course of fertility, mortality, and net migration.[1] The four schedules, Series C, D, E, and F, are based on two main assumptions: that major catastrophes such as wars or epidemics will not occur, and that a relatively high level of economic productivity will be maintained. Although subject to wide margins of error, population projections are less vulnerable to error than are the supposed need and demand for health services, which are dependent upon other social-psychological variables.

The projections were derived using the cohort-component method, which involves carrying forward estimates of current population age by age, for each sex, to future years on the basis of each of the components of population change (that is, births, deaths, and net immigration). The Series C projections, in which high rates of fertility are postulated, also provide the highest population estimates. The Series F projections are based on the assumption of relatively low rates of fertility and provide the lowest population estimates. The completed cohort fertility (the average number of children born by the end of the childbearing period) was estimated for Series C at 2.8 in the year 2020. For Series F, this rate was estimated at 1.8.

The estimated population increase for the United States for each series at selected points in time through 2020 is presented in Table 9.2. All series assume slightly declining mortality and 400,000 annual net immigration. It is important to note the magnitude of the difference for Series C and Series F. In 1990 the difference is expected to be approximately 27 million persons, and by 2020 the difference increases to appoximately 128 million. Such differences are crucial in the estimation of future needs that may be predicated on assumptions concerning population growth.

In addition to absolute population increase, consideration should be given to factors related to changes in population composition, where long-term changes may affect the need for specific types of specialists and facilities. For example, a population that has a long-term increase in the proportion of persons aged 65 and older may require proportionately more specialists in geriatrics or increases in facilities for long-term convalescence.

Speculation concerning future growth trends and composition is, of course, subject to error caused by under- or overestimation

Table 9.2   Estimated population (thousands) for selected years
by census series, with percent increase:
United States, 1970 to 2020

Year	Series			
	C	D	E	F
1970	204,879	204,879	204,879	204,879
1980	230,955	228,676	224,132	221,848
1990	266,238	258,692	246,639	239,084
2000	300,406	285,969	264,430	250,686
2010	344,094	318,156	281,968	259,332
2020	392,030	351,368	297,746	264,564
Percent Increase (1970-2020)	91.3	71.5	45.3	29.1

Source: Bureau of the Census, Series P-25, No. 493,
Washington, 1972.

according to the different components used in the projections. The
major source of error for projections in the United States is with
respect to the birth rate. Because of such variations, Bogue has
stated: "Before 1965, there was a tendency to make predictions that
were too low; after 1965 there seems to have developed the opposite
tendency, that is, to anticipate more population growth than eventually takes place."[6]

Projections of the age structure to the year 2000 become increasingly uncertain because of the unpredictable future course of
fertility. There is considerable variation in the absolute number of
individuals in certain age categories for each series of projections, and
in the percentage distribution as well. For example, Series C
estimates show no substantial increase, while the Series F estimates
show a decrease, for the age group under 15 years (Table 9.3). For
the 15-29 age category there is a small decrease for Series C and a
slightly greater decrease for Series F. The 30-44 category shows an
increase for both series, that for Series F being larger. For Series C a
slight decline in the proportions of the population in the 45-64 and

Table 9.3   Percent distributions of the estimated
populations: United States, 1972 and 2000 -
Series C and Series F

Age	Year		
	1972	Series C 2000	Series F 2000
Total	100.0	100.0	100.0
Under 15	27.2	27.6	20.2
15-29	25.6	23.6	21.2
30-44	16.8	19.9	23.9
45-64	20.4	19.4	23.2
65 and over	10.0	9.6	11.5

Source: Bureau of the Census, Series P-25, No. 493,
Washington, 1972.

the 65 and older categories is projected; however, for Series F increases in these proportions occur.

Changes in the demographic composition, such as age structure, median age, and life expectancy, are of course related to variations in mortality and morbidity rates by diagnosis or condition, as pointed out previously. The interaction of such processes will in the long run be expected to have considerable impact on the estimation of future service and personnel requirements.

Trends in Utilization

Estimates of the need for health services and facilities may be based on changes in patterns of utilization. Utilization is viewed as reflecting the demand for health services, where demand may be a result of illness, perception of illness, or the interaction of illness and social processes. Health service utilization studies, reports, or theories have been presented that demonstrate the utility of a wide number of demographic, social, and illness-related variables in the prediction of utilization patterns.[16-21]

With respect to trends in utilization, there has been a long-term increase. For example, it has been estimated that for any period of twelve consecutive months during 1928-31, approximately 48 percent of the population surveyed saw a physician.[22] By 1969, the proportion had increased to 69 percent.[23] During 1928-31, there were 2.6 physician visits per person per year.[22] By 1969, the average number of visits had increased to 4.3 per person.[23] Similarly, hospital admission rates for general and specialized hospital care increased from 74 per 1,000 in 1940 to 152 in 1970.[2]

Although the proportion of persons seeing a dentist increased from 21 percent in 1930 to 47 percent in 1963, the full impact of increased utilization on the need for dentists and dental personnel may not be felt until some form of insurance or prepayment plans is implemented on a large scale.[8,22]

If trends of increasing utilization continue for physician, hospital, and dental services (holding other factors constant), there will be pressure to increase manpower and facilities. It seems reasonable to assume that utilization will continue to increase as a result of the higher general economic level of the population, more widespread health insurance coverage, and changes in the demographic structure of the population. Since increases in utilization can be made up of both increases in the number of services per person per visit and increases in the total number of visits for health care, a possible result would be a greater demand for professional personnel as well as changes in the delivery of services.

We have attempted to demonstrate in the preceding pages that several factors related to the estimation of requirements for health service needs interact with one another. Changes in mortality rates may be a result of both increasing proportions of persons reaching high-risk ages and improvements in medical care. Similarly, changes for mortality and morbidity rates may influence not only utilization patterns but also the structure and organization of the delivery of services.

Projections of Manpower and Hospital Beds

The ability of a society to respond to the demand for increased manpower, services, or facilities may be approximated by comparing the percentage increase in manpower and facilities to the percentage increase in population size for some specified time period. An occupation or facility that had a larger percentage increase relative to population increase would then be said to be expanding more rapidly than would be expected under assumptions of normal growth with population increase, and vice versa.

Data presented in Table 9.4 show the absolute increase and the percentage increase for selected health service occupations and for hospital beds.[24][25] The occupational categories presented accounted for approximately 65 percent of primary health-related personnel in 1967.[25] Since the population of the United States increased by approximately 35 percent from 1950 through 1970, only the supply of dentists and hospital beds has not kept pace with population increase.[26] The largest increases have been in medical auxiliaries and in aides, orderlies, and attendants.

Alternately, by dividing the percentage increase in manpower by the population percentage increase, an index of relative growth is obtained. Dental auxiliaries, registered nurses, and practical nurses have increased at rates of 1.8, 2.4, and 4.7 times faster than the United States population (Table 9.5). The index for the other categories is interpreted similarly: aides, orderlies, and attendants, and medical auxiliary personnel have increased very rapidly, while primary professional personnel (physicians and dentists) have shown a relatively slow rate of growth. Thus manpower needs resulting from greater utilization of health services have been met more by increases in auxiliary personnel than by corresponding increases in primary professional personnel. Finally, the supply of hospital beds also has shown a relatively slow rate of growth. However, the overall figure in this case masks an increase in general hospital beds and a rather substantial decline in mental hospital beds.

The response of the American health care system has been a gradual increase at professional levels, dentists and hospital beds excluded, and substantial increases in auxiliary workers augmenting professional personnel. Even so, many authorities in this country feel that there are serious deficiencies in the health care system. The major criticism is directed at the current organization and delivery of health services and less at the current ratios of facilities and personnel to population. Faith is expressed, however, that reorganization of services (implicitly along the lines of group practice prepayment plans) may increase productivity and hence reduce the necessity of maintaining a constant resource-population ratio. The National Advisory Commission on Health Manpower has pointed to some of the more evident disadvantages of our present health care situation: long delays in seeing a physician for routine care, impersonal attention, difficulty in obtaining care on weekends, the uneven distribution of hospital beds and other resources and services, and financial barriers that inhibit the seeking of care.[27] The kinds and

Table 9.4 Health manpower and hospital beds, with percentage increases: United States, 1950-1970

Year	Physicians (M.D. & D.O.)	Dentists	Dental auxiliaries[a]	Registered nurses[b]	Practical nurses[c]	Aides, orderlies, and attendants[d]	Medical auxiliaries[e]	Hospital beds[f]
1950	232,697	87,164	84,200	375,000	137,500	221,000	60,800	1,436,000
1960	274,834	101,947	--	504,000	206,000	375,000	128,000	1,658,000
1970	348,328	118,175	138,000	700,000	370,000	815,000	210,000	1,535,000
Percent increase (1950-1970)	49.7	35.6	63.9	86.7	169.1	268.7	245.4	6.9

Source: Public Health Service, Health Resources Statistics, 1968, Washington, 1968, and Health Resources Statistics, 1971, Washington, 1971.

[a]Includes dental hygienists (active), dental assistants (employed), dental laboratory technicians (employed).
[b]Full-time and part-time.
[c]Number of nurses in practice.
[d]Employed in hospitals.
[e]Includes radiologic technologists and clinical laboratory personnel.
[f]Includes both short-stay and long-term hospitals.

Table 9.5   Index of relative growth for
health manpower by type, and
hospital beds: United States,
1970 versus 1950

Category	Index
Physicians (M.D. and D.O)	1.4
Dentists	1.0
Dental auxiliaries	1.8
Registered nurses	2.4
Practical nurses	4.7
Aides, orderlies, and attendants	7.5
Medical auxiliaries	6.9
Hospital beds	0.2

range of problems enumerated by the Advisory Commission imply that no simplistic solution is possible to cure all the ills of the health service system.

Hopefully, advances in technology ranging from computer-based linked records to computer diagnostics and multiphasic screening centers will improve the overall quality of services delivered. However, advances are likely to be less effective than anticipated unless concerted efforts are made to integrate them within a comprehensive health delivery system.

Projections of future health service requirements may be made in several ways. It may be assumed, for example, that a particular growth rate is needed in order to achieve an optimum level of health care by a certain date. Still, the concept of optimum defies measurement. Or manipulation of current health service information may be projected in time, assuming constant ratios to population growth. In this chapter we have chosen to examine current ratios based on the quantity or number in particular health service categories; these quantities in turn were divided by current population estimates, then multiplied by a constant. Such a procedure yields the familiar physician, dentist, nurse, or hospital bed ratios. The data for the various health service and hospital bed ratios were abstracted from Bureau of the Census and Public Health Service reports.[2],[24],[25]

Each ratio was used in turn with the four series of population growth prepared by the Census Bureau to yield estimates of future needs. In order to calculate the projected number of dentists at some future time, for example, the following equation is solved:

$$\text{number of dentists in year } X = \frac{(\text{ratio in 1970}) (\text{population in year } X)}{100,000}$$

The estimates obtained according to each population series then give some idea of a range of requirements for the future, assuming a constant ratio over the years.

The projected numbers of physicians, dentists, nurses, and hospital beds through 2020, using 1970 as the base year, are presented in Tables 9.6 and 9.7. It can be seen that the numerical range of personnel and beds varies considerably according to which series of projections is used. For instance, the differences between the Series C estimates and the Series F estimates based on the U.S. ratio are approximately 183,000 for physicians, 60,000 for dentists, 436,000 for nurses, and 956,000 for hospital beds.

The estimates presented in the left panels of Table 9.6 (based on U.S. ratios) assume of course that current ratios will be maintained in the future. It may be argued, however, that rather than attempting to maintain current ratios, efforts should be directed toward increasing manpower and facilities to some optimum level. While the definition of optimum level implies some knowledge beyond the scope of this chapter concerning desired health levels in relation to mortality and morbidity, we have taken as a crude measure of desired manpower and facilities the highest state ratio for each of the four stipulated categories. These ratios have been projected through the year 2020; the estimates appear in the right-hand panels of Tables 9.6 and 9.7.

As with the previous projections, the range of the differences between Series C and Series F is considerable for each category and somewhat larger than the differences when the United States ratio was used. The differences are approximately 288,000 for physicians, 87,000 for dentists, 583,000 for nurses, and 1,288,000 for hospital beds.

While total projected estimates are useful in describing the relative range and magnitude of the problem of adequate manpower and

Table 9.6   Projected number of physicians and dentists (thousands) based
             on specified population estimates and on (a) current U.S.
             ratios to population and (b) highest state ratios:
             United States, 1970 to 2020

Component and year	U. S. ratio				Highest state ratio			
	Series C	Series D	Series E	Series F	Series C	Series D	Series E	Series F
Physicians								
1970	294	294	294	294	294	294	294	294
1975	309	308	306	305	487	487	483	482
1980	330	327	321	317	522	517	507	501
1990	381	370	353	342	602	585	558	540
2000	430	409	378	358	679	646	598	567
2010	492	455	403	371	778	719	637	586
2020	561	502	426	378	886	794	673	598
Dentists								
1970	95	95	95	95	95	95	95	95
1975	101	101	100	100	147	146	145	145
1980	109	107	105	104	157	155	152	151
1990	125	122	116	112	181	176	168	163
2000	141	134	124	118	204	194	180	170
2010	162	150	133	122	234	216	192	176
2020	184	165	140	124	267	239	202	180

Note: The following categories and their respective United States
ratios were used in these projections: (a) active non-federal
physicians (M.D. and D.O.) - 143/100,000; (b) active non-federal dentists - 47/100,000. Use of ratios limited to active professionals in
each category corrects for the overestimation commonly found in such
ratios because inactive or retired personnel do not provide care.
Corresponding 1970 ratios are: for all physicians - 176, and all dentists - 58.
   In selecting state ratios the District of Columbia was excluded
from consideration. The following ratios and states were used:
(a) physicians, New York - 226; (b) dentists, New York - 68.

facilities, an alternate approach is to observe the average numbers of
personnel and beds which need to be produced each year in order to
reach by 2020 the projected levels shown in Tables 9.6 and 9.7. As is
often the case, summary measures may obscure some important
considerations. In the present instance the average rate will tend to
overestimate requirements in the early years of projections and to
underestimate requirements for the later years. Within each series of
projections the differences in annual growth rates are relatively large.
As summarized in the difference between Series C and Series F
estimates for each category at the bottom of Table 9.8, the figures

Table 9.7 Projected number of nurses and hospital beds (thousands) based on specified population estimates and on (a) current U.S. ratios to population and (b) highest state ratios: United States, 1970 to 2020

Component and year	U. S. ratio				Highest state ratio			
	Series C	Series D	Series E	Series F	Series C	Series D	Series E	Series F
Nurses								
1970	700	700	700	700	700	700	700	700
1975	738	736	732	730	1,157	1,154	1,146	1,144
1980	790	782	767	759	1,238	1,226	1,201	1,189
1990	911	885	844	818	1,427	1,387	1,322	1,281
2000	1,027	978	904	857	1,610	1,533	1,417	1,344
2010	1,177	1,088	964	887	1,844	1,705	1,511	1,390
2020	1,341	1,202	1,018	905	2,101	1,883	1,596	1,418
Hospital beds								
1970	1,535	1,535	1,535	1,535	1,535	1,535	1,535	1,535
1975	1,619	1,615	1,604	1,600	2,180	2,175	2,161	2,155
1980	1,732	1,715	1,681	1,664	2,332	2,310	2,264	2,241
1990	1,997	1,940	1,850	1,793	2,689	2,613	2,491	2,415
2000	2,253	2,145	1,983	1,880	3,034	2,888	2,671	2,532
2010	2,581	2,386	2,115	1,945	3,475	3,213	2,848	2,619
2020	2,940	2,635	2,233	1,984	3,960	3,549	3,007	2,672

Note: The following categories and their respective United States ratios were used in these projections: (a) registered nurses in practice - 342/100,000; (b) hospital beds - 7.5/1,000.
    In selecting state ratios the District of Columbia was excluded from consideration. The following ratios and states were used: (a) registered nurses, Connecticut - 536; (b) hospital beds, South Dakota, Massachusetts - 10.1/1,000.

range from a low of 1,200 for dentists based on the United States ratio to a high of 25,760 for hospital beds for the highest state ratio.

A word of caution is in order. Annual growth figures presented in Table 9.8 refer only to the number of new personnel and facilities, and do not take into account attrition for the manpower estimates or obsolescence of hospital beds. In addition, the data are projected on the basis of active registered nurses and active nonfederal physicians and dentists. The estimates would have to be revised upward according to the expected impact of attrition and with an additional allowance for federal positions if the total number of graduates required each year is the figure desired.

Table 9.8   Average annual growth in number of physicians, dentists,
nurses, and hospital beds, based on United States and
state ratios for Series C to Series F projections:
United States, 1970-2020

Series and ratios	Active non- federal physicians	Active non- federal dentists	Registered nurses	Hospital beds
Series C				
U.S. ratio	5,340	1,780	12,820	28,100
State ratio	11,840	3,440	28,020	48,500
Series D				
U.S. ratio	4,160	1,400	10,040	22,000
State ratio	10,000	2,880	23,660	40,280
Series E				
U.S. ratio	2,640	900	6,360	13,960
State ratio	7,580	2,140	17,920	29,440
Series F				
U.S. ratio	1,680	580	4,100	8,980
State ratio	6,080	1,700	14,360	22,740
Difference (C-F)				
U.S. ratio	3,660	1,200	8,720	19,120
State ratio	5,760	1,740	13,660	25,760

Material presented thus far has been based only on selected
categories. In the following section projected estimates of manpower
for medical auxiliary and paramedical personnel will be presented,
but unlike the previous estimates, state data were not available for all
of the categories. Thus the data as presented in Table 9.9 are ratios
for the United States, used in conjunction with Series C and Series F
projections of population growth.

Net increases, presented at the bottom of the table, show considerable differences by series. Under Series C estimates, the total net
increase is approximately 1,400,000 for all personnel; for Series F,
the total increase is approximately 446,000.

In summary, the projections presented thus far indicate a need for
a long-term increase in the absolute numbers of manpower and
facilities for the future. The actual extent of such increases will, of
course, also be affected by factors not controlled in this chapter:
changes in the scope of delivery of services, a shift to prepayment
plans, alterations in insurance plans, marked reductions in mortality,

Table 9.9 Projected numbers (thousands) of allied health personnel manpower: United States, 1970 to 2020

Year	Dental auxiliaries		Practical nurses		Aides, orderlies, attendants		Medical auxiliaries	
	Series C	Series F	Series C	Series F	Series C	Series F	Series C	Series F
1970	138		370		815		210	
1975	145	143	391	386	859	849	220	218
1980	155	149	418	402	919	883	236	226
1990	178	160	482	433	1,060	951	271	244
2000	201	168	544	454	1,196	998	306	256
2010	231	174	623	469	1,369	1,032	351	265
2020	263	177	710	479	1,560	1,053	400	270
Net increase (1970-2020)	125	39	340	109	745	238	190	60
Difference (Series C - Series F)		86		231		507		130

Source: National Center for Health Statistics, Health Resources Statistics, Washington, 1971, and Bureau of the Census, Series P-25, No. 493, Washington, 1972.

Note: The following ratios were obtained using the resident population of the United States as the denominator: (a) dental auxiliaries (hygienists, assistants, laboratory technicians) - 67; (b) practical nurses - 181; (c) aides, orderlies, and attendants - 398; (d) medical auxiliaries (clinical laboratory and radiologic technology) - 102. All ratios are per 100,000 population.

and decreases or increases in birth rate. Obviously, some degree of caution should be used in interpretation of the projections.

Utilization and the Need for Services and Facilities

Thus far we have attempted to assess the range of future needs in selected areas with respect to manpower and facilities. These assessments have been based primarily on assumptions concerning population growth and constant ratios of supply to population. In this section we will again focus on population increase in conjunction with projections of three selected measures of utilization: dental visits, physician visits, and hospital discharges. These measures in turn will be discussed with respect to trends in mortality and morbidity.

These particular measures of utilization were selected because they represent the range of health services with which most people are likely to be involved at some point in their lives. In contrast to dentist and physician visits, which are primarily free-standing components of health service use, hospital discharges may be viewed as a summary measure for a relatively large number of health service personnel and facilities with which a patient may come in contact either directly or indirectly: physician, nurses, aides and orderlies, laboratory personnel. Each of the three measures of utilization will be broken down into categories that reflect differences in utilization: (a) physician visits by activity limitation status, (b) hospital discharges by condition for which the patient was hospitalized, and (c) dental visits by type of service received.

The basic procedure used in the following tables takes selected rates or measures of utilization by age categories and projects them at the specified year rate to 2000 according to Series C and Series F projections. Although both age and sex are important considerations in terms of differences in utilization, sex was excluded from the projections because there was very little difference in the projected sex ratios.

The projected distributions of the number of physician visits for Series C and Series F appear in Table 9.10. As will be the case for the subsequent tables, percentage changes reflect changes in the age composition of the populations. Where the Series C population has an expected median age of 29.1 in the year 2000, the Series F population has an expected median age of 35.8.

Since the population age structure for Series C is similar to the

Table 9.10   Percent distribution of physician visits by age
              and activity limitation: United States,
              1969 and 2000 - Series C and Series F

Limitation[a] and age	1969	Series C 2000	Series F 2000
No limitation	100.0	100.0	100.0
Under 5	15.6	15.6	10.8
5-14	16.5	13.7	10.9
15-24	16.8	16.9	14.8
25-44	25.1	27.5	33.2
45-64	18.9	17.4	21.6
65 and over	7.1	8.9	8.7
Visits (thousands)	(635,460)	(1,002,000)	(806,000)
Some limitation [b]	100.0	100.0	100.0
Under 5	1.8	1.9	1.0
5-14	4.3	3.8	2.7
15-24	6.1	6.4	4.7
25-44	18.8	21.1	21.5
45-64	34.7	32.3	33.9
65 and over	34.2	34.5	36.2
Visits (thousands)	(204,146)	(313,000)	(298,000)

Source: C.S. Wilder, Physician Visits, 1969,
Washington, 1972, and U.S. Bureau of the Census, Series P-25,
No. 493, Washington, 1972.

[a]Major activity limitation refers to ability to work,
keep house, or engage in school or preschool activities.
[b]Includes the following categories: limited but not in
major activity, limited in amount or kind of major activity,
and unable to carry on major activity.

Note: Percentages may not add to 100.0 due to rounding.

1972 age structure as seen in Table 9.3, the proportion of visits by age in Series C varies only in the range from 0 to 2.8 percent from 1969 for both categories of activity limitation. However, greater changes in the proportion of visits for Series F are present. For the age categories under 25 there is a decrease in the proportion of visits, while for the older categories there are increases in the proportion of visits. With respect to changes in the proportion of visits for Series F, where there is "some limitation" of activity, only small differences from 1969 appear in the range from 0.8 to 2.7 percent.

The effect of changes in the total percentage increase in visits with

1969 as the base year is evident for both series. For the "no limitation" category, the percentage increase is 58 percent for Series C and 27 percent for Series F; for visits in which persons have "some limitation" of activity, the corresponding percentage increases are 53 and 46.

If, as Sanders suggests, the prevalence of chronic conditions increases as a result of better health care, then the estimates for physician visits for chronic conditions would be increased; there will be an intensified demand for more physicians and hospital facilities, and services would presumably increase.[9] Furthermore, an increase in chronic conditions—particularly those that involve limitations in activity—would undoubtedly have its impact on the need for services and manpower. In recent years the place of visit for physicians' services has shifted. The trend has been toward an increase in the proportion of visits in physicians' offices, a substantial decline in home visits, and a slight decline in the proportion of hospital clinic visits. For persons disabled to the extent that they were unable to carry on their major activity, however, 10 percent of their visits were made by a doctor in the home.[23] Thus a large increase in chronic conditions of this kind would require some increase in manpower or a change in the method of delivery of services.

A second measure of utilization is the number of short-stay hospital discharges by the condition for which persons were hospitalized. The data are presented in Table 9.11 for eight major categories representing 80 percent of all discharges. The majority (92 percent) of increases or decreases in proportions by age relative to 1968 for both Series C and F were in the range of ±3 percent. Larger differences are discussed below.

For the "all conditions" category there should be a moderate increase (3.4 percent) in the portion of discharges in the 15-44 category for Series C and a large decrease (5.6 percent) in the under 15 category for Series F. With respect to Series C, moderate increases for the 15-44 age group are observed for the digestive system (3.1 percent), the genito-urinary system (3.4 percent), and injuries (3.6 percent). Differences in the proportion of discharges for Series F relative to 1968 are generally greater than those for Series C. For example, decreases in the proportion of discharges in the under 15 category are present for the nervous system (6.0 percent), respiratory system (13.3 percent), digestive system (5.2 percent), genito-urinary system (3.6 percent), and injuries (7.2 percent). Other Series F changes in proportion are observed in the 65 and older category for

Table 9.11　Percent distribution of short-stay hospital discharges by age for selected conditions for which hospitalized[a]: United States, 1968 and 2000 - Series C and Series F

Condition and age	1968	Series C 2000	Series F 2000
All conditions			
Under 15	14.2	12.6	8.6
15–44	42.8	46.2	44.9
45–64	23.2	21.4	24.1
65 and over	19.6	19.7	22.2
	(28,070)	(44,002)	(39,101)
Neoplasms			
Under 15	3.5	3.2	2.1
15–44	32.9	35.5	32.7
45–64	35.8	33.3	35.4
65 and over	27.8	27.8	29.6
	(1,927)	(3,006)	(2,822)
Nervous system and sense organs			
Under 15	15.0	13.6	9.0
15–44	16.9	18.7	17.5
45–64	25.0	23.6	25.6
65 and over	42.9	44.0	47.7
	(1,542)	(2,365)	(2,180)
Circulatory system			
Under 15	2.4	2.2	1.4
15–44	16.2	17.7	15.9
45–64	36.2	33.9	35.1
65 and over	45.2	46.0	47.6
	(2,669)	(4,116)	(3,981)
Respiratory system			
Under 15	47.3	44.2	34.0
15–44	21.5	24.3	26.4
45–64	15.3	14.8	18.7
65 and over	15.7	16.5	20.7
	(3,272)	(4,881)	(3,884)
Digestive system			
Under 15	13.4	12.0	8.2
15–44	34.3	37.4	35.8
45–64	31.3	29.2	32.4
65 and over	20.9	21.2	23.6
	(3,986)	(6,174)	(5,574)
Genito-urinary system			
Under 15	8.9	7.9	5.3
15–44	48.7	52.1	50.1
45–64	26.4	24.0	26.8
65 and over	15.9	15.8	17.6
	(2,647)	(4,181)	(3,756)

(cont.)

Table 9.11   Percent distribution of short-stay hospital
discharges by age for selected conditions
for which hospitalized[a]: United States,
1968 and 2000 - Series C and Series F (cont.)

Condition and age	1968	Series C 2000	Series F 2000
Pregnancy			
Under 15	0.4	0.3	0.3
15-44	99.3	99.6	99.5
45-64	0.3	0.1	0.2
65 and over	---	---	---
	(4,183)	(7,045)	(6,089)
Injuries			
Under 15	18.7	16.6	11.5
15-44	45.2	48.8	49.3
45-64	20.8	19.1	21.7
65 and over	15.2	15.3	17.3
	(2,886)	(4,518)	(3,988)

Source: A. L. Ranofsky, Inpatient Utilization of
Short-Stay Hospitals by Diagnosis, 1968, Washington, 1973.
U.S. Bureau of the Census, Series P-25, No. 493,
Washington, 1972.
[a]Number of discharges (thousands) in parentheses.
Note: Percentages may not add to 100.0 due to
rounding.

the nervous system, an increase of 4.8 percent, and the 15-44 category for injuries, an increase of 4.1 percent. Diseases of the respiratory system show increases of 4.9, 3.4, and 5.0 percent respectively for the 15-44, 45-64, and 65 and older categories.

Table 9.12 shows the percentage increase in discharges by condition for hospitalization for both Series C and F from the base year 1968. The percentage increase is, as expected, greater for Series C than for Series F because of the greater population increase for the former. Overall, if we compare "all conditions," Series C has an increase of 56.7 percent and Series F has an increase of 39.2 percent. The differences between the estimates of increases by condition are, in descending order: respiratory system (30 percent), pregnancy (23 percent), injuries (18 percent), genito-urinary system (16 percent), digestive system (15 percent), nervous system (12 percent), neoplasms (10 percent), and circulatory system (5 percent).

Although the ranks of the percentage increases for both series are similar, there are three differences: (*a*) pregnancy ranks first in Series

Table 9.12   Projected percent increase in hospital discharges
by hospitalized condition: United States,
1968 to 2000 - Series C and Series F

Condition	Series C	Series F
All conditions	56.7	39.2
Neoplasms	55.9	46.4
Nervous system and sense organs	53.3	41.3
Circulatory system	54.2	49.1
Respiratory system	49.1	18.7
Digestive system	54.8	39.8
Genito-urinary system	57.9	41.6
Pregnancy	68.4	45.5
Injuries	56.5	38.1

C and third in Series F, (b) injuries rank third in Series C and seventh in Series F, and (c) circulatory system ranks sixth in Series C and first in Series F. These shifting patterns may thus specify points at which the delivery of health services and facilities should be altered in order to meet the demand. Analysis of the data in Table 9.12 suggests that there will be increased demand of significant proportions primarily for the care of malignant neoplasms, diseases of the nervous system, and diseases of the circulatory system.

Finally, a third measure of utilization is the number of dental visits by the type of dental service received. The data are presented in Table 9.13 for five major types of services and for all services combined. For the "all services" category Series C estimates vary very little from the base year data, while Series F shows considerable variation—a decrease in the proportions in the under 25 and the 65 and over age categories and an increase in the 25-44 and the 45-64 age categories.

For the "all services" category, Series C percentage differences relative to 1971, do not change notably for the under 25 and 45-64 age categories, while the 25-44 and 65 and older groups have an increase of 5 percent and a decrease of 5 percent respectively. For

Table 9.13   Percent distribution of dental visits by age
for types of dental service[a]: United States,
1971 and 2000 - Series C and Series F

Type of service and age	1971	Series C 2000	Series F 2000
All services			
Under 25	45.8	46.2	39.6
25-44	25.9	30.6	29.7
45-64	21.8	21.5	28.5
65 and over	6.4	1.5	2.1
	(312,000)	(441,000)	(333,000)
Fillings			
Under 25	46.5	45.5	38.2
25-44	28.5	32.3	32.3
45-64	19.8	19.1	25.4
65 and over	5.1	2.9	3.9
	(93,000)	(136,000)	(102,000)
Extractions			
Under 25	39.9	35.6	30.4
25-44	32.0	35.6	32.6
45-64	21.5	20.3	26.0
65 and over	6.4	8.5	10.8
	(38,000)	(59,000)	(46,000)
Cleanings			
Under 25	43.9	43.2	37.0
25-44	25.9	29.6	27.4
45-64	23.3	22.2	29.0
65 and over	6.7	4.9	6.4
	(56,000)	(81,000)	(62,000)
Examinations			
Under 25	54.0	49.1	41.5
25-44	24.3	26.2	25.8
45-64	17.6	15.2	20.2
65 and over	4.1	9.3	12.3
	(74,000)	(118,000)	(89,000)
Denture work			
Under 25	12.2	11.1	7.4
25-44	29.3	33.3	27.7
45-64	41.5	38.0	44.4
65 and over	17.1	17.4	20.3
	(41,000)	(63,000)	(54,000)

Source: R.W. Wilson, Current Estimates, 1971,
Washington, 1973, and U.S. Bureau of the Census, Series P-25,
No. 493, Washington, 1972.
   [a]Number of visits (thousands) in parentheses.

Note: Percentages may not add to 100.0 due to rounding.

Series F, decreases are observed for those under 25 years of age (6 percent) and those 65 and older (4 percent). Increases of approximately 4 percent and 7 percent are found respectively for those 25-44 and 45-64.

In Series C, decreases of more than 3 percent relative to 1971 occur in the under 25 age category for extractions (4 percent) and examinations (5 percent), and for denture work (4 percent) for those aged 45-64. Increases in the range of 3 to 4 percent for the 25-44 age category are present for fillings, extractions, cleaning, and denture work.

Large declines from 1971 to 2000 for Series F in the range of 4 to 13 percent occur in the under age 25 category for each dental service: fillings (8 percent), extractions (10 percent), cleanings (7 percent), examinations (13 percent), and denture work (5 percent). Increases for ages 45-64 are present for fillings (6 percent), cleanings (6 percent), and extractions (5 percent). Other increases for extractions (4 percent) and examinations (8 percent) occur for the 65 and over category.

In terms of the projected total numbers of dental visits, the percentage increases with respect to the base year for the "all services" category were 41 for Series C and 7 for Series F. As shown in Table 9.14, the largest increase in Series C was for examinations, whereas for Series F the largest increase was for denture work; this reflects the younger population of Series C and the older population of Series F.

Table 9.14   Projected percent increase in dental
visits by type of dental service:
United States, 1971 to 2000 -
Series C and Series F

Type of service	Series C	Series F
All services	41.3	6.7
Fillings	46.2	9.6
Extractions	55.2	21.0
Cleanings	44.6	10.7
Examinations	59.4	20.2
Denture work	50.0	28.5

Although the findings in Table 9.14 indicate a substantial increase in the number of dental visits over time, there is the possibility that the need for additional dental personnel will decrease because of changes in utilization patterns. One such change may result from an increase in the proportion of persons drinking fluoridated water. The number of such persons has grown from approximately 47 million in 1960 to approximately 88 million at the beginning of 1970.[28,29] Recent findings reported by Upton and Silverman indicate that fluoridation may reduce the demand for dental services by 57 percent.[30] Furthermore, their results imply that while the number of visits per person per year may decline because of increased intervals between visits, the proportion of persons making dental visits will not necessarily decline. Thus the projected number of dentists and dental auxiliary personnel based on United States dentist-population ratios may be sufficient to meet future needs.

Discussion

Requirements for future health service needs · and services have been discussed in this chapter with respect to the independent and interactive effects of morbidity and mortality patterns, organization of the health care system, demographic processes, and patterns of utilization. Throughout much of the discussion attention has been given to population growth and changes in the age structure of the population and the impact of such changes on morbidity and mortality.

Whether future demands are met in the long run depends primarily on the health system's ability to respond to change in any of the four areas mentioned in the previous paragraph. Certainly our society has the capability to respond in terms of graduating more doctors, dentists, or nurses, or building new facilities. The crucial test may very well depend on changes in the organization and delivery of services, but even the range of organizational forms that may be appropriate is literally as open-ended as the potential consumption of resources if they are provided. We are unable by systematic and scientific criteria to defer to any particular organizational forms; hence we prefer to stress relative abundance of resources within which delivery methods can be fashioned.

The projections presented in this chapter should serve to indicate potential requirements for manpower and facilities, as a range of possibilities in terms of future utilization of health services, given alternate assumptions concerning population growth and composition. If an increased demand for health services is brought about by increases in population size, changes in the age structure, or further increases in life expectancy, then the problem of future needs certainly becomes more complex as, indeed, it seems reasonable to predict. Given the increase in size of the population for those ages requiring long-term and relatively expensive care as a result of chronic conditions, it seems likely that this will be the area of the greatest future need and possibly the area of greatest controversy in the face of new life-prolonging techniques and transplants. The meeting of such needs may depend on the overall responsiveness of the health system to increased costs and utilization at all levels, as well as the influence of public policies and programs enacted at the governmental level.

Projections of population with the assumption of constant ratios between health facilities and personnel, taking into account age composition and its translation into contemporary patterns of use, is an interesting exercise to reveal what would happen "if." Adding any more variables—such as continuing medical discoveries, further changes in life style that may be deleterious to health, and organizational innovations in delivering services such as the much-acclaimed use of health screening and computers—probably increases the chance of error until the projections become a game. We have no idea what society in the future may regard as satisfactory tradeoffs between more technologically elaborate homes and hospitals; conceivably, more and more resources may be poured into "cathedrals" of healing and life prolongation. Certainly, we see no possibility of proportionally fewer facilities and personnel in relation to population than we have now.

The "need-demand" aspect of health services and the discretionary judgment required by professionals in handling it is so open-ended as to defy a rational structuring of need-demand and resources, except for a few highly specified diseases such as diabetes. Furthermore, we do not see a necessary reduction in the proportion of diseases that can be specified, because other diseases will emerge by changes in perception and definition. Disease and illness states are highly volatile. There will always be a disease pattern of some kind; to believe that there can be a disease-free society is utopian. Rene Dubos has written convincingly on the foregoing views.[31]

To sum up the general direction that health services will need to take: there will be more disease, more medical technology, more people, and, if the economists are right, more money. For us, these predictions spell expansion.

APPENDIX TABLES AND FIGURES
REFERENCES
INDEX

Table A.5.1 Death rates per 100,000 population for all causes by age, sex, and color: United States and each geographic division, 1959-61

Color, sex, and geog. division	All ages	Under 5	5-14	15-24	25-34	35-44	45-54	55-64	65-74	75-84	85 & over
White male											
United States	1,084.9	622.2	52.9	143.3	161.3	329.1	917.6	2,200.0	4,764.7	10,181.7	21,611.6
New England	1,173.7	597.2	48.9	115.1	131.6	306.1	909.1	2,304.1	5,050.4	10,604.7	22,055.6
Middle Atlantic	1,200.5	581.7	48.7	121.4	137.5	312.7	953.4	2,356.1	5,197.4	10,965.8	22,383.6
E. No. Central	1,100.7	596.6	51.3	141.4	148.4	312.1	898.5	2,175.7	4,883.4	10,455.3	22,440.6
W. No. Central	1,151.8	595.4	55.3	154.6	159.4	292.9	811.0	1,946.1	4,316.8	9,741.2	21,756.4
So. Atlantic	1,000.5	653.1	56.5	142.5	178.3	374.2	1,002.1	2,302.3	4,584.3	9,691.6	20,407.6
E. So. Central	1,023.5	673.9	55.1	164.9	206.6	383.6	938.3	2,086.4	4,420.8	9,899.2	21,444.7
W. So. Central	975.9	674.5	59.7	158.8	181.3	346.1	896.4	2,067.6	4,452.0	9,577.1	20,251.7
Mountain	958.7	726.7	61.4	193.4	209.3	366.9	882.8	2,099.3	4,452.5	9,641.5	20,617.7
Pacific	1,017.0	627.1	48.8	142.1	166.3	325.9	902.6	2,178.6	4,639.0	9,765.9	20,918.0
White female											
United States	793.2	471.2	34.3	54.3	85.5	187.4	456.6	1,063.1	2,755.4	7,619.7	19,271.9
New England	941.0	445.6	32.8	43.0	78.2	181.5	474.6	1,142.4	2,974.0	7,962.5	19,657.2
Middle Atlantic	915.1	445.4	31.5	48.5	83.0	193.7	498.5	1,232.7	3,203.8	8,472.0	20,282.9
E. No. Central	811.1	450.4	34.0	51.6	81.9	187.9	466.5	1,098.5	2,878.6	7,886.3	19,816.4
W. No. Central	835.5	445.8	34.0	55.4	82.0	165.6	399.8	922.5	2,463.3	7,113.2	19,113.6
So. Atlantic	694.2	486.7	34.9	53.4	86.5	187.9	437.6	988.6	2,540.4	7,308.2	18,637.8
E. So. Central	726.0	545.3	38.8	59.3	92.4	184.7	409.8	940.6	2,556.2	7,615.2	19,134.7
W. So. Central	658.9	520.7	37.8	62.2	88.1	179.7	394.3	896.2	2,326.1	6,834.7	17,524.2
Mountain	630.1	537.4	41.8	73.8	101.1	196.7	469.1	985.5	2,474.3	6,911.7	18,268.1
Pacific	736.9	466.4	32.0	57.6	89.9	196.3	478.5	1,016.2	2,484.5	6,961.2	18,535.7

Nonwhite male

United States	1,127.4	1,213.9	73.5	213.5	387.9	724.1	1,508.6	3,073.3	5,537.2	8,408.6	14,776.3
New England	998.4	1,110.0	72.8	143.0	261.8	612.0	1,291.5	2,812.9	5,851.3	10,200.3	16,207.2
Middle Atlantic	1,137.0	1,270.5	72.9	195.3	387.0	762.6	1,622.5	3,088.3	5,671.4	9,318.5	16,635.3
E. No. Central	1,038.0	1,049.6	65.6	176.5	334.9	642.9	1,435.4	2,957.7	5,748.3	9,108.2	15,228.0
W. No. Central	1,317.1	1,230.4	70.0	234.6	378.0	726.2	1,546.2	3,109.9	5,868.3	9,244.0	16,079.3
So. Atlantic	1,182.8	1,309.9	78.3	230.8	451.7	868.6	1,803.6	3,740.3	5,959.4	7,892.4	13,351.7
E. So. Central	1,283.0	1,299.8	78.9	232.2	439.7	764.0	1,491.2	3,042.0	5,520.5	8,671.7	16,582.4
W. So. Central	1,174.9	1,212.9	70.3	226.8	422.5	670.4	1,351.8	2,842.0	5,261.7	7,807.4	12,739.4
Mountain	1,024.3	1,562.1	87.3	356.3	536.0	758.8	1,336.9	2,267.2	4,015.9	8,043.1	14,026.7
Pacific	781.6	903.4	64.1	155.0	236.2	464.6	932.6	1,979.2	4,217.8	8,169.1	17,163.6

Nonwhite female

United States	858.8	974.7	51.6	109.2	252.2	538.4	1,122.1	2,360.4	3,907.1	6,626.2	12,776.6
New England	748.8	792.1	55.6	86.2	222.2	437.5	828.4	1,971.3	3,762.3	8,001.9	17,124.7
Middle Atlantic	821.2	1,000.4	48.5	101.7	253.1	517.4	1,063.4	2,172.9	3,862.9	7,551.0	14,716.8
E. No. Central	786.5	866.5	40.9	98.6	220.5	498.4	1,110.1	2,338.5	4,000.6	7,204.3	14,207.0
W. No. Central	997.0	1,010.7	51.4	105.8	234.2	536.5	1,208.4	2,339.9	4,063.4	7,370.6	14,487.6
So. Atlantic	908.4	1,038.4	55.7	112.5	296.0	633.9	1,280.8	2,810.9	4,154.6	6,031.5	11,148.9
E. So. Central	1,030.0	1,058.5	60.0	128.0	306.2	619.5	1,145.8	2,390.8	4,039.2	7,100.3	14,282.6
W. So. Central	912.6	992.3	51.6	115.2	244.1	513.3	1,105.9	2,262.3	3,739.0	5,989.2	10,879.3
Mountain	699.0	1,273.7	61.0	172.0	284.4	512.9	890.5	1,632.4	3,129.4	6,142.7	11,523.3
Pacific	519.6	702.5	41.8	78.1	148.1	329.1	712.5	1,384.7	2,831.1	6,324.3	14,161.0

Table A.5.2   Age-adjusted death rates per 100,000 population for
all causes by color and sex: United States, each
geographic division and state, 1959-61

Geographic division and state	White		Nonwhite	
	Male	Female	Male	Female
United States	906.3	549.7	1,185.4	878.5
New England	920.3	569.4	1,127.8	803.8
Connecticut	875.5	551.7	1,173.6	832.6
Maine	950.6	579.2	1,220.5*	703.6*
Massachusetts	930.7	574.8	1,081.9	790.5
New Hampshire	947.6	560.7	1,521.6*	478.3*
Rhode Island	915.3	582.3	1,247.9	831.8*
Vermont	948.3	563.0	575.2*	730.9*
Middle Atlantic	946.0	604.6	1,232.4	872.1
New Jersey	929.7	595.3	1,210.8	891.4
New York	940.0	603.2	1,243.3	850.8
Pennsylvania	963.9	612.2	1,215.8	893.9
East North Central	908.1	563.2	1,152.1	872.2
Illinois	935.0	573.6	1,226.6	917.2
Indiana	903.5	552.3	1,175.9	880.5
Michigan	908.0	562.8	1,026.6	815.5
Ohio	906.6	569.0	1,164.9	860.9
Wisconsin	854.1	537.2	1,025.7	803.1
West North Central	839.1	502.6	1,227.7	909.8
Iowa	832.7	496.7	1,050.5	903.1
Kansas	813.9	484.8	1,024.0	808.3
Minnesota	823.7	501.5	1,098.5	753.5
Missouri	883.8	525.7	1,266.0	923.9
Nebraska	812.0	483.7	1,363.2	929.0
North Dakota	795.7	494.9	1,352.1*	1,074.1*
South Dakota	838.3	486.7	1,544.0	1,197.4
South Atlantic	915.7	525.2	1,323.9	957.7
Delaware	923.0	573.2	1,364.7	996.3
District of Columbia	1,046.7	583.2	1,304.0	910.2
Florida	842.5	468.3	1,252.7	934.7
Georgia	941.3	511.1	1,365.6	984.7
Maryland	968.8	590.1	1,319.8	964.9
North Carolina	929.5	518.5	1,318.1	927.9
South Carolina	1,003.1	552.6	1,441.9	1,030.4
Virginia	924.5	539.5	1,305.6	961.3
West Virginia	943.5	574.4	1,211.2	862.0

(continued)

Table A.5.2 Age-adjusted death rates per 100,000 population for
all causes by color and sex: United States, each
geographic division and state, 1959-61 (continued)

Geographic division and state	White		Nonwhite	
	Male	Female	Male	Female
East South Central	900.8	532.4	1,214.2	933.2
Alabama	917.9	518.9	1,240.2	957.7
Kentucky	902.6	553.7	1,319.7	965.7
Mississippi	895.4	510.8	1,147.8	880.8
Tennessee	889.8	531.2	1,211.1	950.0
West South Central	877.2	494.7	1,118.4	841.5
Arkansas	848.3	477.2	1,040.9	813.2
Louisiana	960.9	533.5	1,174.4	891.0
Oklahoma	869.2	484.3	1,054.6	795.0
Texas	865.2	491.5	1,110.2	817.3
Mountain	898.0	529.7	1,095.2	776.4
Arizona	958.2	520.7	1,118.3	790.5
Colorado	860.0	526.1	988.4	652.3
Idaho	846.6	501.4	1,108.5*	782.8*
Montana	947.0	544.3	1,276.8	1,099.9
Nevada	1,082.8	595.3	1,109.1	990.7*
New Mexico	884.2	556.9	1,021.2	656.4
Utah	823.4	509.3	1,182.8	713.1*
Wyoming	911.0	523.7	1,139.2*	1,178.9*
Pacific	887.4	524.0	871.5	624.7
Alaska	931.6	549.2	1,019.6	894.2
California	888.5	525.8	900.1	644.0
Hawaii	991.8	638.2	701.7	503.9
Oregon	883.1	512.4	1,146.1	761.6
Washington	882.3	517.7	1,056.5	689.1

Table A.5.3 Age-adjusted death rates per 100,000 population for all causes by color and sex, for metropolitan and non-metropolitan counties: United States and each geographic division, 1959-61

Sex and geographic division	White				Nonwhite	
	Metropolitan counties			Non-metropolitan counties	Metropolitan counties Total	Non-metropolitan counties
	Total	With central city	Without central city			
Males						
United States	923.0	938.0	858.9	882.5	1,190.8	1,184.7
New England	919.4	925.3	861.2	920.6	1,132.6	1,093.4
Middle Atlantic	946.4	977.0	870.6	942.3	1,239.3	1,117.4
E. No. Central	931.8	943.2	862.3	871.0	1,166.4	999.2
W. No. Central	893.6	917.3	812.7	809.9	1,223.9	1,223.8
South Atlantic	907.2	929.8	855.5	925.4	1,345.1	1,307.7
E. So. Central	936.0	930.6	977.0	888.5	1,278.9	1,170.5
W. So. Central	905.9	912.1	848.6	860.5	1,177.2	1,074.1
Mountain	897.8	911.8	789.1	900.2	1,089.2	1,094.0
Pacific	892.3	902.1	828.6	874.9	868.8	901.3
Females						
United States	562.3	567.4	541.1	528.2	877.5	886.7
New England	572.8	577.0	531.5	556.6	815.0	693.2*
Middle Atlantic	607.7	624.8	564.9	591.9	873.8	836.8
E. No. Central	574.9	579.6	546.0	543.1	877.8	805.5
W. No. Central	521.9	527.3	505.5	490.2	900.9	927.0
South Atlantic	522.5	526.6	518.8	527.8	981.9	937.3
E. So. Central	533.7	526.9	586.2	532.2	976.4	903.2
W. So. Central	509.0	512.1	477.9	482.5	871.5	820.4
Mountain	526.2	531.9	487.0	532.9	767.7	778.7
Pacific	527.3	530.8	503.6	510.2	614.9	674.1

Table A.5.4   Death rates per 100,000 population for all causes by age, color, and sex for metropolitan and non-metropolitan counties: United States, 1959-61

Sex and age	White				Nonwhite	
	Metropolitan counties			Non-metro-politan counties	Metro-politan counties Total	Non-metro-politan counties
	Total	With central city	Without central city			
Males						
Age-adjusted, all ages	923.0	938.0	858.9	882.5	1,190.8	1,184.7
All ages, crude	1,054.6	1,106.5	856.4	1,135.9	1,086.4	1,200.5
Under 5	602.4	620.6	539.4	656.6	1,134.5	1,353.5
5-14	48.6	49.5	45.5	59.7	67.5	82.3
15-24	122.4	122.1	124.0	174.9	190.7	247.1
25-34	144.5	149.4	125.7	193.6	359.8	458.9
35-44	318.0	331.9	269.4	350.4	708.8	761.9
45-54	942.5	974.6	815.6	873.7	1,543.4	1,438.2
55-64	2,297.2	2,348.8	2,061.2	2,034.2	3,132.0	2,964.3
65-74	5,010.0	5,062.0	4,748.4	4,399.8	5,765.4	5,231.8
75-84	10,464.8	10,505.9	10,260.8	9,831.6	8,658.3	8,132.8
85 & over	21,476.6	21,507.4	21,333.8	21,760.5	14,486.6	15,048.8
Females						
Age-adjusted, all ages	562.3	567.4	541.1	528.2	877.5	886.7
All ages, crude	786.4	819.8	655.6	805.1	817.7	934.5
Under 5	456.0	472.1	400.2	497.5	909.9	1,088.9
5-14	32.3	33.0	30.0	37.6	45.5	60.9
15-24	49.9	50.0	49.1	61.5	100.1	124.9
25-34	84.2	87.0	74.1	87.8	238.2	288.2
35-44	191.2	197.9	166.6	180.0	524.0	573.3
45-54	477.6	487.2	436.2	417.9	1,127.6	1,111.1
55-64	1,112.7	1,122.5	1,065.5	973.8	2,373.8	2,336.2
65-74	2,864.4	2,871.9	2,826.4	2,574.0	4,035.5	3,731.4
75-84	7,782.8	7,785.9	7,767.6	7,377.5	6,838.9	6,359.6
85 & over	19,294.2	19,411.1	18,738.1	19,239.5	12,512.6	13,078.8

Table A.5.5 Age-adjusted[a] death rates per 100,000 population for all causes for selected age-sex-color groups: United States, each state and each state economic area[b], 1959-61

Division, state, and state economic area (SEA)	White, age 45-64			White, age 35-74		White, both sexes, 45-74	Nonwhite, both sexes, 45-74
	Male	Female	M/F Ratio	Male	Female		
United States	1,474.1	719.8	2.05	1,525.8	814.1	1,663.3	2,520.3
New England	1,514.4	764.4	1.98	1,577.8	865.0	1,750.7	2,312.8
Connecticut	1,409.2	733.5	1.92	1,503.3	839.0	1,683.0	2,371.0
SEA 1 (Northwest)	1,319.1	681.5	1.94	1,445.6	769.1	1,590.9	*
SEA 2 (East)	1,402.8	688.0	2.04	1,519.2	797.2	1,663.4	1,873.0#
SEA A Bridgport-Stamford Norwalk	1,403.4	750.3	1.87	1,513.3	859.8	1,703.9	2,395.2
SEA B New Haven-Waterbury	1,469.7	764.5	1.92	1,541.9	869.4	1,736.0	2,544.5
SEA C Hartford-New Britain-Bristol	1,378.1	721.7	1.91	1,458.5	825.6	1,640.0	2,359.8
Maine	1,518.2	763.9	1.99	1,582.6	866.6	1,745.9	2,180.0
SEA 1 (North)	1,355.3	800.8	1.69	1,461.0	889.7	1,656.9	*
SEA 2 (Central)	1,494.9	737.9	2.03	1,575.5	831.9	1,710.8	*
SEA 3 (East)	1,588.0	712.6	2.23	1,570.1	835.9	1,708.9	*
SEA 4 (South)	1,511.4	779.6	1.94	1,596.9	888.4	1,784.4	*
SEA A Portland	1,574.3	795.0	1.98	1,634.7	887.7	1,798.1	*
Massachusetts	1,560.8	780.0	2.00	1,610.9	878.9	1,780.8	2,237.0
SEA 1 Franklin Co.	1,247.5	692.2	1.80	1,379.3	808.1	1,561.6	*
SEA 2 (Southeast)	1,569.4	691.2	2.27	1,585.2	771.1	1,677.0	2,211.2#
SEA A Springfield-Holyoke	1,496.0	759.6	1.97	1,558.9	859.9	1,728.4	2,372.3
SEA B Worcester	1,477.0	728.0	2.03	1,538.7	838.3	1,709.3	1,550.9#

SEA	C	Boston-Lawrence-Lowell	1,604.6	797.1	2.01	1,646.4	888.9	1,812.2	2,199.3
SEA	D	Brockton	1,434.7	748.0	1.92	1,543.5	869.0	1,709.8	2,710.4#
SEA	E	Fall River-New Bedford	1,563.9	800.8	1.95	1,607.7	915.6	1,811.2	2,520.0#
SEA	F	Pittsfield	1,528.6	756.5	2.02	1,589.5	888.8	1,774.9	2,629.3#
		New Hampshire	1,519.7	728.9	2.08	1,579.1	835.8	1,739.5	1,851.4
SEA	1	(North)	1,491.6	738.9	2.02	1,576.1	870.5	1,744.4	*
SEA	2	(South)	1,430.8	729.3	1.96	1,502.1	818.6	1,683.7	*
SEA	A	Manchester	1,677.2	720.2	2.33	1,696.0	830.4	1,817.1	*
		Rhode Island	1,556.7	790.4	1.97	1,600.7	890.9	1,799.1	2,689.8
SEA	1	(South)	1,419.5	739.1	1.92	1,466.7	834.6	1,678.5	2,741.7#
SEA	A	Providence	1,575.0	797.2	1.98	1,619.9	898.6	1,815.3	2,677.2
		Vermont	1,468.5	743.1	1.98	1,558.6	826.1	1,697.5	1,784.4
SEA	1	NW (Northwest)	1,489.5	780.0	1.91	1,611.8	865.9	1,750.5	*
SEA	2	SE (Southeast)	1,458.5	724.2	2.01	1,531.8	805.1	1,671.3	*
		Middle Atlantic	1,562.1	817.1	1.91	1,624.7	928.0	1,830.9	2,512.3
		New Jersey	1,545.6	820.4	1.88	1,606.8	923.9	1,820.6	2,492.0
SEA	1	(North)	1,516.5	820.9	1.85	1,555.3	903.9	1,771.0	2,420.4
SEA	2	(South)	1,723.3	840.4	2.05	1,672.6	942.4	1,877.9	2,409.1
SEA	A	Warren Co.	1,567.1	907.5	1.73	1,650.4	980.3	1,885.7	*
SEA	B	Newark	1,489.5	785.3	1.90	1,582.5	902.3	1,784.9	2,577.1
SEA	C	Trenton	1,669.2	747.0	2.23	1,722.6	899.2	1,883.7	**2,445.4**
SEA	D	Burlington-Camden-Gloucester Co.	1,522.4	845.6	1.80	1,597.4	942.1	1,833.8	2,405.7
SEA	E	Atlantic City	1,577.0	899.9	1.75	1,631.6	949.8	1,851.1	2,370.6
SEA	F	Salem Co.	1,396.5	967.5	1.44	1,559.7	996.9	1,836.0	2,258.1
SEA	G	Patterson-Clifton-Passaic	1,386.1	737.1	1.88	1,462.7	852.8	1,674.2	2,439.9
SEA	H	Jersey City	1,928.9	1,009.4	1.91	1,937.8	1,098.6	2,159.0	2,652.2

(Continued)

Table A.5.5 Age-adjusted[a] death rates per 100,000 population for all causes for selected age-sex-color groups: United States, each state and each state economic area[b], 1959-61 (Continued)

Division, state, and state economic area (SEA)	White, age 45-64 Male	White, age 45-64 Female	White, age 45-64 M/F Ratio	White, age 35-74 Male	White, age 35-74 Female	White, both sexes, 45-74	Nonwhite, both sexes, 45-74
New York	1,542.3	805.2	1.92	1,606.8	915.2	1,808.3	2,434.7
SEA 1 (Northwest)	1,308.3	673.0	1.94	1,397.0	786.7	1,564.0	2,547.3#
SEA 2 (West Central)[c]	1,323.4	735.3	1.80	1,474.5	813.8	1,641.3	1,790.0#
SEA 3 (Southwest)	1,466.5	779.7	1.88	1,552.1	854.6	1,711.6	2,178.6#
SEA 4 (North Central)	1,581.4	778.4	2.03	1,608.4	916.1	1,806.9	*
SEA 5 (North Central)	1,521.7	825.7	1.84	1,615.4	917.4	1,830.4	*
SEA 6 (South Central)	1,490.1	739.0	2.02	1,505.9	831.5	1,676.2	*
SEA 7 (Northeast)	1,601.3	823.9	1.94	1,671.5	940.8	1,860.5	1,371.0#
SEA 8 (East Central)	1,634.9	805.3	2.03	1,667.4	925.6	1,847.1	*
SEA 9 (Southeast)[c]	1,547.7	760.2	2.04	1,592.3	865.7	1,759.1	1,986.8
SEA A Buffalo	1,616.7	827.6	1.95	1,702.8	962.6	1,914.0	2,523.6
SEA B Rochester	1,371.0	712.8	1.92	1,488.6	809.9	1,660.8	2,391.0
SEA C Syracuse	1,531.8	787.1	1.95	1,582.4	899.7	1,789.5	2,417.8#
SEA D Utica-Rome	1,467.7	759.8	1.93	1,555.1	877.2	1,753.7	1,923.6#
SEA E Binghamton	1,472.6	731.4	2.01	1,529.0	847.7	1,722.2	2,316.6#
SEA F Albany-Schenectady-Troy	1,669.6	815.9	2.05	1,740.0	917.6	1,909.3	2,428.8
SEA G New York City	1,552.9	819.1	1.90	1,612.7	931.6	1,823.2	2,452.2
Pennsylvania	1,603.0	835.1	1.92	1,662.7	951.0	1,872.4	2,640.8
SEA 1 (Northwest)	1,403.2	745.2	1.88	1,473.5	858.2	1,655.0	2,167.8
SEA 2 (Northeast)	1,451.9	739.3	1.96	1,572.4	850.7	1,707.1	*
SEA 3 (Central, North Central)	1,414.5	814.8	1.74	1,465.5	904.9	1,703.9	*
SEA 4 (Southwest)	1,497.5	841.6	1.78	1,547.1	938.7	1,758.8	2,578.1
SEA 5 (South Central)	1,548.6	804.5	1.92	1,590.8	923.6	1,794.2	1,894.2#
SEA 6 (East Central)	1,831.1	920.3	1.99	1,902.0	1,076.3	2,131.9	2,258.9#
SEA 7 (South Central, East)	1,406.1	784.0	1.79	1,450.5	887.0	1,670.3	2,089.5#

SEA	A	Erie	1,662.1	834.4	1.99	1,687.2	896.8	1,863.6	3,714.1#
SEA	B	Philadelphia	1,648.8	847.7	1.95	1,696.8	958.1	1,907.5	2,628.1
SEA	C	Scranton	2,015.2	983.6	2.05	2,066.6	1,178.6	2,308.4	*
SEA	D	Pittsburgh	1,598.5	851.6	1.88	1,664.0	966.1	1,884.9	2,701.6
SEA	E	Johnstown	1,537.6	840.4	1.83	1,632.9	944.7	1,833.6	2,102.1#
SEA	F	Altoona	1,602.3	800.9	2.00	1,617.9	898.0	1,810.0	*
SEA	G	Wilkes-Barre, Hazelton	2,033.5	909.7	2.24	2,109.6	1,107.5	2,309.0	4,897.4#
SEA	H	Harrisburg	1,631.0	775.8	2.10	1,632.3	872.6	1,800.3	2,767.7
SEA	J	York	1,353.7	776.9	1.74	1,429.8	850.1	1,638.3	2,673.9#
SEA	K	Lancaster	1,336.4	661.2	2.02	1,401.3	791.5	1,580.8	2,799.1#
SEA	L	Reading	1,427.2	813.6	1.75	1,514.1	907.1	1,736.2	2,604.4#
SEA	M	Allentown, Bethlehem, Easton	1,464.3	794.6	1.84	1,597.0	922.4	1,806.1	3,480.6#
East North Central			1,452.7	740.7	1.96	1,525.5	842.1	1,689.2	2,493.3#
Illinois			1,519.4	762.8	1.99	1,592.7	869.0	1,753.1	2,675.5
SEA	1	(Northwest)	1,247.1	662.2	1.88	1,395.6	759.4	1,527.4	2,282.8#
SEA	2	Boone Co.	1,258.2	637.4	1.97	1,267.4	720.9	1,429.6	*
SEA	3	(Northwest Central)	1,301.3	674.9	1.93	1,381.4	758.2	1,510.2	1,651.7#
SEA	4	(West Central)	1,322.8	640.2	2.07	1,386.7	738.3	1,503.7	2,882.9#
SEA	5	(Northeast)c	1,296.3	725.1	1.79	1,410.6	810.7	1,572.0	1,220.3#
SEA	6	(East Central)	1,333.7	665.6	2.00	1,395.9	743.6	1,520.2	2,472.8
SEA	7	(Southwest)c	1,210.3	638.0	1.90	1,303.8	723.1	1,435.0	2,135.7#
SEA	8	(South Central)	1,360.7	597.0	2.28	1,394.4	702.6	1,510.0	2,234.3#
SEA	9	(Southeast)	1,415.6	676.2	2.09	1,424.3	800.0	1,588.1	*
SEA	10	(South Central, South)	1,542.6	720.9	2.14	1,615.2	820.7	1,723.9	2,105.1#
SEA	11	(South)	1,352.7	698.7	1.94	1,489.1	823.4	1,612.8	2,449.7
SEA	A	Rock Island, Moline	1,471.1	707.8	2.08	1,446.9	821.2	1,623.3	2,395.7#
SEA	B	Rockford	1,317.0	679.4	1.94	1,413.2	766.9	1,551.3	2,443.6#
SEA	C	Chicago	1,627.5	819.4	1.99	1,708.9	942.1	1,890.9	2,730.1
SEA	D	Peoria	1,350.5	713.3	1.89	1,473.5	794.0	1,608.9	2,366.6#
SEA	E	Springfield	1,585.4	758.4	2.09	1,690.3	828.0	1,802.1	2,407.0#
SEA	F	East St. Louis	1,483.8	690.4	2.15	1,557.0	791.6	1,685.4	2,759.4
SEA	G	Decatur	1,363.1	669.2	2.04	1,399.1	748.2	1,546.3	2,492.3#

(Continued)

Table A.5.5 Age-adjusted[a] death rates per 100,000 population for all causes for selected age-sex-color groups: United States, each state and each state economic area[b], 1959-61 (Continued)

Division, state, and state economic area (SEA)	White, age 45-64			White, age 35-74		White, both sexes, 45-74	Nonwhite, both sexes, 45-74
	Male	Female	M/F Ratio	Male	Female		
Indiana	1,437.1	712.9	2.02	1,510.1	809.2	1,650.1	2,554.8
SEA 1 (North)[c]	1,308.1	646.8	2.02	1,425.1	790.8	1,588.2	1,385.7#
SEA 2 (North Central, West)	1,371.0	793.6	1.73	1,439.8	833.1	1,615.5	*
SEA 3 (Northeast)	1,367.0	686.2	1.99	1,481.3	781.9	1,602.6	*
SEA 4 (East Central)[c]	1,498.0	698.1	2.15	1,576.4	800.3	1,694.8	2,335.1
SEA 5 (Central)	1,330.1	696.5	1.91	1,425.8	768.1	1,562.3	2,219.3#
SEA 6 (Southwest)	1,410.3	681.9	2.07	1,459.4	785.9	1,580.6	1,916.7#
SEA 7 (South Central)	1,362.5	609.8	2.23	1,390.9	749.4	1,508.0	*
SEA 8 (Southeast)[c]	1,431.0	680.6	2.10	1,443.9	788.0	1,569.2	*
SEA 9 (West Central)	1,464.3	712.1	2.06	1,506.3	808.1	1,665.6	1,976.3#
SEA A Gary, Hammond, East Chicago	1,427.8	819.2	1.74	1,585.3	940.0	1,811.6	2,781.7
SEA B South Bend	1,286.6	737.6	1.74	1,427.1	853.2	1,624.9	2,184.8
SEA C Fort Wayne	1,327.2	711.1	1.87	1,438.8	769.8	1,586.7	2,249.0#
SEA D Indianapolis	1,631.3	709.7	2.30	1,675.0	805.5	1,760.6	2,564.4
SEA E Evansville	1,552.5	688.2	2.26	1,564.4	776.6	1,675.1	3,360.5
SEA F Clark & Floyd Cos.	1,356.1	708.9	1.91	1,465.8	832.7	1,604.6	2,551.3#
SEA G Terre Haute	1,733.0	849.8	2.04	1,740.8	934.3	1,877.7	2,636.0#
SEA H Muncie	1,538.4	765.5	2.01	1,639.3	797.5	1,726.4	2,333.4#
Michigan	1,432.8	745.6	1.92	1,519.7	843.6	1,690.5	2,326.8
SEA 1 (Upper West)	1,560.9	803.9	1.94	1,652.8	925.9	1,837.1	*
SEA 2 (Upper East)	1,481.4	872.9	1.70	1,526.7	961.0	1,769.1	*
SEA 3 (Northwest)[c]	1,390.6	746.8	1.86	1,433.7	835.9	1,624.5	2,299.5#
SEA 4 (North)	1,366.9	699.8	1.95	1,460.8	843.5	1,638.3	2,193.4#
SEA 5 (East Central)	1,334.7	747.8	1.78	1,437.7	820.3	1,611.6	*

SEA 6 (Southwest)	1,357.0	675.9	2.01	1,454.4	776.7	1,593.5	2,123.3
SEA 7 (Central)[c]	1,284.0	707.2	1.82	1,413.0	805.0	1,578.9	*
SEA 8 (Southeast)	1,514.7	837.6	1.81	1,561.7	913.9	1,772.0	2,284.2#
SEA 9 (South Central)	1,360.1	669.4	2.03	1,468.5	784.4	1,600.1	2,187.5
SEA A Saginaw	1,327.3	748.8	1.84	1,426.2	877.4	1,646.2	2,565.7
SEA B Grand Rapids	1,462.2	685.4	1.94	1,403.3	788.0	1,571.2	2,183.5
SEA C Bay City	1,450.3	787.0	1.86	1,496.2	923.8	1,752.5	*
SEA D Flint	1,352.0	800.6	1.81	1,504.2	857.8	1,698.0	2,426.1#
SEA E Lansing	1,494.0	698.1	1.94	1,453.9	804.2	1,603.1	2,217.4#
SEA F Detroit	1,379.6	768.8	1.94	1,590.3	867.8	1,760.8	2,366.3
SEA G Kalamazoo[c]	1,480.0	704.2	1.96	1,477.0	783.0	1,628.5	2,052.3#
SEA H Jackson[c]	1,226.4	773.5	1.91	1,568.5	843.8	1,723.1	2,010.0#
SEA J Ann Arbor[c]		633.5	1.94	1,329.9	713.0	1,469.2	1,862.5#
Ohio	1,467.6	753.5	1.95	1,528.9	852.4	1,700.6	2,470.4
SEA 1 (Northwest)	1,297.4	668.7	1.94	1,410.6	770.2	1,555.7	1,875.6#
SEA 2 (West Central, North)	1,300.7	728.2	1.79	1,394.5	829.7	1,587.1	1,908.8#
SEA 3 (West Central, South)	1,326.2	692.8	1.91	1,367.2	776.7	1,533.2	2,207.7#
SEA 4 (North Central)	1,429.9	679.4	2.10	1,446.2	798.8	1,603.8	2,113.0
SEA 5 (Northeast)	1,380.3	752.7	1.83	1,490.7	854.4	1,670.8	2,108.5#
SEA 6 (East Central)	1,420.4	806.3	1.76	1,481.2	875.2	1,667.6	2,428.8
SEA 7 (South West)[c]	1,275.9	669.7	1.91	1,368.0	811.9	1,526.2	1,647.7#
SEA 8 (Southeast)	1,427.0	726.4	1.97	1,422.7	827.7	1,567.5	1,952.2#
SEA A Toledo	1,627.0	765.4	2.13	1,658.6	874.9	1,804.2	2,415.3
SEA B Columbus	1,602.6	804.0	1.99	1,618.4	885.5	1,793.1	2,483.5
SEA C Dayton	1,446.4	698.4	2.07	1,534.0	794.2	1,669.9	2,480.0
SEA D Hamilton, Middletown	1,443.0	695.1	2.08	1,411.0	830.5	1,600.0	2,913.7
SEA E Cleveland	1,579.2	799.9	1.97	1,647.3	914.7	1,840.1	2,478.3
SEA F Akron	1,423.6	716.8	1.99	1,490.2	812.4	1,645.8	2,303.8
SEA G Canton	1,429.6	739.7	1.93	1,503.1	816.8	1,661.0	2,753.1
SEA H Youngstown	1,418.8	789.9	1.80	1,525.7	905.2	1,742.1	2,360.8
SEA J Belmont Co.	1,479.9	774.2	1.91	1,541.6	885.7	1,744.5	2,433.8#
SEA K Cincinnati	1,505.0	763.0	1.97	1,592.8	851.6	1,745.2	2,701.9
SEA L Lawrence Co.	1,716.2	831.2	2.06	1,761.6	922.8	1,865.6	2,506.3#
SEA M Lorain, Elyria	1,477.9	771.8	1.82	1,513.8	862.1	1,704.1	2,469.6
SEA N Springfield		721.5	2.05	1,524.3	797.8	1,661.0	2,456.1#
SEA O Lima[c]	1,586.2	749.3	2.12	1,587.4	815.9	1,711.2	1,644.5#

(Continued)

Table A.5.5 Age-adjusted^a death rates per 100,000 population for all causes for selected age-sex-color groups: United States, each state and each state economic area^b, 1959-61 (continued)

Division, state, and state economic area (SEA)	White, age 45-64			White, age 35-74		White, both sexes, 45-74	Nonwhite, both sexes, 45-74
	Male	Female	M/F Ratio	Male	Female		
Wisconsin	1,309.0	679.4	1.93	1,386.2	786.0	1,551.6	2,159.5
SEA 1 (North)	1,362.8	714.0	1.91	1,441.1	836.7	1,600.8	2,015.6#
SEA 2 (West Central)	1,148.7	590.0	1.95	1,219.1	697.4	1,365.2	*
SEA 3 (Southwest)	1,326.9	602.3	2.20	1,391.2	734.5	1,502.5	*
SEA 4 (North Central)	1,213.8	590.4	2.06	1,256.3	716.1	1,418.3	**
SEA 5 (South Central)	1,327.1	708.2	1.87	1,331.1	786.6	1,481.2	*
SEA 6 (Northeast)	1,166.4	642.1	1.82	1,271.7	744.5	1,434.5	1,612.0#
SEA 7 (East Central)	1,277.9	667.4	1.91	1,366.4	774.7	1,527.8	1,777.7#
SEA 8 (Southeast)	1,252.7	682.1	1.84	1,329.4	771.5	1,502.7	2,006.8#
SEA A Superior	1,519.0	874.9	1.74	1,559.4	1,036.0	1,821.0	*
SEA B Madison	1,265.0	586.1	2.16	1,292.5	682.0	1,407.1	*
SEA C Milwaukee	1,473.9	747.1	1.97	1,575.1	860.2	1,743.3	2,299.2
SEA D Racine	1,316.0	717.3	1.83	1,380.5	790.0	1,575.6	2,404.0#
SEA E Kenosha	1,154.7	668.0	1.73	1,315.1	797.5	1,525.9	*
SEA F Waukesha Co.	1,212.6	695.1	1.74	1,412.8	798.3	1,586.5	*
West North Central	1,303.6	626.6	2.08	1,364.3	718.6	1,480.7	2,602.5
Iowa	1,293.5	613.1	2.11	1,348.3	704.9	1,460.0	2,280.6
SEA 1 (West)	1,191.3	598.3	1.99	1,254.4	670.6	1,372.5	*
SEA 2 (North Central)	1,236.8	570.4	2.17	1,310.5	675.3	1,406.0	*
SEA 3 (South Central)	1,288.2	594.1	2.17	1,311.7	683.4	1,411.6	*
SEA 4 (Northeast)	1,192.4	558.6	2.13	1,237.5	668.4	1,359.0	**
SEA 5 (East Central)	1,215.4	599.3	2.03	1,276.0	684.4	1,393.4	3,027.7#
SEA 6 (Southeast)	1,355.4	626.4	2.16	1,418.0	719.7	1,516.1	2,705.7#
SEA A Sioux City	1,449.3	646.7	2.24	1,531.7	816.2	1,670.0	2,269.1#
SEA B Council Bluffs	1,407.0	710.2	1.98	1,484.0	805.6	1,616.3	*

SEA C	Des Moines	1,492.6	671.8	2.22	1,539.3	749.1	1,633.2	2,272.1
SEA D	Davenport	1,452.0	667.5	2.18	1,530.9	751.8	1,648.5	2,176.8#
SEA E	Waterloo	1,215.4	691.1	1.76	1,272.4	751.1	1,454.2	2,495.1#
SEA F	Cedar Rapids	1,356.7	634.9	2.14	1,399.4	719.2	1,503.0	*
Kansas		1,259.8	592.3	2.13	1,306.6	684.3	1,411.8	2,237.8
SEA 1	(Southwest)	1,394.4	591.3	2.36	1,414.2	646.0	1,448.0	*
SEA 2	(Northwest)	1,181.4	526.4	2.24	1,246.9	649.5	1,337.7	1,339.0#
SEA 3	(Central)	1,183.5	581.8	2.03	1,243.7	666.1	1,358.9	2,083.9#
SEA 4	(North Central)	1,165.0	565.8	2.06	1,218.6	660.1	1,333.2	*
SEA 5	(East South Central)	1,170.3	556.9	2.10	1,248.7	677.7	1,343.5	2,331.7#
SEA 6	(Northeast)c	1,275.5	660.3	1.93	1,314.8	747.7	1,448.5	2,218.7
SEA 7	(East Central)	1,124.4	516.7	2.18	1,192.4	646.3	1,305.0	2,116.3#
SEA 8	(Southeast)	1,406.7	669.5	2.10	1,491.1	734.7	1,562.5	2,413.8#
SEA A	Wichita	1,382.1	620.7	2.23	1,376.8	674.1	1,470.3	1,898.2
SEA B	Kansas City	1,353.5	624.8	2.17	1,404.5	711.3	1,515.6	2,416.0
SEA C	Topekac	1,362.0	576.7	2.36	1,423.3	713.6	1,520.1	2,192.2
Minnesota		1,253.7	646.3	1.94	1,328.6	729.0	1,466.7	2,112.2
SEA 1	(Northwest)	1,174.5	591.0	1.99	1,250.3	676.8	1,366.8	*
SEA 2	(Northeast)	1,302.6	617.8	2.11	1,376.1	745.4	1,494.8	1,979.2#
SEA 3	(West Central, North)	1,032.0	597.2	1.73	1,105.1	691.7	1,271.7	1,757.1#
SEA 4	(East Central, North)	1,033.4	669.3	1.54	1,178.9	762.2	1,378.0	*
SEA 5	(West Central)	1,053.8	551.3	1.91	1,151.2	646.6	1,264.7	*
SEA 6	(East Central, South)	1,120.8	612.2	1.83	1,207.5	696.6	1,344.0	*
SEA 7	(Southeast)	1,102.8	560.1	1.97	1,214.2	654.8	1,329.4	*
SEA 8	(Southwest)	1,036.0	597.7	1.73	1,160.9	667.7	1,318.3	*
SEA A	Duluth	1,489.7	766.9	1.94	1,534.8	847.0	1,698.2	*
SEA B	Minneapolis, St. Paul	1,403.9	684.0	2.05	1,460.9	756.3	1,590.7	2,281.1

(Continued)

Table A.5.5 Age-adjusted[a] death rates per 100,000 population for all causes for selected age-sex-color groups: United States, each state and each state economic area[b], 1959-61 (Continued)

Division, state, and state economic area (SEA)	White, age 45-64			White, age 35-74		White, both sexes, 45-74	Nonwhite, both sexes, 45-74
	Male	Female	M/F Ratio	Male	Female		
Missouri	1,424.1	657.3	2.17	1,475.9	756.9	1,585.5	2,741.1
SEA 1 (Northwest)	1,346.1	600.3	2.24	1,399.7	705.0	1,477.8	2,840.9
SEA 2 (Northeast)	1,255.4	586.1	2.14	1,328.7	678.7	1,414.7	2,563.8
SEA 3 (West Central)	1,164.2	645.3	1.80	1,290.1	716.0	1,408.5	2,210.6#
SEA 4 (Southwest)	1,529.3	703.1	2.18	1,537.3	792.8	1,661.8	2,023.7#
SEA 5 (Central)	1,244.1	555.6	2.24	1,267.4	655.5	1,362.7	*
SEA 6 (East Central)	1,225.8	605.1	2.03	1,304.3	683.8	1,410.9	2,279.0#
SEA 7 (West Ozarks)	1,171.8	509.0	2.30	1,235.7	661.2	1,313.9	*
SEA 8 (East Ozarks)	1,416.2	629.9	2.25	1,484.3	736.8	1,545.0	*
SEA 9 (Southeast)	1,470.8	629.9	2.33	1,553.8	778.9	1,616.9	2,426.9
SEA A Kansas City	1,586.3	684.2	2.32	1,613.8	777.4	1,702.7	2,786.8
SEA B St. Louis	1,531.7	717.3	2.14	1,597.3	828.0	1,745.1	2,808.4
SEA C Springfield	1,406.0	625.8	2.25	1,529.5	691.8	1,542.9	2,767.4#
Nebraska	1,228.9	588.6	2.09	1,304.5	681.2	1,412.9	2,773.7
SEA 1 (Northwest)	1,079.7	519.0	2.08	1,191.9	620.0	1,298.9	*
SEA 2 (Southwest)	1,211.5	595.8	2.03	1,223.0	718.8	1,384.0	3,289.0#
SEA 3 (Central)	1,210.6	560.9	2.16	1,270.7	663.0	1,367.3	*
SEA 4 (South Central, West)	1,059.6	599.4	1.77	1,127.2	667.7	1,262.3	*
SEA 5 (South Central, East)	1,001.4	538.2	1.86	1,127.7	647.7	1,257.0	*
SEA 6 (Northeast)	1,009.8	536.5	1.88	1,147.4	658.2	1,282.6	3,966.9#
SEA 7 (Southeast)	1,150.1	584.4	1.97	1,244.6	670.9	1,364.5	*
SEA A Lincoln[c]	1,219.6	544.1	2.24	1,329.5	641.8	1,388.4	1,847.7#
SEA B Omaha	1,573.6	686.7	2.29	1,636.3	759.8	1,723.4	2,842.7
North Dakota	1,163.0	605.2	1.92	1,255.6	693.0	1,387.7	2,568.1
SEA 1 (Southwest)	1,184.8	731.9	1.62	1,316.5	861.9	1,558.1	2,725.2#

SEA 2 (West Central)	1,199.8	609.2	1.97	1,258.3	697.6	1,400.6	*
SEA 3 (Central)	1,112.1	598.5	1.86	1,210.0	672.5	1,337.5	2,506.1#
SEA 4 (East)	1,226.6	548.3	2.24	1,316.1	654.9	1,398.0	*
SEA 5 (Southeast)	1,089.4	605.7	1.80	1,168.4	636.6	1,293.1	*
South Dakota	1,257.6	587.0	2.14	1,320.0	685.3	1,417.5	2,628.7
SEA 1 (West)	1,409.2	539.5	2.61	1,432.2	658.3	1,453.3	2,558.8
SEA 2 (North Central)	1,304.1	574.1	2.27	1,358.1	658.9	1,423.8	2,905.6#
SEA 3 (South Central)	1,218.0	550.2	2.21	1,300.6	658.1	1,401.8	3,239.6#
SEA 4 (Northeast)	1,097.2	591.3	1.86	1,215.9	683.6	1,335.5	2,894.1#
SEA 5 (Southeast)	1,206.6	654.8	1.84	1,257.0	745.7	1,433.0	*
South Atlantic	1,566.3	676.7	2.31	1,563.4	762.6	1,639.8	2,882.8
Delaware	1,524.1	764.9	1.99	1,594.8	873.5	1,769.0	2,919.4
SEA 1 (South)	1,447.6	723.9	2.00	1,530.8	825.0	1,687.8	2,640.9
SEA A Wilmington	1,553.1	781.3	1.99	1,621.3	893.8	1,803.1	3,100.4
Washington, D.C.	1,918.4	765.1	2.51	1,846.7	853.8	1,862.2	2,730.5
Florida	1,503.4	638.5	2.35	1,439.5	674.2	1,479.9	2,807.9
SEA 1 (Northwest)	1,609.1	588.8	2.73	1,551.7	752.5	1,625.4	2,600.7
SEA 2 (Central North)	1,561.0	693.1	2.25	1,582.6	777.0	1,658.5	3,007.2
SEA 3 (North Central)c	1,485.0	670.8	2.21	1,570.4	764.7	1,627.5	2,571.4
SEA 4 (East Central)	1,441.6	626.5	2.30	1,372.0	660.5	1,408.3	2,713.8
SEA 5 (Central South)	1,403.7	611.7	2.29	1,368.4	642.1	1,394.6	2,715.5
SEA 6 (Southwest)	1,449.1	626.1	2.31	1,342.1	624.3	1,362.0	2,966.0
SEA A Jacksonville	1,731.8	719.1	2.41	1,721.0	807.4	1,789.4	3,128.8
SEA B Tampa, St. Petersburg	1,540.9	628.9	2.45	1,472.2	653.3	1,490.0	3,115.5
SEA C Miami	1,532.6	685.0	2.24	1,485.2	722.3	1,550.7	2,505.1
SEA D Pensacola	1,602.8	628.3	2.55	1,559.7	718.9	1,610.1	3,075.0
SEA E Orlando	1,401.3	595.3	2.35	1,381.2	639.5	1,420.0	2,759.8
SEA F West Palm Beach	1,448.6	623.3	2.32	1,354.1	633.3	1,387.0	2,612.2
SEA G Ft. Lauderdale	1,413.3	581.8	2.43	1,307.0	603.8	1,354.1	2,739.5

(Continued)

Table A.5.5 Age-adjusted[a] death rates per 100,000 population for all causes, for selected age-sex-color groups: United States, each state and each state economic area[b], 1959-61 (Continued)

Division, state, and state economic area (SEA)	White, age 45-64			White, age 35-74		White, both sexes, 45-74	Nonwhite, both sexes, 45-74
	Male	Female	M/F Ratio	Male	Female		
Georgia	1,582.2	646.0	2.45	1,606.0	728.1	1,645.0	3,034.9
SEA 1 (Northwest)	1,492.9	665.1	2.24	1,554.6	788.2	1,639.1	2,928.5
SEA 2 (Northeast)	1,287.3	558.6	2.30	1,302.5	688.1	1,365.8	2,958.5#
SEA 3 (North Central)	1,303.4	571.8	2.28	1,372.8	638.0	1,398.3	2,689.4
SEA 4 (Central, North)[c]	1,599.1	617.5	2.59	1,626.0	681.4	1,620.2	2,834.9
SEA 5 ("Fall Line")	1,404.1	586.0	2.40	1,633.4	708.9	1,609.5	2,595.8
SEA 6 (Central, South)	1,754.6	614.6	2.85	1,730.2	773.6	1,717.6	2,707.1
SEA 7 (Southwest)	1,694.1	644.2	2.63	1,674.3	688.0	1,677.1	2,972.0
SEA 8 (South Central)	1,665.5	667.7	2.49	1,654.5	771.0	1,705.0	2,946.7
SEA 9 (Southeast)	1,668.1	699.6	2.38	1,779.4	793.6	1,792.9	3,224.1
SEA A Walker Co.	1,462.9	654.0	2.24	1,432.6	688.3	1,490.6	2,568.3#
SEA B Atlanta	1,567.5	656.2	2.39	1,594.5	735.4	1,658.2	3,139.9
SEA C Columbus	1,691.0	712.1	2.37	1,730.2	787.8	1,798.4	2,909.5
SEA D Augusta[c]	1,961.8	726.1	2.70	1,979.9	798.5	1,981.4	3,534.8
SEA E Savannah	1,790.1	739.9	2.42	1,837.3	837.4	1,909.9	3,702.8
SEA F Macon	1,837.4	703.7	2.61	1,905.1	786.7	1,884.5	3,234.5
SEA G Houston Co.	1,414.8	678.9#	2.08	1,457.2	770.4#	1,581.2	3,050.4
Maryland	1,619.6	783.7	2.07	1,677.8	900.0	1,842.8	2,860.2
SEA 1 (West)	1,765.2	840.5	2.10	1,767.6	943.3	1,875.5	3,186.1#
SEA 2 (Northeast)	1,637.5	763.3	2.15	1,650.7	890.4	1,809.0	2,672.1
SEA 3 (South Central)	1,471.3	637.7	2.31	1,506.9	749.3	1,570.7	2,552.5
SEA 4 (Eastern Shore)	1,559.3	702.8	2.22	1,538.1	803.6	1,651.3	2,611.1
SEA A Baltimore	1,755.6	844.9	2.08	1,824.6	968.5	1,998.7	3,006.3
SEA B Montgomery Co., Prince George Co.	1,342.5	678.8	1.98	1,451.4	784.9	1,610.8	2,298.2
SEA C Carroll Co., Howard Co.	1,339.2	777.3	1.72	1,469.1	845.9	1,639.1	2,447.1#

North Carolina

	1,551.8	620.6	2.50	1,569.4	738.5	1,622.2	2,721.4
SEA 1 (Southwest)	1,179.8	576.3	2.05	1,238.9	697.6	1,334.0	2,125.0
SEA 2 (Northwest)	1,508.3	560.3	2.69	1,461.3	672.6	1,496.3	2,311.5
SEA 3 (West North Central)	1,447.7	531.7	2.72	1,450.7	682.3	1,494.0	2,385.5
SEA 4 (West Central)	1,365.9	584.3	2.34	1,443.3	733.8	1,539.6	2,613.5
SEA 5 (West South Central)	1,559.5	597.5	2.61	1,545.9	711.0	1,605.3	2,617.1
SEA 6 (Central)	1,754.6	634.4	2.77	1,782.3	828.4	1,828.9	2,613.4
SEA 7 (East North Central)	1,870.0	662.5	2.82	1,839.4	737.4	1,826.4	2,433.5
SEA 8 (East Central)	1,789.9	693.5	2.58	1,850.4	829.4	1,892.3	2,741.6
SEA 9 (South Central)	1,846.1	729.1	2.53	1,810.4	830.6	1,865.2	2,684.4
SEA 10 (Northeast)	1,818.4	644.0	2.82	1,830.3	775.6	1,810.6	2,576.6
SEA 11 (Southeast)	1,770.7	676.5	2.62	1,773.9	801.1	1,794.3	2,875.4
SEA A Asheville	1,557.3	663.7	2.35	1,548.3	747.5	1,591.1	3,180.2
SEA B Winston-Salem	1,408.3	679.2	2.07	1,496.2	732.1	1,586.3	3,199.1
SEA C Greensboro, High Point	1,520.3	634.1	2.40	1,536.0	720.1	1,596.3	2,979.7
SEA D Charlotte	1,574.2	610.2	2.58	1,627.9	701.6	1,641.8	3,224.0
SEA E Raleigh^c	1,671.4	677.6	2.47	1,632.5	752.7	1,690.7	2,646.3
SEA F Durham	1,694.6	675.3	2.51	1,718.9	755.6	1,721.1	2,843.4

South Carolina

	1,700.1	705.0	2.41	1,740.6	818.2	1,808.6	3,223.9
SEA 1 (Northwest)	1,366.5	602.9	2.27	1,546.0	700.5	1,581.5	2,465.5
SEA 2 (Northwest Central)	1,567.4	673.0	2.33	1,616.8	786.3	1,702.5	3,212.6
SEA 3 (North Central)	1,674.8	669.3	2.50	1,707.6	805.7	1,766.8	2,949.9
SEA 4 (West Central)	1,699.6	619.7	2.74	1,682.9	705.9	1,671.9	2,819.4
SEA 5 (East North Central)	1,900.8	771.0	2.34	1,671.0	944.6	1,880.4	3,122.6
SEA 6 (East Central)	1,844.8	777.0	2.45	1,960.8	874.7	2,016.7	3,251.8
SEA 7 (Northeast)	1,651.8	786.3	2.35	1,944.6	917.2	1,996.9	3,278.8
SEA 8 (Southeast)	1,670.1	831.6	1.99	1,622.9	872.0	1,758.6	3,199.2
SEA A Columbia^c	1,711.3	653.7	2.55	1,753.4	755.9	1,786.4	3,034.1
SEA B Aiken Co.		642.2	2.66	1,743.3	863.9	1,860.6	3,422.9
SEA C Charleston	1,937.8	791.6	2.45	1,859.7	936.8	1,974.5	4,009.3
SEA D Greenville	1,764.2	723.5	2.44	1,822.8·	825.3	1,878.3	3,077.4

(Continued)

Table A.5.5 Age-adjusted[a] death rates per 100,000 population for all causes for selected age-sex-color groups: United States, each state and each state economic area[b], 1959-61 (Continued)

Division, state, and state economic area (SEA)	White, age 45-64			White, age 35-74		White, both sexes, 45-74	Nonwhite, both sexes, 45-74
	Male	Female	M/F Ratio	Male	Female		
Virginia	1,525.6	671.2	2.27	1,562.6	780.2	1,665.1	2,872.8
SEA 1 (West)	1,708.0	788.0	2.17	1,684.4	847.9	1,758.6	2,702.7#
SEA 2 (Southwest)	1,339.0	642.3	2.08	1,415.8	798.4	1,553.2	2,154.8#
SEA 3 (West Central)	1,513.2	671.9	2.25	1,592.8	825.4	1,688.1	3,016.8
SEA 4 (Northwest Central)	1,568.3	640.3	2.45	1,617.7	752.3	1,676.0	2,893.7
SEA 5 (North Central)	1,506.1	690.7	2.18	1,569.3	808.4	1,656.9	2,479.5
SEA 6 (Central)	1,473.9	556.5	2.65	1,470.1	722.7	1,540.5	2,397.1
SEA 7 (South Central)	1,441.7	620.5	2.32	1,454.1	706.0	1,523.2	2,680.7
SEA 8 (East Central)	1,358.2	564.2	2.41	1,378.0	702.0	1,464.0	2,656.3
SEA 9 (East)	1,878.8	738.3	2.54	1,881.2	854.0	1,949.6	3,132.1
SEA 10 (Southeast)	1,633.6	729.8	2.24	1,692.8	817.9	1,774.4	2,917.6
SEA A Roanoke[c]	1,478.4	697.0	2.12	1,536.4	775.4	1,626.7	2,806.5
SEA B Northern Va. Met.	1,282.3	600.9	2.13	1,372.6	723.2	1,514.5	2,421.2
SEA C Richmond	1,714.1	702.8	2.44	1,712.9	799.2	1,803.6	3,132.1
SEA D Norfolk, Portsmouth	1,814.4	795.2	2.28	1,836.1	879.8	1,948.7	3,375.2
SEA E Newport News, Hampton	1,592.2	723.4	2.20	1,686.5	810.9	1,801.7	2,925.5
SEA F Lynchburg	1,471.9	607.8	2.42	1,591.2	710.9	1,614.3	2,938.1
West Virginia	1,537.9	732.7	2.10	1,579.3	845.5	1,693.4	2,447.3
SEA 1 (Northwest)	1,522.2	765.9	1.99	1,550.5	851.2	1,696.1	2,213.4#
SEA 2 (West Central)[c]	1,312.6	691.5	1.90	1,385.2	811.5	1,498.7	*
SEA 3 (North Central)	1,474.0	716.6	2.06	1,519.0	828.1	1,656.6	2,472.2#
SEA 4 (South)	1,763.4	768.8	2.29	1,774.1	882.5	1,848.0	2,433.2
SEA 5 (East)	1,456.6	755.4	1.93	1,520.3	863.1	1,658.8	1,964.3#
SEA 6 (Northeast)[c]	1,733.8	826.0	2.10	1,829.1	918.2	1,942.4	2,554.0#
SEA A Wheeling	1,617.6	778.7	2.08	1,607.1	900.3	1,804.8	2,880.5#

SEA B	Huntington	1,450.0	656.7	2.21	1,554.3	791.5	1,626.9	2,884.1
SEA C	Charleston	1,605.2	717.9	2.24	1,687.3	841.1	1,767.1	2,520.0
East South Central		1,436.5	640.1	2.24	1,478.3	745.2	1,559.3	2,534.6
Alabama		1,474.0	616.8	2.39	1,519.0	715.8	1,564.3	2,686.4
SEA 1	(Northwest)	1,338.1	594.2	2.25	1,370.8	693.8	1,441.3	2,851.2
SEA 2	(Northeast)	1,336.7	583.0	2.29	1,434.1	666.9	1,455.8	2,547.1#
SEA 3	(North Central)	1,468.0	633.1	2.32	1,524.4	739.6	1,582.8	2,687.6
SEA 4	(East Central)	1,362.7	524.8	2.60	1,424.4	677.0	1,456.8	2,749.5
SEA 5	(West Central, North)	1,346.6	607.2	2.22	1,449.4	700.0	1,479.1	2,105.8
SEA 6	(West Central}	1,590.9	569.6	2.79	1,592.7	656.2	1,573.1	2,567.9
SEA 7	(West Central, South)	1,317.7	538.0	2.45	1,474.3	675.1	1,478.9	1,795.9
SEA 8	(Southwest)	1,497.6	564.2	2.65	1,546.4	725.5	1,581.7	2,394.8
SEA 9	(Southeast)	1,458.6	632.8	2.30	1,528.4	711.7	1,548.8	2,567.8
SEA A	Birmingham	1,573.6	612.4	2.57	1,627.2	728.5	1,667.9	2,892.8
SEA B	Russell Co.	2,229.0	682.5	3.27	1,998.9	925.6	2,011.0	3,035.8
SEA C	Montgomery^c	1,852.5	675.6	2.74	1,730.8	748.8	1,776.8	2,992.6
SEA D	Mobile	1,640.5	737.3	2.23	1,710.2	802.7	1,770.7	2,828.4
SEA E	Tuscaloosa^c	1,394.0	559.2	2.49	1,360.3	632.3	1,389.8	2,645.5
SEA F	Huntsville	1,472.4	729.9	2.02	1,525.4	791.9	1,655.0	2,953.3
Kentucky		1,439.9	675.2	2.13	1,476.5	787.6	1,580.3	2,816.7
SEA 1	(West)	1,443.6	530.7	2.72	1,468.7	664.9	1,486.8	2,849.9
SEA 2	(Northwest)	1,383.8	678.3	2.04	1,416.2	739.4	1,523.4	2,777.1
SEA 3	(West Central)	1,244.2	603.2	2.06	1,315.6	735.8	1,435.4	2,427.3
SEA 4	(Southwest Central)	1,265.5	642.0	1.97	1,329.9	722.4	1,430.3	2,518.4
SEA 5	(South Central)	1,263.9	659.8	1.92	1,339.7	791.9	1,468.7	2,456.0
SEA 6	(North Central)	1,305.0	668.7	1.95	1,351.3	796.6	1,495.7	2,516.7
SEA 7	(Central)	1,481.2	721.6	2.05	1,506.4	798.8	1,630.6	2,767.5
SEA 8	(Northeast)	1,169.7	593.6	1.97	1,271.9	739.3	1,353.4	*
SEA 9	(Southeast)	1,517.7	700.4	2.17	1,513.1	795.3	1,567.0	2,375.2
SEA A	Louisville	1,676.2	743.8	2.25	1,728.5	862.2	1,841.9	3,147.7
SEA B	Covington	1,729.0	785.4	2.20	1,761.6	895.4	1,879.8	3,264.2
SEA C	Ashland	1,554.6	704.1	2.21	1,602.5	770.9	1,681.2	3,075.3#
SEA D	Henderson Co.	1,319.9	537.5	2.46	1,439.1	703.1	1,474.4	2,678.3#
SEA E	Lexington^c	1,602.0	695.9	2.30	1,634.4	761.0	1,694.1	2,865.2

(Continued)

Table A.5.5   Age-adjusted[a] death rates per 100,000 population for all causes for selected age-sex-color groups: United States, each state and each state economic area[b], 1959-61 (Continued)

Division, state, and state economic area (SEA)	White, age 45-64			White, age 35-74		White, both sexes, 45-74	Nonwhite, both sexes, 45-74
	Male	Female	M/F Ratio	Male	Female		
Mississippi	1,452.2	598.3	2.43	1,488.7	713.3	1,544.8	2,175.5
SEA 1 (Northwest)	1,556.0	600.9	2.59	1,609.9	719.4	1,635.4	2,331.0
SEA 2 (North Central)	1,417.6	581.1	2.44	1,514.4	657.5	1,511.5	1,964.3
SEA 3 (Southwest)	1,528.6	714.5	2.14	1,578.0	807.3	1,696.1	2,290.8
SEA 4 (Northeast)	1,257.5	558.7	2.25	1,270.5	692.3	1,385.6	2,095.8
SEA 5 (East Central, North)	1,363.2	559.4	2.44	1,457.0	694.2	1,500.3	2,149.6
SEA 6 (East Central)	1,377.0	578.3	2.38	1,427.3	703.2	1,480.7	1,949.0
SEA 7 (South East, North)	1,688.0	634.0	2.66	1,631.5	776.9	1,699.7	2,278.6
SEA 8 (Southeast, South)[c]	1,691.3	658.2	2.57	1,706.8	744.6	1,727.7	2,809.8
SEA A Jackson	1,540.4	538.1	2.86	1,613.3	634.9	1,594.7	2,196.3
Tennessee	1,399.5	642.9	2.18	1,447.1	740.4	1,542.8	2,700.1
SEA 1 (West)	1,249.6	553.8	2.26	1,372.6	629.2	1,407.3	2,163.5
SEA 2 (West Central)	1,105.7	501.5	2.20	1,216.9	646.6	1,309.6	2,354.0
SEA 3 (West Central, East)	1,379.0	603.2	2.29	1,371.5	703.0	1,461.7	2,657.1#
SEA 4 (North Central)	1,253.8	612.7	2.05	1,337.7	745.2	1,445.6	2,747.0
SEA 5 (South Central)	1,268.3	675.9	1.88	1,418.7	713.9	1,509.3	2,737.1
SEA 6 (East Central, West)	1,262.6	624.3	2.02	1,292.7	737.2	1,428.8	2,932.7#
SEA 7 (East Central)	1,408.8	657.2	2.14	1,458.7	748.5	1,534.9	2,229.4#
SEA 8 (East)	1,417.4	691.8	2.05	1,442.9	798.2	1,566.6	2,423.5
SEA A Memphis	1,572.8	678.0	2.32	1,603.5	755.5	1,685.5	2,733.9
SEA B Nashville	1,548.4	645.5	2.40	1,563.5	738.8	1,633.7	3,049.2
SEA C Chattanooga	1,533.3	661.4	2.32	1,596.2	784.5	1,686.4	3,173.4
SEA D Knoxville	1,439.0	635.2	2.27	1,480.2	750.6	1,585.9	2,847.5
West South Central	1,404.6	612.1	2.29	1,453.2	697.2	1,513.4	2,378.5
Arkansas	1,338.3	571.0	2.34	1,394.0	657.5	1,433.5	2,213.4
SEA 1 (Northwest)	1,180.6	578.8	2.04	1,269.9	620.4	1,322.5	*
(North)	1,243.2	605.9	2.05	1,330.5	690.1	1,413.9	2,327.7

SEA 4 (West Central, South)^c	1,435.3	564.0	2.55	1,476.8	696.2	1,499.4	1,977.3
SEA 5 (Southwest)	1,411.9	567.2	2.40	1,424.4	659.6	1,425.0	1,900.6
SEA 6 (South Central)	1,398.4	532.1	2.63	1,453.7	647.3	1,457.4	1,996.9
SEA 7 (Northeast)	1,344.3	606.3	2.24	1,418.4	677.3	1,464.8	2,104.8
SEA 8 (East)	1,415.2	616.3	2.30	1,540.5	662.2	1,553.4	2,314.1
SEA 9 (North Central)	1,079.1	551.8	1.96	1,166.9	628.8	1,254.8	*
SEA A Little Rock^c	1,602.0	578.5	2.77	1,622.1	667.9	1,617.2	2,531.0
Louisiana	1,637.3	683.7	2.39	1,656.0	774.0	1,726.3	2,487.8
SEA 1 (Central)^c	1,754.4	631.4	2.78	1,630.5	734.2	1,690.3	2,153.7
SEA 2 (Northeast)	1,385.6	610.7	2.27	1,444.3	728.4	1,517.3	2,015.3
SEA 3 (East Central)	1,546.7	663.4	2.33	1,652.4	786.7	1,730.9	2,251.4
SEA 4 (North Central)	1,327.9	551.2	2.41	1,330.9	607.4	1,359.3	1,838.2
SEA 5 (East)^c	1,699.3	647.0	2.63	1,738.9	773.1	1,739.1	2,503.0
SEA 6 (South Central)	1,442.4	603.4	2.39	1,532.2	721.6	1,605.2	2,588.9
SEA 7 (Southwest)	1,477.7	779.5	1.90	1,541.4	808.1	1,656.5	2,326.7
SEA 8 (West Central)	1,450.4	662.7	2.19	1,465.3	752.8	1,526.9	1,994.4
SEA A Shreveport	1,697.6	628.4	2.70	1,606.8	678.8	1,625.2	2,293.1
SEA B New Orleans	1,909.2	796.6	2.40	1,939.0	901.2	2,034.8	3,061.3
SEA C Baton Rouge	1,556.2	566.2	2.75	1,609.0	672.0	1,638.5	2,662.1
SEA D Lake Charles	1,461.9	733.9	1.99	1,592.6	711.3	1,639.7	2,281.5
SEA E Monroe	1,619.8	665.2	2.48	1,538.4	759.1	1,628.1	2,477.3
Oklahoma	1,407.6	603.7	2.33	1,439.0	676.8	1,485.2	2,003.4
SEA 1 (Northwest)	1,211.6	500.3	2.42	1,235.9	645.7	1,316.1	2,247.1#
SEA 2 (North Central)	1,299.1	586.3	2.22	1,345.0	683.0	1,426.5	2,407.8#
SEA 3 (Northeast)	1,453.4	631.0	2.30	1,480.7	710.9	1,543.5	1,387.4#
SEA 4 (Southwest)	1,358.9	529.9	2.56	1,419.4	587.0	1,413.0	2,118.7
SEA 5 (Central)	1,360.3	644.9	2.11	1,400.9	668.5	1,456.9	1,832.0
SEA 6 (Central East)	1,397.3	536.1	2.61	1,462.3	646.3	1,453.3	2,151.7
SEA 7 (South)	1,412.4	534.1	2.64	1,512.4	623.4	1,454.9	1,857.4
SEA 8 (East Central)	1,375.3	583.0	2.36	1,423.1	711.2	1,475.9	1,805.8
SEA 9 (South East)	1,407.0	638.7	2.20	1,415.3	646.3	1,454.8	1,673.7
SEA 10 (East Central, North)	1,309.0	621.9	2.10	1,253.8	710.6	1,349.0	2,218.7
SEA A Tulsa	1,511.1	664.4	2.27	1,516.0	723.4	1,596.1	2,229.9
SEA B Oklahoma City	1,497.4	627.7	2.39	1,502.6	702.5	1,553.6	2,222.1
SEA C Creek Co.	1,344.8	780.2	1.72	1,516.3	836.2	1,638.6	1,946.2#
SEA D Canadian Co.	1,218.1	522.1	2.33	1,383.8	593.4	1,360.0	2,125.7#

(Continued)

Table A.5.5 Age-adjusted[a] death rates per 100,000 population for all causes, for selected age-sex-color groups: United States, each state and each state economic area[b], 1959-61 (Continued)

Division, state, and state economic area (SEA)	White, age 45-64			White, age 35-74		White, both sexes, 45-74	Nonwhite, both sexes, 45-74
	Male	Female	M/F Ratio	Male	Female		
Texas	1,355.2	603.6	2.25	1,419.5	692.0	1,485.0	2,419.5
SEA 1 (West)	1,231.2	545.5	2.26	1,320.1	642.3	1,350.3	*
SEA 2 (Central West)	1,226.0	590.3	2.08	1,282.4	664.4	1,350.1	2,480.5
SEA 3 (South West)	1,343.2	730.3	1.84	1,409.2	845.7	1,589.2	2,814.3#
SEA 4 (North West)	1,187.4	554.7	2.14	1,312.4	634.6	1,365.6	1,884.1#
SEA 5 (West Central, North)	1,209.8	540.8	2.24	1,318.0	621.0	1,345.4	1,889.1
SEA 6 (North Central, West)	1,208.5	514.5	2.35	1,298.4	618.8	1,333.4	2,313.1
SEA 7 (North Central)	1,250.9	509.7	2.45	1,296.2	605.3	1,329.7	2,324.1#
SEA 8 (North Central, East)	1,312.2	491.4	2.67	1,357.2	593.4	1,368.1	2,447.0
SEA 9 (Central East)	1,430.2	508.9	2.81	1,382.4	612.0	1,412.7	2,122.0
SEA 10 (Central South)	1,164.6	544.9	2.14	1,243.3	643.0	1,330.5	2,524.1
SEA 11 (Gulf Coast)	1,280.9	740.1	1.73	1,401.5	784.1	1,533.5	2,272.9
SEA 12 (Northeast)	1,324.6	557.3	2.38	1,416.3	643.1	1,433.1	2,165.2
SEA 13 (East Central)	1,280.6	510.5	2.51	1,351.7	590.9	1,352.3	2,079.0
SEA 14 (South East)	1,322.4	581.2	2.28	1,368.0	683.2	1,454.0	2,623.0
SEA 15 (South)	1,170.2	688.3	1.70	1,312.9	803.0	1,473.5	1,936.2#
SEA 16 (West Central, South)	1,317.6	617.7	2.13	1,412.6	739.3	1,511.6	2,612.9#
SEA A El Paso	1,391.7	873.9	1.59	1,490.3	923.9	1,724.0	1,925.2#
SEA B Fort Worth	1,467.2	586.5	2.50	1,519.4	685.1	1,560.3	2,570.8
SEA C Dallas	1,383.8	588.8	2.35	1,462.8	657.1	1,489.8	2,552.7
SEA D Waco[c]	1,399.2	637.6	2.19	1,510.6	714.5	1,576.5	2,355.9
SEA E Austin[c]	1,356.0	556.1	2.44	1,418.0	654.2	1,455.9	1,971.6
SEA F San Antonio	1,395.5	763.5	1.83	1,454.4	821.0	1,610.4	2,663.7
SEA G Houston	1,528.2	647.1	2.36	1,615.9	744.4	1,672.0	2,635.1
SEA H Beaumont, Port Authur	1,504.5	621.1	2.42	1,481.7	761.7	1,587.4	2,661.8
SEA J Amarillo	1,429.1	585.5	2.44	1,483.8	690.0	1,536.1	2,704.0#
SEA K Wichita Falls[c]	1,329.2	584.6	2.27	1,444.3	682.6	1,517.2	2,458.2
SEA L Lubbock	1,408.9	532.6	2.65	1,409.5	579.1	1,396.8	2,443.4

Texas City	1,671.9	731.6	2.29	1,724.1	898.0	1,884.7	2,654.4
SEA N Corpus Christi	1,526.2	685.9	2.23	1,585.4	782.0	1,688.8	2,332.9
SEA O Denton	1,387.5	504.2	2.75	1,518.0	619.4	1,492.0	2,172.7#
SEA P Abilene	1,227.6	450.5	2.72	1,273.3	602.6	1,300.8	2,337.0#
Mountain	1,410.7	693.2	2.04	1,463.7	764.9	1,564.2	1,924.8
Arizona	1,631.0	712.8	2.29	1,624.1	756.6	1,666.7	1,965.4
SEA 1 (North)	1,678.5	689.7	2.43	1,655.7	763.6	1,689.3	1,450.0
SEA 2 (South)	1,512.2	666.5	2.27	1,613.7	746.2	1,635.2	2,608.5
SEA A Phoenix	1,656.4	712.9	2.32	1,604.7	748.4	1,647.3	2,262.0
SEA B Tucson	1,624.3	747.9	2.17	1,666.5	778.3	1,724.7	2,045.4
Colorado	1,344.8	678.1	1.98	1,394.3	756.4	1,515.0	1,865.8
SEA 1 (Northwest)	1,313.8	696.5	1.89	1,451.3	806.2	1,548.0	*
SEA 2 (Southwest)	1,274.2	682.6	1.87	1,390.5	748.4	1,507.2	2,382.5#
SEA 3 (North)	1,175.8	626.2	1.88	1,250.5	698.8	1,338.6	*
SEA 4 (East Central)	1,113.1	548.0	2.03	1,209.3	687.2	1,347.7	*
SEA 5 (South East)c	1,428.7	680.9	2.10	1,392.1	761.2	1,526.4	*
SEA A Denver	1,473.7	714.4	2.06	1,508.7	781.8	1,623.4	1,917.7
SEA B Colorado Springs	1,134.9	627.4	1.81	1,285.8	714.6	1,417.4	1,474.7#
SEA C Puebloc	1,401.0	680.3	2.06	1,402.0	850.0	1,572.3	1,893.0#
SEA D Boulder	1,126.6	614.9	1.83	1,219.5	684.0	1,350.1	*
Idaho	1,253.4	644.3	1.95	1,342.5	724.1	1,451.8	1,844.3
SEA 1 (Central)	1,324.7	766.2	1.73	1,416.2	800.6	1,564.4	*
SEA 2 (Northwest)	1,181.9	627.0	1.89	1,286.9	713.9	1,355.9	2,823.2#
SEA 3 (Southwest)	1,264.2	615.8	2.05	1,362.7	691.2	1,450.8	1,297.8#
SEA 4 (Southeast)	1,227.1	628.5	1.95	1,293.7	748.9	1,442.8	1,844.0#
Montana	1,467.7	724.3	2.03	1,548.1	797.6	1,645.7	2,399.5
SEA 1 (West)	1,576.0	776.0	2.03	1,650.8	849.0	1,742.1	2,975.2#
SEA 2 (North)	1,324.6	736.0	1.80	1,414.6	778.9	1,549.9	2,141.1
SEA 3 (South Central)	1,420.4	592.3	2.40	1,499.7	736.5	1,556.7	2,594.9#
SEA 4 (South East)	1,446.4	580.5	2.49	1,543.0	660.3	1,584.4	*

(Continued)

Table A.5.5   Age-adjusted[a] death rates per 100,000 population for all causes for selected age-sex-color groups: United States, each state and each state economic area[b], 1959-61 (Continued)

Division, state, and state economic area (SEA)	White, age 45-64			White, age 35-74		White, both sexes 45-74	Nonwhite, both sexes 45-74
	Male	Female	M/F Ratio	Male	Female		
Nevada	1,800.7	824.2	2.18	1,824.4	891.2	1,894.5	2,184.1
SEA 1 (all)	1,863.8	822.4	2.27	1,909.3	880.7	1,953.0	2,138.1#
SEA A Las Vegas	1,714.9	828.7	2.07	1,677.7	907.4	1,793.4	2,238.3#
New Mexico	1,318.0	719.2	1.83	1,391.7	803.4	1,530.3	1,548.8
SEA 1 (Northwest)	1,180.5	721.1	1.64	1,335.1	817.4	1,490.5	1,289.8
SEA 2 (Northeast)	1,101.7	690.9	1.59	1,251.0	830.2	1,418.2	1,929.8#
SEA 3 (South)	1,360.9	684.1	1.99	1,432.7	761.8	1,533.4	2,051.6#
SEA A Albuquerque	1,522.3	774.6	1.97	1,505.1	819.4	1,639.2	2,269.9#
Utah	1,279.8	649.6	1.97	1,346.0	727.5	1,466.4	2,013.7
SEA 1 (North)	1,118.1	501.5	2.23	1,248.2	652.9	1,326.6	*
SEA 2 (Central)	1,091.7	685.9	1.59	1,183.2	726.1	1,370.0	*
SEA 3 (South)	1,330.4	638.4	2.08	1,363.5	770.2	1,474.0	2,309.6#
SEA A Salt Lake City	1,365.7	698.0	1.96	1,412.1	754.4	1,539.4	1,839.4#
SEA B Ogden	1,308.3	588.9	2.22	1,405.8	666.5	1,463.8	2,635.6#
Wyoming	1,320.1	666.4	1.98	1,418.6	744.8	1,518.3	2,446.4
SEA 1 (Southwest)	1,366.7	740.7	1.85	1,489.5	783.4	1,611.6	2,573.3#
SEA 2 (Northeast)	1,289.9	619.8	2.08	1,378.0	721.8	1,463.5	2,403.9#
Pacific	1,456.3	711.8	2.05	1,498.2	775.6	1,609.9	1,692.0
Alaska	1,404.1	682.8	2.06	1,529.1	797.1	1,638.4	1,742.5
California	1,469.1	721.3	2.04	1,509.6	782.0	1,622.9	1,796.2

SEA 1 (Northwest)	1,474.5	720.1	2.05	1,562.0	792.1	1,627.0	1,667.2#
SEA 2 (West Central, North)^c	1,592.8	792.5	2.01	1,567.0	800.5	1,665.9	1,168.2#
SEA 3 (West Central)^c	1,458.0	716.0	2.04	1,492.9	766.1	1,585.2	1,473.4
SEA 4 (North Central)	1,523.5	640.1	2.38	1,554.2	754.0	1,627.6	1,864.1#
SEA 5 (Central)	1,481.0	585.2	2.53	1,470.8	659.4	1,502.2	1,875.8#
SEA 6 (Central South)^c	1,435.1	713.2	2.01	1,409.3	784.9	1,522.5	1,712.6#
SEA 7 (Ventura Co.)^c	1,386.9	711.5	1.95	1,453.1	817.2	1,617.0	1,190.5#
SEA 8 (Imperial Co.)	1,450.6	660.5	2.20	1,588.9	793.4	1,684.4	2,645.0#
SEA 9 (Northeast)	1,454.2	725.2	2.01	1,503.9	762.6	1,580.7	1,618.2#
SEA A San Francisco, Oakland	1,521.6	788.2	1.93	1,586.5	841.2	1,721.8	1,806.0
SEA B San Jose	1,329.7	672.3	1.98	1,369.8	702.5	1,475.7	1,204.6#
SEA C Sacramento	1,751.1	758.9	2.31	1,774.8	816.1	1,844.8	2,025.8
SEA D Stockton	1,683.4	673.4	2.50	1,656.5	769.3	1,699.4	1,593.4
SEA E Fresno	1,501.9	644.1	2.33	1,546.7	737.3	1,609.5	2,073.0
SEA F Los Angeles	1,467.7	716.0	2.05	1,512.5	785.5	1,631.4	1,803.1
SEA G San Diego	1,359.2	727.0	1.87	1,387.2	764.4	1,528.6	1,781.9
SEA H San Bernardino, Riverside	1,345.4	673.0	2.00	1,383.2	715.3	1,478.9	1,864.1
SEA J Bakersfield	1,456.8	726.2	2.01	1,558.1	805.3	1,661.4	2,195.0
SEA K Santa Barbara	1,345.3	669.4	2.01	1,384.8	729.8	1,495.4	1,553.0#
Hawaii	1,729.1	989.4	1.75	1,734.0	1,068.4	2,025.4	1,344.8
SEA 1 (all)	1,761.6	1,216.9	1.45	1,957.0	1,360.3	2,293.7	1,298.6
SEA A Honolulu	1,724.7	936.9	1.84	1,686.8	1,003.7	1,956.6	1,371.3
Oregon	1,385.6	668.9	2.07	1,438.6	744.6	1,538.8	2,036.8
SEA 1 (West)	1,435.7	738.0	1.95	1,438.2	808.0	1,579.8	1,691.3#
SEA 2 (Central, West)^c	1,254.6	591.9	2.12	1,349.3	681.3	1,416.7	*
SEA 3 (North Central)^c	1,400.9	613.1	2.28	1,401.0	692.1	1,475.2	3,013.4#
SEA 4 (Southeast)	1,198.1	646.8	1.85	1,315.4	708.8	1,421.6	2,078.8#
SEA A Portland	1,510.5	695.9	2.17	1,546.9	776.5	1,646.2	2,092.9
SEA B Eugene	1,203.7	606.1	1.99	1,316.0	659.3	1,390.2	*

(Continued)

Table A.5.5 Age-adjusted[a] death rates per 100,000 population for all causes for selected age-sex-color groups: United States, each state and each state economic area[b], 1959-61

Division, state, and state economic area (SEA)	White, age 45-64			White, age 35-74		White, both sexes, 45-74	Nonwhite, both sexes, 45-74
	Male	Female	M/F Ratio	Male	Female		
Washington	1,429.1	679.2	2.10	1,474.0	752.1	1,578.0	1,807.4
SEA 1 (West)	1,349.6	723.7	1.86	1,487.7	801.7	1,639.6	2,362.3#
SEA 2 (Northwest)	1,274.2	560.1	2.27	1,300.5	638.4	1,372.4	1,859.5#
SEA 3 (Kitsap Co.)	1,309.0	711.0	1.84	1,316.6	789.1	1,503.4	1,706.1#
SEA 4 (South Central West)	1,346.8	654.4	2.06	1,435.7	740.5	1,504.0	*
SEA 5 (North Central)	1,370.6	615.0	2.23	1,454.4	730.6	1,516.0	2,093.2#
SEA 6 (South Central)	1,323.9	607.4	2.18	1,418.8	680.8	1,482.0	2,450.7#
SEA 7 (Southeast)	1,340.3	599.7	2.23	1,315.4	678.8	1,421.8	1,962.5#
SEA 8 (Northeast)	1,212.0	569.7	2.13	1,292.3	706.9	1,418.3	*
SEA A Seattle	1,527.0	706.1	2.16	1,571.7	787.3	1,676.4	1,649.2
SEA B Tacoma	1,517.1	752.0	2.02	1,531.4	800.7	1,656.1	1,818.5#
SEA C Vancouver, Clark Co.	1,268.0	653.1	1.94	1,355.6	723.2	1,491.1	*
SEA D Spokane	1,523.7	673.5	2.26	1,515.6	715.5	1,587.5	2,051.8#
SEA E Everett	1,395.1	726.7	1.92	1,448.7	788.5	1,573.3	*

[a]Age-adjusted by direct method by 10-year groups to the total U. S. population in the specified age or age-sex group in 1950.

[b]As defined in reference 13 of Chapter 5, and described in text of Chapter 5. See App. Fig. A.5.1.

[c]Rates for the white groups have been calculated on estimated population at risk, excluding populations in resident institutions, essentially as described in reference 27 of Chapter 5. (Rates for the nonwhite group have been calculated without such adjustment.)

* Less than 20 deaths, sum of all age groups included.

Half or more of the age groups had less than 20 deaths each.

Table A.5.6   Coefficients of correlation for specified causes of death among white males aged 35-74:   United States, 509 state economic areas, 1959-61

Cause of death	CVR diseases (330-334,400-468,592-594)	Coronary (420)	Stroke (330-334)	Hypertensive (440-447)	Rheumatic heart disease (400-416)	Other CVR (421-434,450-468,592-594)	Malignant neoplasms (140-205)	Lung cancer (162-163)	Other malignant (140-161,164-205)	Accidents and violence (E800-E999)	Chronic respiratory (241,501,502,525,526,527.1)	All other
All causes	.89*	.79*	.49*	.59*	.03*	.54*	.65*	.60*	.55*	.09*	.28*	.64*
Cardiovascular-renal diseases (330-334,400-468,592-594)		.91*	.60*	.63*	-.05*	.50*	.55	.51	.46	-.11	.07	.33
Coronary heart disease (420)			.34	.43	.02	.19	.63	.54	.55	-.24	.07	.21
"Stroke" (330-334)				.41	-.34	.38	.07	.14	.01	-.10	-.06	.18
Hypertensive heart disease and hypertension (440-447)					-.12	.37	.27	.29	.21	.02	.01	.32
Rheumatic heart disease (400-416)						-.12	.06	-.05	.11	-.23	.13	.06
Other cardiovascular-renal diseases (421-434,450-468,592-594)							.15	.19	.09	.23	.10	.37
Malignant neoplasms (140-205)								.79*	.91*	-.34	.13	.29
Lung cancer (162-163)									.48	-.20	.19	.27
All other malignant neoplasms (140-161,164-205)										-.36	.06	.24
Accidents and violence (E800-E999)											.22	.14
Chronic respiratory diseases (241,501,502,525,526,527.1)												.23

* Correlation of a part with a whole.

Table A.5.7 Coefficients of correlation for specified causes of death among white females aged 35-74: United States, 509 state economic areas, 1959-61

Cause of death	CVR diseases (330-334, 400-468, 592-594)	Coronary (420)	Stroke (330-334)	Hypertensive (440-447)	Rheumatic heart disease (400-416)	Other CVR (421-434, 450-468, 592-594)	Malignant neoplasms (140-205)	Lung cancer (162-163)	Other malignant (140-161, 164-205)	Accidents and violence (E800-E999)	Chronic respiratory (241, 501, 502, 525, 526, 527.1)	All other
All causes	.93*	.83*	.47*	.63*	.46*	.54*	.73*	.27*	.72*	.01*	.13*	.69*
Cardiovascular-renal diseases (330-334, 400-468, 592-594)		.88*	.59*	.69*	.37*	.57*	.55	.21	.54	-.12	.01	.48
Coronary heart disease (420)			.35	.47	.34	.25	.59	.26	.57	-.18	-.03	.38
"Stroke" (330-334)				.27	-.01	.29	.13	.03	.14	-.07	-.06	.17
Hypertensive heart disease and hypertension (440-447)					.10	.50	.31	.10	.31	-.06	.07	.35
Rheumatic heart disease (400-416)						.13	.41	.05	.42	.03	.14	.36
Other cardiovascular-renal diseases (421-434, 450-468, 592-594)							.21	.09	.20	.09	.06	.39
Malignant neoplasms (140-205)								.33*	.99*	-.14	-.01	.41
Lung cancer (162-163)									.19	.05	.04	.14
All other malignant neoplasms (140-161, 164-205)										-.15	-.02	.40
Accidents and violence (E800-E999)											.17	.08
Chronic respiratory diseases (241, 501, 502, 525, 526, 527.1)												.25

* Correlation of a part with a whole.

Table A.5.8 Coefficients of correlation for specified causes of death among white males aged 35-74: United States, 206 metropolitan SEA's (M) and 303 non-metropolitan SEA's (N), 1959-61

Cause of death		CVR diseases (330-334,400-468,592-594)	Coronary (420)	Stroke (330-334)	Hypertensive (440-447)	Rheumatic heart disease (400-416)	Other CVR (421-434,450-468,592-594)	Malignant neoplasms (140-205)	Lung cancer (162-163)	Other malignant (140-161,164-205)	Accidents and violence (E800-E999)	Chronic respiratory (241,501,502,525,526,527.1)	All other
All causes	M	.86*	.71*	.47*	.52*	-.12*	.47*	.61*	.41*	.57*	.16*	.09*	.63*
	N	.90*	.80*	.57*	.63*	-.05*	.65*	.60*	.61*	.41*	.33*	.40*	.62*
Cardiovascular-renal diseases (330-334,400-468,592-594)	M		.90*	.56*	.52*	-.17*	.40*	.50	.35	.46	-.06	-.15	.25
	N		.91*	.69*	.69*	-.04*	.61*	.49	.50	.34	-.05	-.19	.32
Coronary heart disease (420)	M			.32	.34	-.17	.06	.50	.34	.47	-.16	-.18	.17
	N			.43	.46	-.17	.31	.59	.52	.47	-.07	.22	.10
"Stroke" (330-334)	M				.20	.06	.27	.14	.16	.09	.10	-.07	.17
	N				.58	-.36	.45	.10	.20	.00	.08	-.05	.25
Hypertensive heart disease and hypertension (440-447)	M					-.07	.19	.29	.19	.27	.07	.07	.25
	N					-.20	.53	.20	.30	.08	.09	.05	.36
Rheumatic heart disease (400-416)	M						-.12	-.02	-.14	.06	-.30	.00	.13
	N						.11	-.01	-.13	.07	-.13	.24	-.05
Other cardiovascular-renal diseases (421-434,450-468,592-594)	M							.15	.10	.14	.16	.05	.33
	N							.19	.30	.06	.32	.15	.44
Malignant neoplasms (140-205)	M								.71*	.91*	-.24	-.10	.20
	N								.74*	.89*	-.12	-.22	.20
Lung cancer (162-163)	M									.35	-.10	-.03	.06
	N									.34	.06	.29	.29
All other malignant neoplasms (140-161,164-205)	M										-.27	-.12	.24
	N										-.20	.11	.07
Accidents and violence (E800-E999)	M											.35	.13
	N											.31	.38
Chronic respiratory diseases (241,501,502,525,526,527.1)	M												.10
	N												.34

M Metropolitan; correlation of 206 metropolitan SEA's.
N Non-metropolitan; correlation of 303 non-metropolitan SEA's.
* Correlation of a part with a whole.

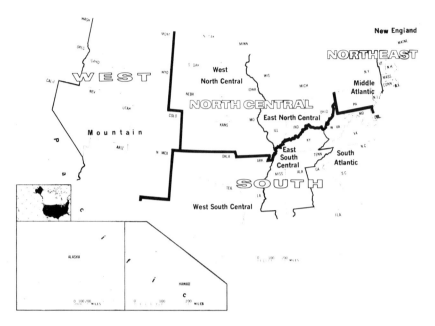

Figure A.5.1 Census regions and geographic divisions of the United States (courtesy of the Bureau of the Census, U. S. Department of Commerce)

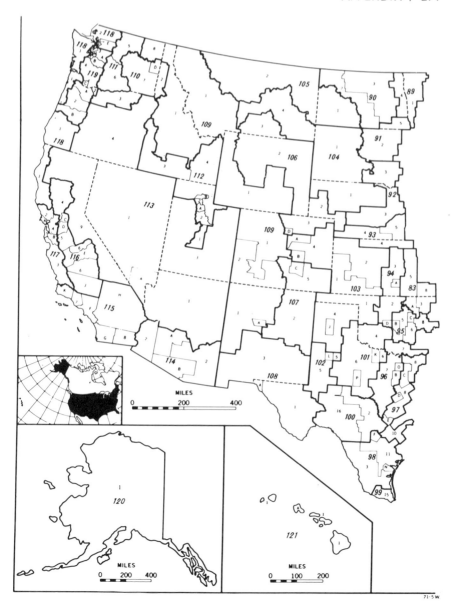

Figure A.5.2 Economic subregions and state economic areas, western half of the United States (see Fig. A.5.3 for legend) (courtesy of the Bureau of the Census, U. S. Department of Commerce)

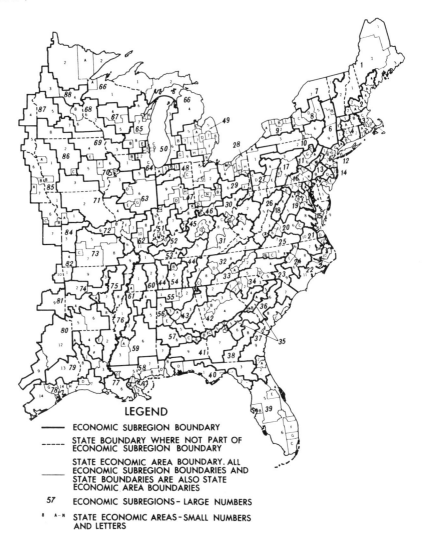

LEGEND

—— ECONOMIC SUBREGION BOUNDARY

- - - - STATE BOUNDARY WHERE NOT PART OF
ECONOMIC SUBREGION BOUNDARY

—— STATE ECONOMIC AREA BOUNDARY. ALL
ECONOMIC SUBREGION BOUNDARIES AND
STATE BOUNDARIES ARE ALSO STATE
ECONOMIC AREA BOUNDARIES

57 ECONOMIC SUBREGIONS – LARGE NUMBERS

ᴬ⁻ᴺ STATE ECONOMIC AREAS – SMALL NUMBERS
AND LETTERS

Figure A.5.3 Economic subregions and state economic areas, eastern half of the United States (courtesy of the Bureau of the Census, U. S. Department of Commerce)

REFERENCES

Chapter 1
Mortality and Longevity in the
United States

1. U.S. Bureau of the Census, *Historical Statistics of the United States, Colonial Times to 1957* (Department of Commerce: 1960), Series B, 155-162, p. 30.

2. Ibid., 163–175, p. 30.

3. I. M. Moriyama, *The Change in Mortality Trend in the United States*, Pub. Health Service Publ. No. 1000, Series 3, No. 1 (National Center for Health Statistics: March 1964).

4. A. J. Klebba, *Mortality Trends in the United States, 1954-1963*, Pub. Health Service Publ. No. 1000, Series 20, No. 2 (National Center for Health Statistics: June 1966).

5. E. M. Kitagawa, "Race Differentials in Mortality in the United States, 1960 (Corrected and Uncorrected)." Paper presented at Annual Meeting of Population Association of America, Boston, April 1968.

6. L. I. Dublin, A. J. Lotka, and M. Spiegelman, *Length of Life* (New York: Ronald Press Co., 1949, rev. ed.), esp. pp. 35, 36, 348, and 351.

7. F. L. Hoffman, "American Mortality Progress during the Last Half Century," in M. Ravenel, ed., *A Half Century of Public Health* (New York: Amer. Pub. Health Assoc., 1921), pp. 94-117.

8. I. Rosenwaike, "On Measuring the Extreme Aged in the Population," *J. Am. Stat. Assoc.* 63:29-40 (March 1968).

9. W. Perks, "On Some Experiments in the Graduation of Mortality Statistics," *J. Inst. Actuaries* 63:12-40 (1932).

10. B. L. Strehler and A. S. Mildvan, "General Theory of Mortality and Aging," *Science* 142:14-21 (July 1, 1960).

11. G. A. Sacher and E. Trucco, "The Stochastic Theory of Mortality," *Ann. N. Y. Acad. Sci.* 96:985-1007 (March 2, 1962).

12. U.S. Bureau of the Census, *Statistical Abstract of the United States: 1972* (Department of Commerce: 1972), pp. 24, 91, and 258.

13. M. Spiegelman, *Introduction to Demography* (Cambridge, Mass.: Harvard University Press, 1968, rev. ed.), esp. pp. 249-252.

14. P. H. Jacobson, "The Changing Role of Mortality in American Family Life," *Lex et Scientia* 3:117-124 (April-June 1966).

15. L. I. Dublin and A. J. Lotka, *The Money Value of a Man* (New York: Ronald Press Co., 1946, rev. ed.).

Chapter 2
Mortality in the United States by Cause

1. I. M. Moriyama, D. E. Krueger, and J. Stamler, *Cardiovascular Diseases in the United States* (Cambridge, Mass.: Harvard University Press, 1971).

2. A. M. Lilienfeld, M. L. Levin, and I. I. Kessler, *Cancer in the United States* (Cambridge, Mass.: Harvard University Press, 1972).

3. National Center for Health Statistics, *Eighth Revision—International Classification of Diseases, Adapted for Use in the United States*, Pub. Health Service Publ. No. 1693 (Dec. 1968).

4. M. M. Faust and A. B. Dolman, "Comparability of Mortality Statistics for the Sixth and Seventh Revision: United States, 1958," *Vital Statistics—Special Reports*, 51 (No. 4) (National Center for Health Statistics: March 1965).

5. S. Shapiro, E. R. Schlesinger, and R.E.L. Nesbitt, Jr., *Infant, Perinatal, Maternal, and Childhood Mortality in the United States* (Cambridge, Mass.: Harvard University Press, 1968).

6. F. Bayo, "United States Life Tables by Causes of Death: 1959-61," *Life Tables: 1959-61*, 1 (No. 6) (National Center for Health Statistics: May 1968).

7. M. Spiegelman, "The Curve of Human Mortality," Proceedings of Seminars, 1965-69, Council on Aging and Human Development (Durham, N.C.: Duke University, Nov. 1969), pp. 286-298.

Chapter 3
International Comparisons of Mortality and Longevity

1. Statistical Office, *Demographic Yearbook, 1966* (New York: United Nations, 1967), p. 1.

2. Statistical Office, *Demographic Yearbook, 1968* (New York: United Nations, 1969), Table 1.

3. Ibid., Table 21.

4. E. Adams, "International Migration Trends Affecting Europe in the 1960's," *International Population Conference, London, 1969, Vol. IV* (International Union for the Scientific Study of Population, Liège, 1971).

5. S. Shapiro, E. R. Schlesinger, and R.E.L. Nesbitt, Jr., *Infant, Perinatal, Maternal, and Childhood Mortality in the United States* (Cambridge, Mass.: Harvard University Press, 1968), esp. pp. 114-132.

6. C. L. Erhardt and H. Abramson, "Anoxia and Perinatal Mortality," in H. Abramson, ed., *Resuscitation of the Newborn Infant* (New York: C. V. Mosby Co., 1973, 3rd ed.).

7. M. Spiegelman, "Recent Mortality in Countries of Traditionally Low Mortality," *Proc. World Pop. Conf., 1965*, II (New York: United Nations, 1967), p. 375.

8. M. Spiegelman, "Why Do These Mortality Curves Cross?," *N.Y. Statistician* 18(8):1 (April 1967).

9. M. Spiegelman, *Introduction to Demography* (Cambridge, Mass.: Harvard University Press, 1968, rev. ed.), chap. 6.

10. M. Spiegelman, "Mortality Trends for Causes of Death in Countries of Low Mortality," *Demography* 2:115-125 (1965).

11. H. C. Chase, *International Comparison of Perinatal and Infant Mortality*, Pub. Health Service Publ. No. 1000, Series 3, No. 6 (National Center for Health Statistics: March 1967).

12. M. Spiegelman, "Mortality Trends and Projections," *Trans. Soc. Actuaries* 19:D449-D469 (Oct. 1967).

13. I. M. Moriyama, D. E. Krueger, and J. Stamler, *Cardiovascular Diseases in the United States* (Cambridge, Mass.: Harvard University Press, 1971).

14. Department of Public Health, *Trends in Cancer Mortality for Selected Sites in 24 Countries, 1950-59* (Sendai, Japan: Tohoku University School of Medicine, July 1963).

15. World Health Organization, *Epidemiological and Vital Statistics Report*, 18 (No. 7) (Geneva: 1965), p. 316.

16. World Health Organization, *Epidemiological and Vital Statistics Report*, 18 (No. 10) (Geneva: 1965), p. 386.

17. A. L. Lilienfeld, M. L. Levin, and I. I. Kessler, *Cancer in the United States* (Cambridge, Mass.: Harvard University Press, 1972).

18. World Health Organization, *Epidemiological and Vital Statistics Report*, 20 (No. 1) (Geneva: 1967), p. 88.

19. A. M. Lowell, L. B. Edwards, and C. E. Palmer, *Tuberculosis* (Cambridge, Mass.: Harvard University Press, 1969).

20. C. C. Dauer, R. F. Korns, and L. M. Schuman, *Infectious Diseases* (Cambridge, Mass.: Harvard University Press, 1968).

21. H. F. Dorn and I. M. Moriyama, "Uses and Significance of Multiple Cause Tabulations for Mortality Statistics," *Am. J. Pub. Health* 54:400-406 (March 1964).

22. A. I. Mendeloff and J. P. Dunn, *Digestive Diseases* (Cambridge, Mass.: Harvard University Press, 1971).

23. M. Kramer, E. S. Pollack, R. W. Redick, and B. Z. Locke, *Mental Disorders/Suicide* (Cambridge, Mass.: Harvard University Press, 1972).

24. A. P. Iskrant and P. V. Joliet, *Accidents and Homicide* (Cambridge, Mass.: Harvard University Press, 1968).

25. G. Stolnitz, "A Century of International Mortality Trends: I," *Pop. Studies* 9:24-55 (July 1955).

26. G. Stolnitz, "A Century of International Mortality Trends: II," *Pop. Studies* 10:17-42 (July 1956).

Chapter 4
Morbidity in the United States

1. B. MacMahon and T. F. Pugh, *Epidemiology: Principles and Methods* (Boston: Little, Brown and Co., 1970), p. 66.

2. E. Balamuth, *Health Interview Responses Compared with Medical Records*, Pub. Health Service Publ. No. 1000, Series 2, No. 7 (National Center for Health Statistics: July 1965).

3. W. G. Madow, *Interview Data on Chronic Conditions Compared with Information Derived from Medical Records*, Pub. Health Service Publ. No. 1000, Series 2, No. 23 (National Center for Health Statistics: May 1967).

4. C. F. Cannell, F. J. Fowler and K. H. Marquis, *The Influence of Interviewer and Respondent: Psychological and Behavioral Variables on the Reporting in Household Interviews*, Pub. Health Service Publ. No. 1000, Series 2, No. 26 (National Center for Health Statistics: March 1968).

5. T. Parsons, "Definitions of Health and Illness in the Light of American Values and Social Structure," in E. G. Jaco, ed., *Patients, Physicians, and Illness* (Glencoe, Ill.: The Free Press, 1958), pp. 165-187.

6. National Center for Health Statistics, *Health Survey Procedure: Concepts, Questionnaire Development, and Definitions in the Health Interview Survey*, Pub. Health Service Publ. No. 1000, Series 1, No. 2 (May 1964), pp. 4, 42, and 45.

7. L. D. Haber, "Identifying the Disabled: Concepts and Methods in the Measurement of Disability," *Soc. Sec. Bull.* 30:17-34 (Dec. 1967), p. 22.

8. P. S. Lawrence et al., *Medical Care, Health Status, and Family Income*, Pub. Health Service Publ. No. 1000, Series 10, No. 9 (May 1964), Sec. IV, Table 4.

9. G. A. Gleeson, *Limitation of Activity and Mobility Due to Chronic Conditions, United States, July 1957-June 1958*, Pub. Health Service Publ. No. 584, Series B., No. 11 (Public Health Service: July 1959), Table A.

10. C. S. Wilder, *Limitation of Activity and Mobility Due to Chronic Conditions, United States, July 1965-June 1966*, Pub. Health Service Publ. No. 1000, Series 10, No. 45 (National Center for Health Statistics: May 1968), Tables A and B.

11. A. L. Ranofsky, *Utilization of Short-Stay Hospitals, Summary of Nonmedical Statistics, United States—1967*, Vital and Health Statistics, Series 13, No. 9 (National Center for Health Statistics: May 1972), Tables 7, 9, and Appendix Table II.

12. C. Namey and R. W. Wilson, *Age Patterns in Medical Care, Illness, and Disability, United States, 1968-1969*, Vital and Health Statistics, Series 10, No. 70 (National Center for Health Statistics: April 1972).

13. M. Kramer, E. S. Pollack, R. W. Redick, and B. Z. Locke, *Mental Disorders/Suicide* (Cambridge, Mass.: Harvard University Press, 1972).

14. H. J. Dupuy et al., *Selected Symptoms of Psychological Distress, United States*, Pub. Health Service Publ. No. 1000, Series 11, No. 37 (National Center for Health Statistics: Aug. 1970).

15. C. A. Taube, *Characteristics of Patients in Mental Hospitals, United States, April-June 1963*, Pub. Health Service Publ. No. 1000, Series 12, No. 3 (National Center for Health Statistics: Dec. 1965).

16. E. S. Johnson, J. E. Kelly, and L. E. Van Kirk, *Selected Dental Findings in Adults by Age, Race and Sex, United States, 1960-1962*, Pub. Health Service Publ. No. 1000, Series 11, No. 7 (National Center for Health Statistics: Feb. 1965).

17. J. E. Kelly, L. E. Van Kirk, and C. Garst, *Total Loss of Teeth in Adults, United States, 1960-1962*, Pub. Health Service Publ. No. 1000, Series 11, No. 27 (National Center for Health Statistics: Oct. 1967).

18. W. J. Pelton et al., *The Epidemiology of Oral Health* (Cambridge, Mass.: Harvard University Press, 1969).

Chapter 5

Geographic Variation in Mortality and Morbidity

1. L. Shattuck, "Art. XVI—Report to the Committee of the City Council (Boston 1846)," reviewed in *Am. J. Med. Sci.* 12:177-178 (July 1846).

2. L. Shattuck et al., *Report of Sanitary Commission of Massachusetts, 1850* (Cambridge, Mass.: Harvard University Press, 1948).

3. National Office of Vital Statistics (1949-59) and National Center for Health Statistics (1960-67), *Vital Statistics of the United States*, annual volumes (Government Printing Office: 1951-69).

4. F. E. Linder and R. D. Grove, *Vital Statistics Rates in the United States 1900-1940* (Bureau of the Census: 1943).

5. R. D. Grove and A. M. Hetzel, *Vital Statistics Rates in the United States 1940-1960*, Pub. Health Service Publ. No. 1677 (National Center for Health Statistics: 1968).

6. E. A. Duffy and R. E. Carroll, *United States Metropolitan Mortality, 1959-1961*, Pub. Health Service Publ. No. 999, Series AP, No. 39 (National Center for Air Pollution Control: 1967).

7. T. D. Woolsey, "An Investigation of Low Mortality in Certain Areas," *Pub. Health Rep.* 64:909-920 (July 22, 1949).

8. P. E. Enterline and W. H. Stewart, "Geographic Patterns in Deaths from Coronary Heart Disease," *Pub. Health Rep.* 71:849-855 (Sept. 1956).

9. P. E. Enterline, A. E. Rikli, H. I. Sauer, and M. Hyman, "Death Rates for Coronary Heart Disease in Metropolitan and Other Areas," *Pub. Health Rep.* 75:759-766 (Aug. 1960).

10. E. F. Winton and L. J. McCabe, Jr., "Studies of Water Mineralization and Health," *Water Conditioning* 11(9):12-18 (Nov. 1969).

11. H. A. Schroeder, "Relation between Mortality from Cardiovascular Disease and Treated Water Supplies," *J. A. M. A.* 172:1902-1908 (April 23, 1960).

12. P. E. Sartwell, "Trends in Epidemiology," in E. T. Stewart, ed., *Trends in Epidemiology: Application to Health Service Research and Training* (Springfield, Ill.: Charles C Thomas, 1972).

13. U.S. Bureau of the Census, *U.S. Census of Population, 1960, Number of Inhabitants, United States Summary, Final Report*, PC(1)-1A (Government Printing Office: 1961), pp. 1-16.

14. National Office of Vital Statistics, "Death Rates for Selected Causes by Age, Color, and Sex: United States and Each State, 1949-51, All Causes," *Vital Statistics—Special Reports,* 49 (No. 1) (Dec. 19, 1959).

15. C. A. Hill, Jr., "Measures of Longevity of American Indians," *Pub. Health Rep.* 85:233-239 (March 1970).

16. D. J. Bogue, B. D. Misea, and D. P. Dandekar, "A New Estimate of the Negro Population and Negro Vital Rates in the United States, 1930-1960," *Demography* 1:339-358 (1964).

17. National Center for Health Statistics, *Report of the Fifteenth Anniversary Conference of the United States National Committee on Vital and Health Statistics*, Pub. Health Service Publ. No. 1000, Series 4, No. 4 (June 1966), p. 5.

18. T. Z. Hambright, *Comparability of Age on the Death Certificate and Matching Census Record, United States, May-August 1960*, Pub. Health Service Publ. No. 1000, Series 2, No. 29 (National Center for Health Statistics: June 1968).

19. H. I. Sauer, "Adequacy of Age Data for Age-Specific Death Rates." Paper presented at Annual Meeting of Population Association of America, New York, April 1966.

20. H. I. Sauer, "Migration and the Risk of Dying," Proceedings of the Social Statistics Section, American Statistical Association (1967), pp. 399-407.

21. H. I. Sauer and H. D. Donnell, Jr., "Age and Geographic Differences in Death Rates," *J. Geront.* 25:83-86 (1970).

22. H. I. Sauer, "Geographic Differences in the Risk of Premature Death," *Business & Government Rev.* (University of Missouri–Columbia), 11(3):19-26 (May-June 1970).

23. U.S. Bureau of the Census, *U.S. Census of Population: 1960, Selected Area Reports, State Economic Areas, Final Report*, PC(3)-1A (Government Printing Office: 1963).

24. Committee on Forms and Methods of Statistical Practice, "Age Adjustment of the Crude Death Rate," *Am. Pub. Health Assoc. Year Book, 1939-40*, Supplement to *Am. J. Pub. Health* 30:123-131 (Feb. 1940).

25. H. I. Sauer, "Geographic Patterns of Nonwhite Mortality." Paper presented at Population Association of America, Atlanta, April 17, 1970.

26. H. I. Sauer, "Epidemiology of Cardiovascular Mortality—Geographic and Ethnic," *Am. J. Pub. Health* 52:94-105 (Jan. 1962).

27. H. I. Sauer, G. H. Payne, C. A. Council, and J. C. Terrell, "Cardiovascular Disease Mortality Patterns in Georgia and North Carolina," *Pub. Health Rep.* 81(5):455-465 (May 1966).

28. C. G. Bennett, G. H. Tokuyama, and T. C. McBride, "Cardiovascular-Renal Mortality in Hawaii," *Am. J. Pub. Health* 52:1418-1431 (Sept. 1962).

29. C. L. Chiang, "Standard Error of the Age-Adjusted Death Rate," *Vital Statistics–Special Reports*, 47 (No. 9) (National Vital Statistics Division: Aug. 17, 1961).

30. R. C. Geary, "The Contiguity Ratio and Statistical Mapping," *The Incorp. Statistician* 5:115-145 (1954). Summarized in O.D. Duncan, R.P. Cuzzort, and B. Duncan, *Statistical Geography Problems in Analyzing Areal Data* (Glencoe, Ill.: The Free Press, 1961), pp. 131-136.

31. M. Gover, "Statistical Studies of Heart Disease. IV. Mortality from Heart Disease (All Forms) Related to Geographic Section and Size of City," *Pub. Health Rep.* 64:439-456 (April 8, 1949).

32. H. I. Sauer, J. E. Banta, and W. W. Marshall, Jr., "Cardiovascular Diseases Mortality Patterns Among Middle-Aged White Males in Missouri," *Missouri Med.* 61:921-926, 929 (Nov. 1964).

33. H. I. Sauer, H. L. Rickman, G. H. Payne, and E. A. Rogers, "Mortality Patterns of Middle-Aged Whites in Nebraska," *Nebraska Med. J.* 51:393-398 (Oct. 1966).

34. D. E. Krueger and I. M. Moriyama, "Mortality of the Foreign Born," *Am. J. Pub. Health* 57:496-503 (March 1967).

35. I. M. Moriyama, D. E. Krueger, and J. Stamler, *Cardiovascular Diseases in the United States* (Cambridge, Mass.: Harvard University Press, 1970).

36. A. M. Lilienfeld, M. L. Levin, and I. I. Kessler, *Cancer in the United States* (Cambridge, Mass.: Harvard University Press, 1972).

37. S. L. Syme, "Implications and Future Prospects," suppl. to *Milbank Mem. Fund Quart.* 45:175-180 (April 1967).

38. H. I. Sauer and P. E. Enterline, "Are Geographic Variations in Death Rates for the Cardiovascular Diseases Real?," *J. Chron. Dis.* 10:513-524 (Dec. 1959).

39. G. D. Friedman, "Cigarette Smoking and Geographic Variation in Coro-

nary Heart Disease Mortality in the U.S.," *J. Chron. Dis.* 20:769-779 (Oct. 1967).

40. L. Guralnick, "Mortality by Occupation and Industry Among Men 20 to 64 Years of Age: U.S. 1950," *Vital Statistics—Special Reports*, 53 (No. 2) (National Vital Statistics Division: Sept. 1962).

41. J. L. Steinfeld, *The Health Consequences of Smoking, A Report of the Surgeon General, 1972* (Government Printing Office: 1972).

42. B. MacMahon and T. F. Pugh, *Epidemiology: Principles and Methods* (Boston: Little, Brown and Co., 1970).

43. T. Gordon, *Blood Pressure of Adults by Race and Area, United States, 1960-1962*, Pub. Health Service Publ. No. 1000, Series 11, No. 5 (National Center for Health Statistics: July 1964).

44. C. S. Wilder, *Bed Disability Among the Chronically Limited, United States, July 1957-June 1961*, Pub. Health Service Publ. No. 1000, Series 10, No. 12 (National Center for Health Statistics: Sept. 1964).

45. L. E. Bollow and G. A. Gleeson, *Persons Hospitalized by Number of Hospital Episodes and Days in a Year, United States, July 1960-June 1962*, Pub. Health Service Publ. No. 1000, Series 10, No. 20 (National Center for Health Statistics: June 1965).

46. C. S. Wilder, *Chronic Conditions and Limitations of Activity and Mobility, United States, July 1965-June 1967*, Pub. Health Service Publ. No. 1000, Series 10, No. 61 (National Center for Health Statistics: Jan. 1971).

47. C. S. Wilder, *Health Characteristics by Geographic Region, Large Metropolitan Areas, and Other Places of Residence, United States, July 1963-June 1965*, Pub. Health Service Publ. No. 1000, Series 10, No. 36 (National Center for Health Statistics: April 1967).

48. M. G. Kovar, *Acute Conditions, Geographic Distribution, United States, July 1958-1959*, Pub. Health Service Publ. No. 584, Series B, No. 23 (Division of Public Health Methods: Oct. 1960).

49. C. S. Wilder, *Acute Conditions, Geographic Distribution, United States, July 1960-June 1961*, Pub. Health Service Publ. No. 584, Series B, No. 34 (National Center for Health Statistics: June 1962).

50. C. S. Wilder, *Acute Conditions, Incidence and Associated Disability, United States, July 1961-June 1962*, Pub. Health Service Publ. No. 1000, Series 10, No. 1 (National Center for Health Statistics: May 1963).

51. C. S. Wilder, *Acute Conditions, Incidence and Associated Disability, United States, July 1962-June 1963*, Pub. Health Service Publ. No. 1000, Series 10, No. 10 (National Center for Health Statistics: June 1964).

52. C. S. Wilder, *Acute Conditions, Incidence and Associated Disability, United States, July 1963-June 1964*, Pub. Health Service Publ. No. 1000, Series 10, No. 15 (National Center for Health Statistics: April 1965).

53. C. S. Wilder, *Acute Conditions, Incidence and Associated Disability, United States, July 1967-June 1968*, Pub. Health Service Publ. No. 1000, Series 10, No. 54 (National Center for Health Statistics: June 1969).

54. H. H. Hechter and N. O. Borhani, "Mortality and Geographic Distribution of Arteriosclerotic Heart Disease," *Pub. Health Rep.* 80:11-24 (Jan. 1965).

55. M. A. McCarthy, *Comparison of the Classification of Place of Residence on Death Certificates and Matching Census Records, United States, May-August*

1960, Pub. Health Service Publ. No. 1000, Series 2, No. 30 (National Center for Health Statistics: Jan. 1969).

56. S. L. Syme, "Stress and Coronary Heart Disease, Preventive Implications," *Post-Grad. Med.* 48:123-127 (July 1970).

57. G. M. Sternberg, *Malaria and Malarial Diseases* (New York: William Wood & Co., 1884), p. 31.

Chapter 6
The Aged: Health, Illness, Disability,
and Use of Medical Services

1. E. Shanas, *The Health of Older People: A Social Survey* (Cambridge, Mass.: Harvard University Press, 1962), p. 180.

2. E. Suchman, B. Phillips, and G. Streib, "An Analysis of the Validity of Health Questionnaires," *Social Forces* 36:223-232 (March 1958).

3. E. Shanas, P. Townsend, D. Wedderburn, H. Friis, P. Milhøj, and J. Stehouwer, *Old People in Three Industrialized Societies* (New York: Atherton Press, 1968).

4. Public Health Service, *Health in the Later Years of Life* (National Center for Health Statistics: 1971).

5. M. Nielson, et al., "Older Persons After Hospitalization: A Controlled Study of Home Aide Service," *Am. J. Pub. Health* 62:1094-1101 (Aug. 1972).

6. R. Morgan, *Nursing and Personal Care Services Received by Residents of Nursing and Personal Care Homes, United States, May-June 1964*, Pub. Health Service Publ. No. 1000, Series 12, No. 10 (National Center for Health Statistics: Sept. 1968).

7. J. N. Agate, "Old People: Diseases of Deprivation," *Proc. Roy. Soc. Med.* 61:919-922 (Sept. 1968).

Chapter 7
Variations in Mortality, Morbidity, and
Health Care by Marital Status

1. A. J. Klebba, *Mortality from Selected Causes by Marital Status: United States, Part B*, Pub. Health Service Publ. No. 1000, Series 20, No. 8b (National Center for Health Statistics: Dec. 1970), p. 19.

2. R. D. Grove and A. M. Hetzel, *Vital Statistics Rates in the United States, 1940-1960*, Pub. Health Service Publ. No. 1677 (National Center for Health Statistics: 1968), Table 67.

3. Ibid., Table 39.

4. M. Kramer, "Epidemiology, Biostatistics and Mental Health Planning," *Psychiatric Research Report 22* (Am. Psychiat. Assoc.: April 1967), pp. 25-44.

5. D. S. Thomas and B. Z. Locke, "Marital Status, Education, and Occupational Differentials in Mental Disease," *Milbank Mem. Fund Quart.* 41:145-160 (April 1963).

6. B. M. Rosen, T. W. Anderson, and A. K. Bahn, "Psychiatric Services for the Aged: A Nationwide Survey of Patterns of Utilization," *J. Chron. Dis.* 21:167-177 (June 1968).

7. M. D. Blumenthal, "Mental Health Among the Divorced: A Field Study of Divorced and Never Divorced Persons," *Arch. Gen. Psychiat.* 16:603-608 (May 1967).

8. L. Srole, T. S. Langer, S. T. Michael, M. K. Opler, and T. A. C. Rennie, "Mental Health in the Metropolis," *Intern. J. Psychiat.* 1:64-76 (Jan. 1965).

9. R. F. Klein, A. Dean, and M. D. Bogdanoff, "The Impact of Illness upon the Spouse," *J. Chron. Dis.* 20:241-248 (April 1967).

10. B. MacMahon and T. F. Pugh, "Suicide in the Widowed," *Am. J. Epidemiol.* 81:23-31 (Jan. 1965).

11. C. M. Parkes, "Recent Bereavement as a Cause of Mental Illness," *Brit. J. Psychiat.* 110:198-204 (March 1964).

12. Z. Stein and M. Susser, "Widowhood and Mental Illness," *Brit. J. Prev. Soc. Med.* 23:106-110 (May 1969).

13. C. Parkes, C. Murray, B. Benjamin, and R. G. Fitzgerald, "Broken Heart: A Statistical Study of Increased Mortality Among Widowers," *Brit. Med. J.* 1:740-743 (March 22, 1969).

14. H. H. Avnet, *Physician Service Patterns and Illness Rate* (New York: Group Health Insurance, Inc., 1967), Tables 13, 34, 37, 61, 69, 70, 75, 80, 85, 95, 105, 115, and 142.

15. R. Morgan, *Marital Status and Living Arrangements Before Admission to Nursing and Personal Care Homes, United States, May-June 1964*, Pub. Health Service Publ. No. 1000, Series 12, No. 12 (National Center for Health Statistics: May 1969).

Chapter 8
Infant Mortality in the United States

1. I. M. Moriyama, "Recent Change in Infant Mortality Trend," *Pub. Health Rep.* 75:391-405 (May 1960).

2. S. Shapiro and I. M. Moriyama, "International Trends in Infant Mortality and Their Implications for the United States," *Am. J. Pub. Health* 53:747-760 (May 1963).

3. H. C. Chase, *International Comparison of Perinatal and Infant Mortality*, Pub. Health Service Publ. No. 1000, Series 3, No. 6 (National Center for Health Statistics: March 1967).

4. S. Shapiro, E. R. Schlesinger, and R. E. L. Nesbitt, Jr., *Infant and Perinatal Mortality in the United States*, Pub. Health Service Publ. No. 1000, Series 3, No. 4 (National Center for Health Statistics: Oct. 1965).

5. S. Shapiro, E. R. Schlesinger, and R. E. L. Nesbit, Jr., *Infant, Perinatal, Maternal, and Childhood Mortality in the United States* (Cambridge, Mass.: Harvard University Press, 1968).

6. National Center for Health Statistics, "Births, Marriages, Divorces, and Deaths . . . ," *Monthly Vital Statistics Report* (monthly issues).

7. U.S. Bureau of the Census (to 1945), National Office of Vital Statistics (1945-59), National Vital Statistics Division (1960-62), and National Center for Health Statistics (1963 to present), *Vital Statistics of the United States* (Government Printing Office: annual volumes).

8. F. E. Linder and R. D. Grove, *Vital Statistics Rates in the United States 1900-1940* (Bureau of the Census: 1943).

9. R. D. Grove and A. M. Hetzel, *Vital Statistics Rates in the United States 1940-1960*, Pub. Health Service Publ. No. 1677 (National Center for Health Statistics: 1968).

10. J. Loeb, "Weight at Birth and Survival of Newborn, by Age of Mother and Total-Birth Order: United States, Early 1950," *Vital Statistics—Special Reports*, 42 (No. 2) (National Office of Vital Statistics: Aug. 1958).

11. H. C. Chase, "Infant Mortality and Weight at Birth: 1960 United States Birth Cohort," *Am. J. Pub. Health* 59:1618-1628 (Sept. 1969).

12. R.J. Armstrong, *A Study of Infant Mortality from Linked Records. By Birth Weight, Period of Gestation, and Other Variables*, Vital and Health Statistics, Series 20, No. 12 (National Center for Health Statistics: May 1972).

13. H. C. Chase, *A Study of Infant Mortality from Linked Records: Comparison of Neonatal Mortality from Two Cohort Studies. United States, January-March 1950 and 1960*, Vital and Health Statistics, Series 20, No. 13 (National Center for Health Statistics: June 1972).

14. B. MacMahon, M. G. Kovar, and J. J. Feldman, *Infant Mortality Rates: Socioeconomic Factors*, Vital and Health Statistics, Series 22, No. 14 (National Center for Health Statistics: March 1972).

15. B. MacMahon, M. G. Kovar, and J. J. Feldman, *Infant Mortality Rates: Relationship With Mother's Reproductive History, United States*, Vital and Health Statistics, Series 22, No. 15 (National Center for Health Statistics: April 1973).

16. F. D. Norris and P. W. Shipley, "A Closer Look at Race Differentials in California's Infant Mortality, 1965-67," *HSMHA Health Rep.* 86:810-814 (Sept. 1971).

17. M. Susser, F. A. Marolla, and J. Fleiss, "Birth Weight, Fetal Age and Perinatal Mortality," *Am. J. Epidemiol.* 96:197-204 (Sept. 1972).

18. J. A. Heady and M. A. Heasman, *Social and Biological Factors in Infant Mortality*, General Register Office, Studies in Medical and Population Subjects No. 15 (London: Her Majesty's Stationery Office, 1959).

19. E. R. Schlesinger, S. M. Mazumdar, and V. M. Logrillo, "Long-term Trends in Perinatal Deaths among Offspring of Mothers with Previous Child Losses," *Am. J. Epidemiol.* 96:255-262 (Oct. 1972).

Chapter 9
Projections of Health Service Personnel
and Facilities

1. U.S. Bureau of the Census, "Projections of the Population of the United States, By Age and Sex: 1972 to 2020," *Current Population Reports*, Series P-25, No. 493 (Department of Commerce: Dec. 1972).

2. U.S. Bureau of the Census, *Statistical Abstract of the United States, 1972* (Department of Commerce, 1972), p. 74.

3. U.S. Bureau of the Census, *Historical Statistics of the United States, 1900-1957* (Department of Commerce: 1958).

4. I. M. Moriyama, *The Change in Mortality Trend in the United States*, Pub. Health Service Publ. 1000, Series 3, No. 1 (National Center for Health Statistics: March 1964).

5. M. Lerner and O. W. Anderson, *Health Progress in the United States, 1900-1960* (Chicago: University of Chicago Press, 1963).

6. D. J. Bogue, *Principles of Demography* (New York: John Wiley, 1969), p. 883.

7. C. S. Wilder, *Acute Conditions, Incidence and Associated Disability, United States, July 1966-June 1967*, Pub. Health Service Publ. No. 1000, Series 10, No. 44 (National Center for Health Statistics: March 1968).

8. M. H. Wilder, *Current Estimates From the Health Interview Survey, United States, 1970*, Vital and Health Statistics, Series 10, No. 72 (National Center for Health Statistics: May 1972).

9. B. Sanders, "Measuring Community Health Levels," *Am. J. Pub. Health* 54:1063-1070 (July 1964).

10. Department of Economic and Social Affairs, *Population Bulletin of the United Nations*, No. 6—1962 (United Nations: 1963).

11. G. A. Gleeson, *Age Patterns in Medical Care, Illness and Disability, United States, July 1963-June 1965*, Pub. Health Service Publ. No. 1000, Series 10, No. 32 (National Center for Health Statistics: June 1966).

12. A. G. Dingfelder, *Chronic Conditions Causing Activity Limitation, United States, July 1963-June 1965*, Pub. Health Service Publ. No. 1000, Series 10, No. 51 (National Center for Health Statistics: Feb. 1969).

13. M. Lerner, "Hospital Use by Diagnosis—A Comparison of Two Experiences," Center for Health Administration Studies, *Research Series 19* (University of Chicago: 1961).

14. O. W. Anderson, "Health Services in a Land of Plenty," Center for Health Administration Studies, *Health Administration Perspectives*, Series A7 (University of Chicago: 1968).

15. Commission on Professional and Hospital Activities, *PAS Reporter* 7 (No. 14) (1969).

16. R. Andersen and O. W. Anderson, *A Decade of Health Services: Social Survey Trends in Use and Expenditure* (Chicago: University of Chicago Press, 1967).

17. R. Anderson, "A Behavioral Model of Families' Use of Health Services," Center for Health Administration Studies, *Research Series 25* (University of Chicago: 1968).

18. G. Wirick, "A Multiple Equation Model of Demand for Health Care," *Health Serv. Res.* 1:301-346 (winter 1966).

19. M. Greenlick, A. Hurtado, C. Pope, E. Saward, and S. Yoshioka, "Determinants of Medical Care Utilization," *Health Serv. Res.* 3:296-315 (winter 1968).

20. P. Feldstein, "The Demand for Medical Care," in *The Cost of Medical Care*, Vol. 1 (Chicago: American Medical Association, 1964), pp. 57-76.

21. A. J. Alderman, *Volume of Dental Visits, United States, July 1963-June 1964*, Pub. Health Service Publ. No. 1000, Series 10, No. 23 (National Center for Health Statistics: Oct. 1965).

22. I. Falk, M. Klem, and N. Sinai, *The Incidence of Illness and the Receipt and Costs of Medical Care Among Representative Families*, Publications of the Committee on the Costs of Medical Care: No. 26 (Chicago: University of Chicago Press, 1933), Table 21 and Appendix Table B-27.

23. C. S. Wilder, *Physician Visits, Volume and Interval Since Last Visit, United States, 1969,* Vital and Health Statistics, Series 10, No. 75 (National Center for Health Statistics: July 1972), p. 3.

24. National Center for Health Statistics, *Health Resources Statistics, 1968,* Pub. Health Service Publ. No. 1509 (Dec. 1968).

25. National Center for Health Statistics, *Health Resources Statistics, 1971,* Public Health Service Publ. No. 1509 (Feb. 1972).

26. R. W. Wilson, *Current Estimates From the Health Interview Survey, United States, 1971,* Vital and Health Statistics, Series 10, No. 79 (National Center for Health Statistics: Feb. 1973).

27. National Advisory Commission on Health Manpower, *Report,* Vols. 1 and 2 (Government Printing Office: Nov. 1967), pp. 1-2.

28. American Dental Association, *Fluoridation Reporter* 8, No. 1 (1970).

29. Division of Dental Health, *Fluoridation Census, 1969* (Department of Health, Education and Welfare: 1970).

30. C. Upton and W. Silverman, "The Demand for Dental Services." Unpublished paper from Graduate School of Business, University of Chicago, 1970.

31. R. Dubos, *Mirage of Health: Utopias, Progress, and Biological Change* (New York: Harper and Row, 1959).

INDEX

Accidents (excluding motor vehicle), 38; decrease in fatalities from, 21, 26; rank as cause of death, by color, sex, and age, 30, 31; probability of death by, 33; international comparisons of death by, 62. *See also* Motor vehicle accidents

Acute conditions, 103, 126; defined, 66, 67, 133; variation by age and sex, 68; disability among persons with, 69–70; specific conditions, 70–71; secular trends, 72; relation to family income, 72–73; among the elderly, 133–135. *See also* Chronic conditions

Africa, 39; expectation of life at birth, 40

Agate, J. N., 157

Age: mortality by, 3–11, 18; rank of causes of death by, 26–31; international comparison of death rates by, 41–46; variation in acute conditions by, 68; variation in chronic conditions by, 75–77; hospital discharge rate by, 85; and geographic variation in mortality and morbidity, 117–118; infant mortality rates by, 191–192

Aged, the, 130–131; health, 132–133; acute conditions, 133–135; chronic conditions, 135–140; in institutions, 140–142; use of medical services, 142–148; use of physician services, 148–150; use of dental services, 150–151; visits to other specialists, 151; expenditure on prescription drugs, 153; use of home care, 153–155; general concerns regarding health, 155–158

Alabama, mortality rates, 111

Anderson, T. W., 180

Arkansas, mortality rates, 108, 111, 112, 128

Arteriosclerosis, 33–35; rank as cause of death, 26, 30; probability of dying from, 31–33, 38. *See also* Cardiovascular-renal diseases

Arthritis and rheumatism, among the elderly, 137

Asia, comparative mortality, 39

Australia, 39; mortality, 41; death from influenza and pneumonia, 58; suicide rate, 60

Avnet, H. H., 185

Bahn, A. K., 180

Belgium: causes of death, 52; cardiovascular-renal mortality, 54; death from tuberculosis and from influenza and pneumonia, 58

Blumenthal, M. D., 180, 183

Bogdanoff, M. D., 181–182

Bogue, D. J., 217

Bureau of the Census, United States, 110, 127, 210; population projections, 216–218, 223, 228–235

California, mortality rates, 108

Canada: crude death rates, 41; causes of death, 52; cardiovascular-renal mortality, 54; death from influenza and pneumonia, 58; suicide rate, 60

Cancer, *see* Malignant neoplasms

Cardiovascular-renal diseases, 33–35, 38, 211; death rate, 21; rank as cause of death, 25–26; rank as cause of death, by color, sex, and age, 30; probability of dying from, 31–33; and cohort mortality, 35–37; international comparisons of death from, 54–56; and geographic variation in mortality and morbidity, 120–122

Carroll, R. E., 105

Cause-specific mortality, 21–23, 38; problems in interpretation, 23–24; rank (1967 and 1900), 24–26; rank by color, sex, and age, 26–31; probability, 31–33; gain in longevity by eliminating, 33–35; and cohort mortality, 35–38; in developed countries, 50–62; and geographic variation in mortality and morbidity, 120–122

Central nervous system, vascular lesions, 23, 30

Chiang, C. L., 114

Chronic conditions, 103; growing importance, 21–23, 38; predominance in mortality rates for developed countries, 51; defined, 66–67, 135; variation by age and sex, 75–77; disability among persons with, 77–78; specific conditions, 78–80; secular trends, 80–82; relation to family income, 82–83; and geographic variation in mortality and morbidity, 124–126; among the elderly, 135–140; and improved health care, 212–230. *See also* Acute conditions

Cirrhosis of the liver: death rate, 21–23; rank as cause of death, by color, sex, and age, 26, 31; and cohort mortality, 38; international comparisons of death from, 60

Cohort mortality, 13–17; specific causes